Critical Care in Internal Medicine

Progress in Critical Care Medicine

Vol. 2

Series Editor
Walter H. Massion, Oklahoma City, Okla.

KARGER

S. Karger · Basel · München · Paris · London · New York · Tokyo · Sydney

Critical Care in Internal Medicine

Volume Editor
D. Robert McCaffree, Oklahoma City, Okla.

15 figures and 54 tables, 1985

KARGER

S. Karger · Basel · München · Paris · London · New York · Tokyo · Sydney

Progress in Critical Care Medicine

National Library of Medicine, Cataloging in Publication
Critical care in internal medicine
Volume editor, D. Robert McCaffree. – Basel; New York: Karger, 1985
(Progress in critical care medicine; vol. 2)
Based on selected papers from an annual course in critical care medicine held in Oklahoma City, 1984, sponsored by the Dept. of Medicine of the University of Oklahoma. Includes index.
1. Critical Care – congresses 2. Internal Medicine – congresses
I. McCaffree, Donald Robert II. University of Oklahoma. Dept. of Medicine III. Series
W1 PR668KM v. 2 [WB 115 C934 1984]
ISBN 3-8055-3900-2

Drug Dosage

The authors and the publisher have exerted every effort to ensure that drug selection and dosage set forth in this text are in accord with current recommendations and practice at the time of publication. However, in view of ongoing research, changes in government regulations, and the constant flow of information relating to drug therapy and drug reactions, the reader is urged to check the package insert for each drug for any change in indications and dosage and for added warnings and precautions. This is particularly important when the recommended agent is a new and/or infrequently employed drug.

Printed in Switzerland by Thür AG Offsetdruck, Pratteln
ISBN 3-8055-3900-2

Contents

Renal System

Digestive System

Metabolism

Infections

Pharmacology and Poisoning

Dedication

To my wife and children – *Mary Anne, Sara and Matthew* –
my Mother – *Cleo McCaffree* –
and in loving memory of my Father – *L.A. McCaffree*

Preface

For more than a decade, the Department of Medicine of the University of Oklahoma has sponsored a very successful annual course in Critical Care Medicine. While the course under Dr. *McCaffree's* direction provided the impetus for this book, it is not a compendium of lectures given at the course. Rather, the book consists of selected and specially prepared discourses.

I call special attention to two unique contributions that exemplify that medicine is a hybrid of the humanities and sciences. One is Dr. *Viner's* report of personal experiences as a critically ill patient, emphasizing in a most compelling way that there is far more to the care of the critically ill than technology. The other is Dr. *Petty's* chapter on ethical considerations in the use of mechanical ventilation.

The material that needs to be addressed is vast, involving the total man, as well as individual organ systems. When I learned of this book, I knew Dr. *McCaffree* could not include all of the relevant subjects. Whenever selection, no matter how thoughtful, is introduced, there are those who would have made different choices. The material is *all* important in the care of the critically ill.

Solomon Papper

MD, Regents' Professor, Former Head, Department of Medicine,
University of Oklahoma Health Sciences Center, College of Medicine and
Staff Physician, VA Medical Center, Oklahoma City, Okla.

Prog. crit. Care Med., vol. 2, pp. 1–2 (Karger, Basel 1985)

Introduction

Over the past decade, remarkable strides have been made in our understanding of the pathophysiologic processes of life-threatening illnesses and our abilities to intervene in these processes to reverse or reduce their effects. In part because of our advancing knowledge and in part because of technologies which have become available for our use, the interest in acute life-threatening illnesses has expanded rapidly. This has been evidenced by the development of intensive care units in virtually every acute care hospital in the country, by the numbers of postgraduate courses on critical illness now available to the practitioner and by the expanding volumes of literature on these topics.

In view of the latter fact, why should yet another volume on critical care be presented? Part of that answer resides in the experience we have gained at the University of Oklahoma in presenting a postgraduate course on critical care medicine for over a decade. The association with physicians across the country who deal with these topics on a daily basis and our own experience have given some perspective on the problems most commonly encountered or most commonly presenting diagnostic and therapeutic difficulties to the physician. We felt that a reference dealing primarily with the diagnosis and therapy of these selected diseases in a concise way would be a useful addition. That selection obviously includes some biases regarding those topics that might be most useful. The most obvious exclusions from these topics are respiratory failure and cardiac emergencies. These topics will be the subject of future volumes of *Progress in Critical Care Medicine.*

The reader will also notice that some of the chapters do not fit into a disease category. We felt that it was important to offer some perspective on the impact of critical illness on the person. The contributions of Drs. *Petty* and *Viner* accomplish this admirably. One gives the perspective developed by an experienced clinician who has worked with many patients over the years and the other the perspective of another accomplished clinician gained from his own intensely personal experience as an ICU patient.

Finally, we had no intention of preparing an encyclopedic textbook. There are already several excellent textbooks on the market. We hope that this volume will prove to be a useful and frequently utilized presentation of problems encountered in critically ill patients by internists, family practitioners and surgeons. If we achieve this goal to even a limited extent, the efforts that were put into this volume are worthwhile.

Prog. crit. Care Med., vol. 2, pp. 3–13 (Karger, Basel 1985)

Life at the Other End of the Endotracheal Tube: A Physician's Personal View of Critical Illness

Edward D. Viner

University of Pennsylvania School of Medicine, Hematology-Oncology Section, Pennsylvania Hospital, Philadelphia, Pa., USA

Introduction

Having considered the technical and scientific aspects of acute lung injury and mechanical ventilation, it is time to pause and remember that there is a living, thinking, feeling, and frightened human being on the other end of that machine. While it is incompatible with our self images as empathetic care providers, having had a serious personal experience with illness, I can assure you that none of us *really* know what we doctors ask our patients to endure, and what a devastating physical and emotional experience it is to be critically ill. The facts of my particular case really do not matter, other than to provide the perspective from which I speak, and to make all of this a little less sterile and academic. Besides the specific medical details of his case, each patient brings his own personality and psychosocial background to his illness, all of which affect that individual's ability to cope with the stress of his ordeal. The physician must be ever mindful of all of this in considering his patient on the other end of the tube, whom illness has reduced to an eye-watering, lip-quivering mass of protoplasm.

Case Presentation

I was a 34-year-old hematologist working with critically ill and dying patients every day, when, on May 2, 1972, at the behest of my then pregnant wife, I went for the first complete physical examination of my adult life. While in every respect I anticipated a purely routine venture, the examining physician communicated an unspoken message of alarm as he paused in examining my liver. Having established that there was marked enlargement of the right lobe, a liver scan was performed the next day. After literally grabbing the scan out of a reluctant radiologist's hand, and seeing for myself the large cold area in the right lobe, I then joined the downcast herd of patients inevitably found in X-ray department waiting rooms. I immediately identified with these unfortunates, whose doctors, like mine, were doing X-rays looking for cancer. As I proceeded to have a chest film, intravenous pyelogram and long upper GI, all in search of the presumed occult primary tumor, I sat there terror stricken, trying to deal with the mental images of my cachectic, end-stage, cancer patients, and my speculation as to whether I would still be alive when our baby came that August. In between studies, I called home to tell my wife about the findings, and that I would be admitted to the hospital. I called my secretary to have her cancel all my patients, *forever,* and called my insurance agent, accountant, and attorney to meet me in my hospital room that afternoon. I, as most doctors, did not have my personal affairs in order, and properly attending to all of this ultimately was to provide me with significant peace of mind in the weeks to come.

The following morning I had a bone marrow examination, proctoscopy and barium enema, all of which were normal. At this point it seemed likely that the lesion was a primary hepatic tumor and a subsequent arteriogram confirmed that it was almost surely a hepatoma. It was decided that exploratory surgery should be performed, but this was delayed by the development of a deep venous phlebitis, which in combination with a low-grade fever, only served to reinforce further my certainty that I indeed had a hepatic malignancy. Finally, on May 16, surgical exploration of my liver through a thoracoabdominal approach was carried out. The lesion fortunately proved to be a huge benign hemangioma, but I really did not believe my doctors were telling me the truth concerning the pathology, even though I was shown the reports firsthand, and ultimately was visited by the chief of pathology. Only weeks later, after being put on the respirator, and realizing that my senior attending surgeon, Dr. *Jonathan Rhoads,* was too sensible to put me through all this, if indeed I had had an inoperable malignancy, did I really become secure that the pathology was truly benign.

The first five postoperative days were spent in the intensive care unit, with tubes coming out of everywhere, but this experience did not prove particularly difficult. However, soon after being transferred out of the unit, I began to have a recurrent spiking fever requiring hours on an ice blanket each day for more than two weeks. Multiple thoracenteses, bronchoscopic examinations, and various scans failed to reveal the cause, and ultimately it was presumed that there must be a subhepatic collection of pus. Accordingly, I was to be operated upon again.

I went to the second surgical procedure again very frightened, not because of fear of malignancy this time, but with a temperature of nearly 105°, I felt too sick to go to surgery safely. My first awareness postoperatively was the bank of lights overhead, indicating that I was back in the intensive care unit and that I was too sick to be brought back to my private room. As the scene unfolded, the large overhead clock, and the darkness outside, told me that it was 3.00 a.m., and the presence of my surgeon further alarmed me since the chairman of surgery does not come in for routine postoperative problems in the middle of the night. I then also realized that I was packed in ice cubes, and from bits and pieces of the conversation that I overheard, I concluded that I had indeed been found to have a large abdominal abscess, that I had developed Gram-negative septicemic shock and, in short, was in *bad trouble.* The subsequent days were to confirm that perception, and more.

The next night with the endotracheal tube in place, I began to vomit. I was awake and alert and wanted to pull the tube and bite block out of my mouth so I could vomit over the side of the bed. I realized that I might aspirate, and indeed, later knew that I was doing so, even though the nurse told me 'everything is under control; you can't be aspirating because of the balloon on the endotracheal tube'. Over the next couple of days I developed a combination of aspiration pneumonia and shock lung, and finally after becoming totally exhausted from the work of breathing, I wrote my wife a note, telling her that I could not last more than a few more hours unless something different could be done. At my request, she called in my close friend, the former head of the hospital's respiratory intensive care unit, who was away on vacation. Dr. *Robert Rogers,* now Chief of the Pulmonary Section of the University of Pittsburgh, responded immediately, and quickly taught me that there is a real *art* to running a respirator. I am still not really sure of all that he did, but within several hours I was breathing infinitely more comfortably and the immediate crisis had passed. There was more yet to come, however. A tracheotomy became necessary, and I subsequently learned that the complication of 'PEEP' is 'POP' as I begun a series of pneumothoraces requiring multiple chest tubes.

The final statistics summarizing my misadventure include 120 days in the hospital, 31 days on the respirator, 10 chest tubes, 13 thoracenteses, 118 arterial blood gases (without benefit of an arterial line, and which I calculated one night trying to while the hours away, required a rough average of 3.2 sticks per specimen), hundreds of hours on the ice blanket, 3 bronchoscopic examinations, and 7 months out of work. It was a year before I really felt well again with no further chest or abdominal pain or overt dyspnea. Along the way, there were many indelible lessons learned, which, until then, I had thought, in a superficial intellectualization, to be self-evident.

Perceptions from the ICU Experience

First of all, we doctors really have no concept of that which we ask our patients to endure physically and emotionally, all at a time when they are most vulnerable, physically and emotionally. Patients would benefit immeasurably if every care provider could experience the preoperative terror of thinking he has an end-stage malignancy, the nostalgia inherent in believing that he will not see his children grow up, and the preterminal mourning over the thought that he is leaving behind everyone whom he knows and loves. It is clear that if the illness is serious enough, even the most resolute patient will meet his match. While I had started out feeling strong, both physically and emotionally, by the end of the 31-day stint on the respirator, I had literally become that labile, eye-watering, lip-quivering mass of protoplasm that we physicians have all seen on the end of the endotracheal tube.

The patient lives in a very circumscribed world. Accordingly, everyone who enters his day assumes a magnified role. While the doctor is theoretically the 'leading man' in the cast of characters, he is there for only a few minutes once, or at most, several times daily. Therefore, it is the nurse with whom the patient literally lives his day, who is really the most important of all. However, the patient's world also includes various paraprofessional and support personnel, on down the hierarchical ladder to the ward clerk, the paperboy and the 'environmental engineer' who mops the floor around the bed. It is unfortunate that these people do not realize the importance of their roles in the patient's life, and are not prepared for this responsibility. A warm smile instead of an air of oblivious indifference makes all the difference to the patient on a respirator.

As stated, it is the nurse, and not the doctor, who is the single most important person in the critically ill patient's life. In turn, the single most important attribute of the nurse is *whether she cares.* I thought I could tell with great accuracy whether an individual nurse did or did not, and I quickly decided that there were basically two types, angels and bitches. However, it also became clear that there was also a third group comprised of nurses who, no doubt, had been excellent, but who had been in the intensive care unit too long. While they were fine technicians when it came to aspirating a patient and doing other procedures, the human qualities had been lost. I lay there trying hard to define just what defines a 'good nurse', and finally decided that it is a combination of warmth and sensitivity with a significant degree of professionalism which are the key ingredients. I learned that there is a remarkable degree of nonverbal communication between the respirator patient and the nurse. Her moods, attitudes, basic intelligence and ability, her personality and her personal problems all interact to affect the bottom line for the patient. I found myself concerned about who was coming on the next shift. Some inspired confidence; with others I could expect a confrontation. I was also surprised with my concern over the personal appearance of my nurses. If her uniform was dirty or sloppy, I became concerned that her care would be similar. I resented undignified behavior in the unit; loud noise and raucous laughter seemed inappropriate and incongruent to my personal situation of being half dead on that machine. Whereas I ordinarily would have smiled at some of the interchanges between a surgical resident and nurse in the middle of the night at the nurses' station, that was not in keeping with the raison d'être of their being there, which from my limited vantage point was to keep me alive.

One of the most frustrating aspects was the custom of rotating the nurses. The rationale seemed to be that no one nurse should get too involved with a given patient, although from the patient's point of view, this boiled down to having one first date after another. By the end of the shift, just when a given nurse had learned how to aspirate and position me in the least painful way possible, she was replaced by someone I had never seen before, and with whom I had to go through the same learning experience all over again. I also got a bit paranoid about why the nurses were being changed all the time. 'Didn't they like me?' 'Did I smell bad?' 'Wasn't I a good patient?'

Many of these feelings also applied to the physicians, particularly the house staff. There was a tremendous difference between how the various surgical residents cared for me. It was obvious that some either refused to get involved, or really did not know how, at a personal level. On the other hand, my senior surgeon who had performed both operations, was caring and totally in charge. I came to realize how vital it was for there to be a steady 'captain of the ship', for it was easy to see how quickly one's care could deteriorate to the level provided when a committee of subspecialists is collectively in charge.

Another basic issue also applies equally to doctors, nurses and all health care providers. It is a problem, on the other hand, with which I have some sympathy, for even now, in spite of the unique learning experience my illness provided, I find myself, nonetheless, forgetting to *listen to the patient.* There were countless examples over the many weeks in the ICU when this basic failure made life difficult and, at times, even dangerous for me. As noted, the night I aspirated what seemed to me a gallon of gastric juice, I was awake and tried to tell the nurse in charge that I was aspirating, and that it would be better if she pulled the endotracheal tube and bite block out and simply let me vomit. I was told, 'My, my, my, don't we know a lot about ourselves'. With the first pneumothorax, I tried to explain that I was short of breath, but the attitude was that I had been short of breath for a week, so what was new? Well, this was new, and different, and I knew something was wrong, although I knew not what. Finally, it was the respiratory therapist, and not a doctor, who recognized that I had a tension pneumothorax (the surgical resident refused to come over from the nursing station to listen to my chest). While on hyperalimentation, an erroneously large dose of insulin was given on one occasion, following which I had the classical symptoms and signs of an acute hypoglycemic episode. I was cold and soaking wet, and felt absolutely bizarre up there on cloud nine. When I tried to explain this to both the nurses and the surgical house staff, I was told that I could not possibly have a hypoglycemic reaction with 50% glucose running. It remained for a physician not involved with my care, who was visiting the patient in the next bed, to recognize that the pleas I was writing on the clipboard were correct, and to speed up the IV enough to raise my blood sugar. In truth though, we will never know if my diagnosis was correct, for I never was able to get anyone to draw the blood sugar which would have vindicated me. The respiratory patient in particular is dependent both on the machine, and on the care provided. Beside the basic frustration inherent in not being in control of one's destiny, it was also frightening to realize that the staff did not always respect one's observations about himself.

While, appropriately enough, great attention was given to the operation of the respirator, my blood gases, and the other parameters by which I was followed, after a time I became rather ambivalent about all of this and really was much more concerned about creature comfort. This is something hard to come by in the ICU situation. Basically, I hesitated to ask for amenities, when others around me were also very ill. I longed for one of those old-fashioned private duty nurses we so irreverently called 'biddies', whose whole purpose would be to fluff my pillow and position me comfortably. Naturally, I was told that type of nurse was not allowed in the ICU, and that such an individual would just be in the way of the more crisis-oriented, and sophisticated, unit staff. I tried to tell them that I really did not care about the machine any more, that the President would have a creature comfort nurse, that I would pay for it, etc., but it was all to no avail.

After a time, having long since lost any ability to control the situation physically, I also began to lose emotional control. At times I was frankly psychotic. Intermittently I realized this, and was both very frightened and embarrassed by it. While intellectually I knew what was happening to me, and that it would pass if I survived, nonetheless, I became quite concerned about whether I would be whole again mentally. I also worried that I would never be able to function as a doctor again. I thought about asking to see a psychiatrist, but decided that he really could not help in view of the existing physical situation. I also was a little embarrassed to acknowledge that I needed this type of help, which was an unfortunate mistake. In coherent moments I could understand the reason for specific delusional ideas, dreams and nightmares. For example, it was not surprising to find myself both insecure and concerned about the lack of privacy when I found myself on the back of a flat-bodied truck in the middle of a corn field at a state fair in Kansas. My demand to be put back in the ICU at the University Hospital where I would be safe, made obvious sense, and my annoyance at being gawked at by the surrounding spectators was understandable in view of the lack of privacy in the ICU situation. I came to know John Kennedy very well as we both sat in the bottom of PT boat 109, a concept engendered by the 'putt putt' sound made by water in the respirator tubing which is not unlike a boat motor. I was repeatedly concerned that the place was being robbed and no one was doing anything about it, perhaps reflecting the stealing away of my health without recourse. Frequently, when the bed sheet was stained with a drop of blood, I asked for a new one. The nurses had trouble understanding that during the night, the werewolves and vultures came and ate any blood spots, leaving me cold and shivering with a cover full of holes. I was appreciative of those who were wise enough to react to my mental aberrations with a sensible, straightforward attempt to reorient me, and angry later with anyone who led me on during one of my 'trips'.

Towards the end of the ICU experience, when sleep deprivation, morphine and the intensity of my physical problems were no longer interacting to produce psychotic thinking, this was replaced by fear that I just would not be able to hack it emotionally until I could escape from the unit. I began to cry at the sight of my wife entering the room, and at the mention of the family dog, let alone our children. On the last day, when there was a retraction of the promise that I could leave the unit that morning, because my blood gases were not adequate, I told my doctor that I just could not stand it there any longer, and that I absolutely had to go. If there is heaven on earth, it is the private room to which I was transferred, where it was clean and quiet, and where my very own private duty nurse could take care of my basic need for comfort, without being a slave to the respirator and its attendant demands.

I am often asked if I suffered much pain during this experience. In actuality I did not, and indeed pain, when it was an issue, seemed readily relieved by morphine. A more important and difficult challenge was being just plain *miserable*. Under this heading, I include the problem of being chronically uncomfortable, with multiple chest tubes making it impossible to move or breathe without a sharp reminder, and the raw post-tonsillectomy feeling in one's throat after a nasogastric tube has been in place for 31 straight days. Also included in the misery category are the problems of nausea, abdominal cramps, and hiccoughs, of feeling dirty, with no decent bath or shampoo for many weeks, the bad taste of an oral fungus infection, and multiple other minor indispositions. Sleep deprivation was also a very difficult contributing problem for me. For the first five days on the respirator, I essentially had no sleep and finally bargained with my doctor to close the curtain around the bed and leave me totally alone for two hours so that I could regain the strength to go on. I remember very vividly telling him that if I died, I died. Time, in general, passed at a snail's pace, and most nights seemed interminable.

The problems of communicating were serious and varied. It was very difficult to write everything laboriously on a clipboard all of those weeks on the respirator. Indeed, one of my very favorite visitors was one of the hospital research staff, who had been totally deaf since early childhood, and as a result, could read lips expertly. For him, communicating with me was no different than with anyone else. With little to divert me, I became terribly tired of thinking about myself incessantly. Finally, Dr. *Rogers* brought me a transistor radio, and I suddenly again became aware of an outside world. There were even those times when the problem of communication was dangerous. On two occasions, the janitor pulled the respirator plug out of the socket without realizing it, leaving me on a closed system with no movement of air. I am told that emergency alarms were supposed to go off, but my only memory was having to detach the respiratory tube from the tracheostomy myself in order to breathe room air.

Another question commonly asked of me concerns whether I thought about dying. This was an all-pervading and relentless issue, though my thoughts ultimately became quite ambivalent. Most of the time I was very frightened that I would, though I derived some comfort, during the long hours I spent preoccupied with this issue, from the fact that I had had the opportunity to arrange my economic affairs in a way that would enable my children to be educated and my wife to be comfortable. There were other times, however, when I was so tired of plugging on, that I wished I would just go to sleep forever. Lastly, at times there were some thoughts about committing suicide. I was frightened by such thoughts, and it took the nurses some time to understand the origin of my occasional questions concerning whether the unit windows were locked. Much of the time was spent thinking nostalgically about my family and about all the everyday things we take for granted, but which now suddenly were to be no more. I would not see the Philadelphia Eagles play again or again drive along the River Drive at cherry blossom time, or see who would win the election. Later, I realized that all this constituted a type of preterminal mourning process. One of the most distressing aspects of my preoccupation with dying was a recurrent dream which I had many times a night even after I was convalescing at home. Simply stated, I was placed on a stretcher, just as I had been for countless excursions to X-ray, the OR, Physical Therapy, etc. This trip, however, took me down into the bowels of the hospital where a door was opened into a room with five tables. On four of the tables were bodies and the fifth one, in the middle, was empty. At that point the morgue attendant indicated that I was to climb up there, and my autopsy began.

There was little opportunity to talk about all of this, and in fairness to my doctors and nurses, I gave little indication of my preoccupation with death and dying. On one Sunday morning, however, I did finally tell the assembled group at the bedside that I was very fearful of that possibility and that I had to talk about it. True to storybook fashion, each person in the retinue physically drew back in response. The distance was perhaps only a quarter inch, but it was perceptible and obvious, and my reaction was to feel somewhat sorry that I had laid such a difficult situation on them. I realized that nowhere in our training at the time, had anyone taught us how to deal with such a statement from a patient. My senior surgeon, Dr. *Rhoads,* however, responded straightforwardly and appropriately to my pleas, communicating openly that the physicians also had been very concerned that I would die, but was then able to point out that each day I was a little better than the day before, and that they were cautiously optimistic that I would survive. This open exchange was very comforting to me and I did not again during my illness have such a compelling need to discuss these issues. However, adding to the total misery of the situation was the never-ending anxiety and resulting depression over my long-term prognosis. Even after it became clear, even to me, that I would survive, it was by no means clearly to any one whether I would be more than a respiratory cripple.

I cannot leave this discussion without acknowledging the tremendous support provided by my wife. While she was pregnant, and ultimately delivered our baby alone, by natural childbirth, four days before I left the hospital, she nonetheless was able to give selflessly throughout my ordeal. Because she had been an intensive care nurse herself, she was what the nursing staff termed a 'good visitor' and thus was allowed to stay after hours. I became totally convinced of the importance of a critically ill patient having his family with him for more time than the negligible visiting hours allowed in most intensive care units, and subsequently, have worked hard to get visiting privileges liberalized in our hospital.

Conclusions

I came away from this experience with great concern about who should receive the type of heroic effort which saved my life. I was naturally very grateful that everyone had worked so intensively to get me through it, yet it was obvious that the patient pays dearly, both physically and emotionally, in such a circumstance. Thus it seems clearly that for the patient who cannot get better by virtue of a diagnosis of end-stage malignancy, or other terminal disease, this type of care is totally inappropriate. I had many conscious thoughts that living was not in itself paramount and that maintenance of dignity and quality of life are truly valid concerns.

Accordingly, in the end, to me the two biggest decisions concerning the respirator are whether to use it at all and, subsequently, when to turn it off if the patient is not salvageable. However, cessation of an aggressive approach does not mean cessation of 'intensive care'. It does involve, though, acceptance of different goals, i.e., comfort for the patient and sensitive support for the family. These lessons from my personal experience led to my becoming involved with the hospice movement, which was just beginning in the United States at that time, for it was clear that the hospice philosophy was much in keeping with these concepts.

I would like to think that my experience has helped me to be a better doctor in a number of basic ways. I hope, and trust, that I now find it easier to listen to the patient. I no longer use machines and other intensive supportive procedures simply because they exist. I am able to talk more easily with sick people now that I have been there, and I understand that these patients are preoccupied with the fear of dying and want to talk about it. I am much more liberal with the use of morphine, when indicated, and can accept comfort as an end in itself. In short, I am able to deal better with the fact that some patients should be allowed to die quietly, with dignity, and without machines.

So, my final message is that we must not become a battery of specialists rendering superior *treatment* while *care* is absent. The patient should be the *beneficiary* of what we are doing, and not the *victim.* We must always keep our perspective, and not get lost in the maelstrom of our technology. We must always keep track of where we are going with our machines, not only medically and scientifically, but also economically, legally, morally and humanly.

E.D. Viner, MD,
Head, Hematology-Oncology Section, Pennsylvania Hospital,
Clinical Professor of Medicine, University of Pennsylvania School of Medicine,
727 Delancey Street, Philadelphia, PA 19107 (USA)

Prog. crit. Care Med., vol. 2, pp. 14–24 (Karger, Basel 1985)

Mechanical Ventilation and Human Ethics

Thomas L. Petty

University of Colorado Health Sciences Center, Denver, Colo., USA

Today all modern hospitals are equipped with mechanical ventilators capable of supporting life in many desperate situations. The mechanical ventilator achieved popularity in the mid-1960s when it became apparent that patients suffering from acute respiratory failure of many different causes could be salvaged by the skillful use of an airway and by life support with a ventilator. Earlier enthusiasm for ventilatory support focused on the problem of sudden respiratory arrest in poliomyelitis affecting young children, which was a dramatic event. The use of mechanical ventilators for this indication has subsided due to the success of polio vaccination. Replacing poliomyelitis, however, are even greater challenges, such as the adult respiratory distress syndrome, the increasing number of patients with self-induced poisonings, problems in the postoperative period or following cardiac arrest and other respiratory emergencies.

Work from our own center has demonstrated that recovery can occur in approximately 75% of all patients requiring mechanical ventilation [1]. This astounding outcome represents a true advance in our ability to care for desperately ill patients. However, all who are seriously involved in respiratory care or intensive care in general (also called critical care), recognize that a great deal of harm and suffering can also be caused by the inappropriate or irresponsible use of mechanical ventilators in hopeless situations. In these instances, the mechanical ventilator does not save life, but rather extends death. When this happens, untold human suffering occurs not only by the patient, but also by the family. The economic impact of this form of torture is massive and responsible for a significant proportion of the $290 billion spent on health care in the United States today. Thus, something must be done to take a more reasonable and responsible approach to the problem.

The medical literature and lay press alike are replete with discussions on legal, moral and ethical aspects of all aspects of medicine including the use of mechanical ventilators. Definitions of brain death, cortical death, rights of the individuals, rights of the family and the responsibility of society are discussed and debated. Physicians, lawyers, judges, theologians and ethicists often cannot agree whether it is right or wrong to discontinue ventilation of an obviously functionally dead or dying patient or whether it is ethical not to intervene with the use of mechanical ventilation before death occurs in certain clinical situations. No one can set down absolute principles to guide every physician with every patient. Since this is true, physicians must either assume the responsibility of caring for their patients in an appropriate and humane manner or else seek consultation from those who are willing. Otherwise, the patient, the family, and society suffer.

This chapter, based on over 20 years of nearly daily experience with ventilator patients, explores some of the issues concerning the ethical use of mechanical ventilators in critically ill patients [2].

Indications and Goals of Mechanical Ventilation

The majority of patients with acute respiratory failure from a variety of causes can be salvaged. At the outset, all patients with adult respiratory distress syndrome, by definition, will require mechanical ventilation. Patients with reversible neuromuscular disorders obviously require mechanical ventilation when their respiratory muscles (the most vital pump) tire or fail. Most notable examples are the Guillain-Barré syndrome, myasthenia gravis in crisis, disease states caused by neuromuscular toxins and neuromuscular blockade from pharmacological agents. On the other hand, patients with emerging amyotrophic lateral sclerosis (motor neuron disease), patients hopelessly ill with progressive multiple sclerosis and patients suffering major cerebral vascular catastrophes from hemorrhage or thrombosis are often inappropriately supported by mechanical ventilation when no hope for recovery exists.

Certainly, all patients with accidental poisoning and those large numbers of disillusioned members of society who overdose with a variety of drugs can and should be ventilated hoping for recovery from the motivating factors leading to the drug overdose in the case of self-ingested poisons.

Intensive psychiatric care is required in the hope of preventing repetition of this tragedy.

In addition, all patients suffering cardiac arrest have reduced respiratory center activity, at least at first, and even though many of these patients will never recover cortical function, one simply cannot be certain in many instances until 24–48 h have passed. Thus, it is appropriate to ventilate all of these patients at least initially if the reasons for resuscitation were sound.

Another situation in which mechanical ventilation is frequently used is the immediate postoperative period following major thoracic or abdominal surgery. In these instances, mechanical ventilatory support is useful in insuring adequate oxygenation and carbon dioxide elimination, usually for short periods, i.e. until the action of anesthetic and neuromuscular blocking agents is reversed and until the patient is awake and alert and able to support his own ventilation. The use of the mechanical ventilator also allows liberal use of narcotic agents to control pain without fear of respiratory depression. Many patients with inoperable carcinoma who have suffered endlessly from the apparent necessity of repeated surgery or following unsuccessful radiotherapy or chemotherapy with or without overwhelming infection, simply should not be ventilated when death begins to intervene. In these instances use of a ventilator is 'extraordinary treatment' and could be considered an assault to the dying patient.

The mechanical ventilator has a role in the management of patients with chronic obstructive pulmonary disease (COPD) *if* there is a treatable reversible feature of the disease. Most patients with acute respiratory failure accompanying COPD can survive these episodes by non-ventilator means, including the use of controlled oxygen, bronchodilating agents, antibiotics and corticosteroids. In some instances, the use of the mechanical ventilator is warranted to 'buy additional time', if the potential for reversibility and a comfortable, meaningful existence remains following this reprieve. Most asthmatics suffering life-threatening status asthmaticus respond to pharmacologic agents, but some require periods of ventilator support and recover. The mechanical ventilator is recognized as a two-edged sword in status asthmaticus since intubation of the airway may evoke additional bronchospasm or cardiac arrhythmia leading to a disastrous outcome [3]. Mechanical ventilation is rarely successful in prolonging happy life in terminal cystic fibrosis. The great majority of patients simply suffer longer if mechanical ventilation is used following a protracted period of insidious deterioration in the final stages of this disease [4].

Thus, it is apparent to all experienced individuals working in the field that the mechanical ventilator, though life saving, is not magic. No one should expect it to do the impossible. It should be our tool in the service of humanity and not a weapon against it.

Deciding Not to Ventilate Patients

There is a danger that the simple availability of mechanical ventilators demands their use in all desperate situations. Why is this the case? It is almost a reflex. Why do we not decide *not to do something* for a change on behalf of suffering patients? The answer to this question is obviously complex. Part of the problem comes from our own hopes for success in medicine. We are gratified by success and disillusioned with failure. The public also carries a high expectation of medical success aided and abetted by dramatic television stories which, although they may sometimes represent true human situations, are often fantasy. In fact, we live in a fantasy world with all of our high technology, where peer and public pressure can easily force us to the limits of the possible and beyond. In this fantasy world in which we may find ourselves, we cannot separate reality from nonsense. As we reflexly apply our technology, we fail to think what we are doing.

Another reason for our endless and inappropriate use of mechanical ventilators is sheer laziness. It is very easy to institute mechanical ventilation or persist with it, rather than consider an alternative. We will not take the time to sit down with the patient and his family and discuss the impossibility of going on with surgery, radiotherapy, chemotherapy in a case of cancer, or face the hopelessness of some cases of stroke or the inevitability of an irreversible neuromuscular disease or advancing COPD which has exhausted all of our abilities and therapies. If we only would face the obvious, which is often well known to patients and families anyway, and discuss the certainty of death and the physical, psychological and psychosocial costs of delaying this final process, we will serve our patients and their families better. We must present death as a natural event, guaranteed to all from the time of birth, in fact, from the time of conception. In our society, we have a very poor ability to deal with what is in fact a natural event! Our job in medicine is to forestall premature morbidity and mortality and at the same time to improve or at least maintain the quality of life. It is wrong in the minds of most reasonable people to continue to forestall mortality if life is miserable. But the argument is, 'who can tell?', 'who will take the responsibility?'. I firmly believe that the patient, his family, and the physician working together can decide and together must face this responsibility. Doing anything less is irresponsible to the patient, the family and to society.

Death itself is discussed as 'the future'; it can be compared to a transition. Death can be likened to sleep and in fact pleasant anticipation can replace fears and anxieties, by emphasizing the restful and renewing features of sleep. Death is a long sleep – perhaps more. By an optimist, death is presented as an adventure in a game we all must play. When these realities are understood and accepted, a great relief often spreads over the patient and the family. It is in a sense a 'détente' which is a reward promising relief of anxiety, depression and despair. Many patients can be sent home to die. Often they feel uplifted at the time of discharge and appear to live longer and happier at home, rather than in the hospital with a constant struggle with futile therapies and unnecessary further studies. The emerging hospice movement is very helpful at this time. In our city, both a home care hospice as well as a hospital service are available. Certainly this form of caring for patients is far preferable to continued suffering in intensive care units tethered to a mechanical ventilator with all of the attendant invasive, and dehumanizing procedures we are painfully aware of. Physicians can still care for their dying patients at home with the liberal use of phone calls and the occasional house-call which certainly must return to today's medical practice.

Discontinuing Mechanical Ventilation in Hopeless Patients

Another situation which leads to conflict and tragedy is failure to discontinue mechanical ventilation when it is only causing harm. Some tragic cases, often highly publicized by the press because of the media's endless need to unsettle and alarm the public, are encountered almost daily by anyone who reads newspapers, listens to radio or watches television. Issues of patients rights, right to live, right to die, legal definitions of brain death, attempts at other definitions of useful life including cortical function, etc., go on and on. *None* of these considerations or definitions are appropriate in every human situation and all have certain inherent inadequacies. Ethicists often cannot decide on what is ethical, moralists debate mortality and theologians cannot agree on the meaning of life or the significance of death.

Judges often cannot judge and the law fails to deal with human suffering because it is not capable of responding to all situations.

Again, the patient, the family and the physician working together ought to be able to decide when it is reasonable, indeed, right and proper to discontinue the mechanical ventilator which is only functioning as a symbol, a monument to man's stupidity over reasonable expectations for the future. In our state, a definition of brain death is a matter to be decided by the responsible physician with full discussions with the family. When it is decided that the patient cannot survive, it is a relatively simple matter to discontinue the mechanical ventilator and often to remove the endotracheal tube. It is well known that many brain-injured patients continue to breathe nonetheless, and in these instances a tracheostomy is sometimes performed to control secretions and a feeding gastrostomy placed, but again these approaches are inappropriate considering the realities of the situation. No one, however, would quarrel with the maintenance of an airway or fluids to avoid dehydration, as ingredients of life. Reasonable people would discontinue antibiotics or pressor agents or even replacement hormones in terminal situations. Thus, 'mechanical last rites' can be avoided [5]. In these situations it should be remembered that the physician must make decisions on behalf of the patient and the family. The family should not be asked to decide whether or not a ventilator should be discontinued. The family does not have the medical experience for this decision and will sometimes face anxieties and guilt after the fact of final somatic death. Thus, the physician should advise on behalf of the patient and the family will hopefully accept this advice. If they will not, things of course become much more difficult, but in almost all instances an adversary relationship between the physician and the family can be avoided with forthright and honest discussions in advance of problems, thus preventing disagreement. When the physician plays this role in deciding what should happen in terms of discontinuing mechanical ventilation or not starting it in the first place, he is not playing God, in fact he is playing doctor!

Dealing with Death and Dying Patients in General

So much of medical tragedy could be avoided by prophylactic means based upon a clear contract between patient and physician and meaningful discussions about all stages of illness, including the final phases resulting in death. Perhaps we will teach this necessity of medical practice better in the future as we face a growing aging population. Today we have no specialists who deal with the event of death like those who prepare for and assist in the moment of birth. It seems so sad that we have left life in such a suspended state in medical practice!

Case Examples

Since it is certain that no set of laws or guidelines will apply in all clinical situations, it must become obvious that the practicing physician and in fact all in the medical profession must develop their own reasoned approach to the problem. The approach must be systematic and one that the individual can utilize in comfort consistent with his own training and beliefs. It is taken for granted that appropriate training was received by all health care workers who may have to decide not to intervene with mechanical ventilators or to discontinue ventilation and that the physicians in charge have sought consultation and conducted whatever diagnostic procedures necessary to be absolutely convinced that all reasonable hopes for recovery must be abandoned. Rather than going into details of training, competence, diagnostic procedures or consultations, it may be preferable to cite some clinical examples where decisions had to be made, often quickly, in the course of 1 month of 'on service' responsibilities while I was responsible for the intensive care unit. These are real-life situations which will be recognized by all in the profession.

Case 1

A 65-year-old woman with longstanding hypertension had suffered a disabling stroke 8 years previously. She was admitted to the coronary care unit from a nursing home following excruciating chest pain. ECG and serum enzyme evidence of massive anterior lateral myocardial infarction was obtained during the first 48 h of admission. The patient was found in ventricular fibrillation on the 4th hospital day and following electroshock and a long resuscitation effort she was intubated and mechanical ventilatory support begun. A deep comatose state was present in the immediate resuscitation period and for 72 h thereafter. Erratic respiratory activity was present during brief periods of T-tube weaning. The patient was maintained on the ventilator for an additional day and respiratory center activity stabilized. Thereafter it was possible to remove the mechanical ventilator and spontaneous respirations continued. Oxygen was administered by nasal cannula and adequate arterial oxygenation and carbon dioxide elimination continued. Intravenous fluids were given and urinary output remained excellent. Because of failure of any cortical recovery, the patient was transferred from the intensive care unit to the ward in preparation for return to the nursing home. She remained monitored by telemetry. 48 h later, asystole was noted and 'code blue' was called. There was a frantic rush to the bedside by at least 11 medical students, interns or houseofficers. The attending physician, responsible for the care of the patient, was seeing another patient in the next room at this moment. In fact, he was the first on the scene of the cardiac arrest. He stood calmly by and counseled the houseofficers as they rushed into the room. Thus no repeat resuscitative efforts were instituted. In the final conference with the family the physician explained that no resuscitative efforts were attempted because of lack of any brain recovery following the earlier resuscitation effort. The family was thankful that death had intervened at this time.

Comment

This is a relatively easy example of nonintervention in a hopeless post-cardiac arrest situation. In the absence of head trauma or sedative drugs, failure to regain brain function following total loss of all integrative function for more than 24 h is an absolute sign that recovery will never occur in my experience and the experience of others. Thus, the adage 'don't just do something stand there' [6] is highly appropriate for this situation. Further agony by the family who had hoped and indeed prayed for death could thus be avoided in this situation.

Case 2

A prominent maître d'hôtel of a popular hotel restaurant was 'found down' by his wife. 2 years earlier he had been resuscitated by an emergency medical team in a similar clinical situation at home on his 74th birthday. He had recovered and had returned to his work but had suffered unstable cardiac rhythms. Nonetheless, he persisted in his work which he dearly enjoyed. On this second occasion the wife had no idea how long the patient had been unresponsive in the bedroom. Nonetheless, the emergency team again instituted counter shock with a slow junctional rhythm as the result. Vasopressors were administered en route to the hospital. The patient was transferred to the intensive care unit and mechanical ventilation continued. After 48 h no purposeful movements or brain stem reflexes were present. Electroencephalogram showed very primitive slow wave activity. Consultation with the neurology service was obtained and it was concluded independently that the chances of recovery of brain function were zero. This fact was discussed with the wife who agreed that it would be in the best interests of everyone to discontinue mechanical ventilation as well as all drugs. Both the mechanical ventilator and the endotracheal tube were removed but spontaneous breathing remained. The patient was transferred to the ward and died 24 h later of an apparent respiratory arrest.

Comment

Even though earlier resuscitation had been successful it was certain on the present occasion that no hope for recovery existed. This fact was presented to the wife following consultation and diagnostic tests which confirmed the obvious. The wife and her son accepted the decision and thanked the nurses and doctors for their kind assistance. Thus, a relatively ideal resolution was obtained. The alternative would have been a period of continued somatic life at great psychological and economic cost to the family.

Case 3

A 78-year-old lady with Huntington's chorea had been cared for by her family at home for several years. She was found with gasping respirations and the '911' emergency medical team was alerted. The patient was intubated and brought to the emergency room. The family reported years of deteriorating state and difficulties of caring for the patient at home. Nonetheless, they insisted that 'everything be done'. Accordingly, the mechanical ventilation instituted by the resuscitation team was continued, vasopressors used and treatment for severe hypothermia (admitting temperature 32 °C) begun. As the body temperature of the patient improved the tremor of Huntington's chorea returned. No cortical responses were present. On this occasion, the attending physician sat down with the family and pointed out that 'everything' had been done for the past 72 h. It was advised that death could occur on extubation, but that the patient might continue to breathe. With this form of support the family was quite satisfied that everything had been done and with full agreement the patient was extubated. She continued to breathe and remained in a semi-vegetative state. We therefore pointed out to the family that the emergency was over and the family could take the patient home once again. They accepted and the patient went back to her previous residence in the care of her family where she died 2 weeks later.

Comment

In this situation, an adversary relationship with the family was avoided by assenting to their initial wishes. Others would have probably preferred not to intervene recognizing the hopelessness of the situation. Gaining the confidence of the family and imparting some more experience with the natural course of the disease was extremely valuable in resolving the situation which otherwise could have led to days, weeks or months of further mechanical ventilatory assistance in the intensive care unit.

Case 4

A 45-year-old man with chronic myelogenous leukemia for 10 years developed a 'blast crisis'. An incomplete hematological remission had been gained with aggressive chemotherapy. The patient was admitted to the intensive care unit for lower gastrointestinal bleeding. Numerous attempts to determine the site of bleeding including repeated endoscopies and radionuclide scans had failed to reveal the source of hemorrhage. Over 11 days, 40 units of either whole blood, fresh frozen plasma or platelets were given but oozing continued. Finally, a third scan suggested bleeding in the cecum and the patient was taken to surgery in a final attempt to stop hemorrhage. Three bleeding ulcers were found on opening the cecum. A right hemicolectomy was completed and the patient transferred to the recovery room and finally to the surgical intensive care unit. The mechanical ventilator which had been used in the immediate postoperative period could easily be removed and spontaneous respiration was satisfactory. He became awake and alert and visited with his family. 5 days later, bleeding returned. As preparation for further diagnostic studies and possible surgery was being made, chills, profound hypotension and diaphoresis occurred. Over the course of the next 12 h, diffuse pulmonary infiltrates appeared in all lung fields indicating an emerging acute lung injury and respiratory distress syndrome. The patient began to feel exhausted and blood gases showed a marked deterioration, with hypoxemia refractory to nasal oxygen and later to oxygen delivered by a reservoir mask. The patient was intubated and the family summoned quickly to the bedside. With the attending physician present it was discussed frankly that hopes for recovery in this situation were nil. Amidst considerable tears and handholding, the attending physician offered the opinion that further suffering was inappropriate. The family and friends then said 'goodby' and the patient was given intravenous morphine for relief of pain. The endotracheal tube was removed and death occurred within 2 h. The family thanked the physicians and nurses for their compassionate care.

Comment

In this situation, hopes for any recovery in a blast crisis following years of chronic myelogenous leukemia and failure of aggressive chemotherapy were nil. A long hospitalization requiring extensive diagnostic tests and surgery had proven unsuccessful and terminal sepsis was present. Further 'life support' would have been assaultive to both the patient and family, a fact which had been discussed in advance of the final event. Bringing the family together for the final goodby helped relieve everyone's anxiety and the patient died peacefully.

Case 5

A 58-year-old woman had suffered progressive muscle weakness finally diagnosed as amyotrophic lateral sclerosis (motor neuron disease). Marked bulbar weakness was present and swallowing became difficult resulting in a 20-lb. weight loss. Since the patient's habitus was rather lean before the rapidly emerging neurological process began, she presented in a very cachectic state. The attending neurologist decided that a feeding gastrostomy was needed to avoid further starvation. No preoperative blood gases or ventilatory function tests were obtained. The gastrostomy was placed very easily by the surgical team, but in the immediate postoperative period the patient was very weak and required a mechanical ventilator. The next morning she was awake and alert and an attempt at extubation was made. Within 3 h, the patient was diaphoretic and suffering anxiety and air hunger. She was therefore reintubated and rested quietly with ventilatory assistance. The use of the feeding gastrostomy tube was begun, but strength did not return. Discussions between the consulting respiratory care team and neurologists then began for the first time. Also the family sought discussions with the consulting respiratory care team. The possibility of a continuing 'life' with ventilatory support had never occurred to either patient or family. Both the patient's daughter, who was in her second trimester of pregnancy, and the patient herself became angry over the 'entrapment', yet neither could face the realities of death. At this writing, the patient remains in a totally paralyzed state and on a mechanical ventilator. The final resolution of this dilemma awaits responsible decision.

Comment

In this unhappy situation neither the family nor the patient's personal physician accepted the inevitability of death. Preparation for the final outcome was therefore postponed or denied. The consulting respiratory care team was sought out for help and assistance, but since the respiratory care physician was not the managing physician, he did not make the decisions that should have been made by the attending neurologist.

Is this patient as well as her family and society served by this inappropriate use of the mechanical ventilator? Doubtless many would debate the issue, but anyone going to the bedside and speaking with the patient would find little to debate.

References

1 Petty, T.L.; Lakshminarayan, S.; Sahn, S.A.; Zwillich, C.W.; Nett, L.M.: Intensive respiratory care unit (review of 10 years' experience). J. Am. med. Ass. *233:* 34–37 (1975).

2 Petty, T.L.: Intensive and rehabilitative respiratory care; 3rd ed. (Lea & Febiger, Philadelphia 1982).

3 Scoggin, C.H.; Sahn, S.A.; Petty, T.L.: Status asthmaticus – a nine year experience. J. Am. med. Ass. *238:* 1158–1162 (1977).

4 Davis, P.B.; di Sant'Agnese, P.: Assisted ventilation for patients with cystic fibrosis. J. Am. med. Ass. *239:* 1851–1854 (1978).

5 Petty, T.L.: Mechanical last 'rights'. Archs intern. Med. *142:* 1442 (1982).

6 Petty, T.L.: Don't just do something – stand there! Archs intern. Med. *139:* 920–921 (1979).

Thomas L. Petty, MD, Professor of Medicine,
Co-Director, Webb-Wuring Lung Institute,
Head, Division of Pulmonary Sciences, University of Colorado
Health Sciences Center, 4200 E Ninth Avenue, Denver, CO 80262 (USA)

Prog. crit. Care Med., vol. 2, pp. 25–35 (Karger, Basel 1985)

Status epilepticus

Peggy J. Wisdom

Department of Neurology, University of Oklahoma Health Sciences Center, Oklahoma City, Okla., USA

Status epilepticus is a serious neurologic disorder. Convulsive status epilepticus is a life-threatening disorder which requires immediate and prudent therapeutic intervention. Prompt recognition of convulsive status epilepticus as a neurologic emergency and the immediate institution of effective therapy reduces acute mortality and morbidity. While nonconvulsive status epilepticus is less common than convulsive status epilepticus, delay in recognition and treatment of complex partial status epilepticus may result in profound residual behavioral disorders [44].

Therapeutic success and prognosis are also dependent upon the cause of status epilepticus. Status epilepticus is associated with acute neurologic and systemic disorders as well as chronic epilepsy. Status epilepticus is reported to occur in 1.3–6.6% of individuals with chronic epilepsy [10, 24, 32]. However, the most common cause of status epilepticus in chronic epilepsy is noncompliance with anticonvulsant therapy. Status epilepticus associated with acute neurologic or systemic disorders is less responsive to therapeutic intervention and is associated with a higher morbidity and mortality.

The purpose of this paper is to review the clinical features, causes, precipitating factors, and therapeutic considerations regarding status epilepticus in the adult.

Clinical Features

Status epilepticus is characterized by either continuous seizure activity or frequently repeated seizures which persist for longer than 30 min. Classification of status epilepticus is based on the international classification of seizures [22]. Subvarieties of convulsive status epilepticus are: tono-clonic status epilepticus, focal status epilepticus, and myoclonic status epilepticus. Nonconvulsive status epilepticus is classified as absence status epilepticus or complex partial status epilepticus (psychomotor status epilepticus).

Convulsive tono-clonic status epilepticus is the most frequent and the most serious type of status epilepticus. Convulsive tono-clonic status epilepticus occurring in adults has a focal onset in 62–72% of cases [3, 9]. Features include focal motor seizure activity or adversive head and eye movement. Adult-onset convulsive tono-clonic status epilepticus, particularly of focal onset, is associated with symptomatic epilepsy from acute central nervous system disorders, metabolic-toxic disorders, or preexisting static central nervous system lesions.

Myoclonic status epilepticus is characterized by repetitive, generalized muscular jerks. There is usually not an associated loss of consciousness; however, there may be an encephalopathy secondary to the underlying cause. Myoclonic status epilepticus may occur with acute or progressive central nervous system disorders. Metabolic and toxic disorders including anoxic encephalopathy are the most common causes.

Focal status epilepticus is characterized by frequent focal motor seizures with preservation of consciousness. It is commonly associated with acute and chronic cerebral infarction and metabolic disorders of the central nervous system [10, 43].

Nonconvulsive status epilepticus is clinically characterized by prolonged episodes of confusion. While not life threatening, there are recent reports of profound memory disorders from prolonged complex partial status epilepticus [44]. Nonconvulsive status epilepticus may be difficult to differentiate from metabolic or toxic encephalopathies without the use of the electroencephalogram.

Metabolic and toxic disorders were identified as common causes of convulsive status epilepticus in studies reported by *Celesia* [10] and *Aminoff and Simon* [3]. Electrolyte imbalance, renal failure, hypoglycemia, hyperosmolar coma, anoxia, alcohol withdrawal, and drug overdose are present in the majority of cases.

Regardless of the underlying cause of convulsive status epilepticus, the majority of cases are precipitated by anticonvulsant incompliance, alcohol abuse, and systemic infections. In cases with preexisting epilepsy, 53% are precipitated by anticonvulsant incompliance, and 22% are precipitated by alcohol withdrawal [3].

Prognosis

Mortality rates from convulsive status epilepticus vary from 6 to 23%, and mortality rates for status epilepticus associated with preexisting epilepsy were recently reported as between 2.5 and 6% [3, 10]. Convulsive status epilepticus from acute neurologic or systemic disorders has a higher mortality.

Neurologic sequelae of status epilepticus are influenced by the presence of preexisting neurologic disease or acute systemic or neurologic disorders in addition to the duration of status epilepticus. *Rowan and Scott* [38] found no neurologic sequelae in those cases which lasted 1.5 h or less and significant neurologic sequelae in those cases which lasted 10 h.

Neurologic sequelae and death are probably the consequences of hypoxemia, hypoglycemia, hyperpyrexia, hypotension, and acidosis which are pathophysiologic changes associated with prolonged status epilepticus [30]. In experimental studies of prolonged status epilepticus, ischemic cell change is found in the neocortex, cerebellum, and hippocampus [29]. Adequate oxygenation may prevent systemic complications during prolonged status epilepticus; however, brain damage or death may occur despite adequate oxygenation [34, 46].

Absence status (spike wave stupor, petit mal status) can occur at any age; however, 30% of the cases are seen in young adults [42]. Although the majority of cases have a previous history of absence seizures, absence status may be the first symptom of epilepsy [35]. In adults, absence status epilepticus may be the only manifestation of epilepsy [4]. Clinical characteristics encompass a spectrum of continuous behavioral disturbances which range from mild impairment of attention to confusion and stupor. Absence status epilepticus may continue for hours to several days. Electroencephalographically generalized spike wave discharges occur throughout the duration of absence status epilepticus.

Complex partial status epilepticus (psychomotor status) occurs less frequently than absence status. Clinical manifestations of complex partial status epilepticus are prolonged confusional states interrupted by total nonresponsiveness, staring, and stereotyped automatisms [16, 18, 44]. Electroencephalographically generalized slowing is noted during the confusional phase, and epileptiform discharge in the temporal lobe is noted during the nonresponsive phase. Case reports are few in number; however, most cases are associated with preexisting epilepsy [16, 18, 28, 40, 48].

Causes and Precipitating Factors

Convulsive status epilepticus is frequently associated with acute neurologic or systemic disorders in the nonepileptic patient and with chronic neurologic disorders in the epileptic. Causes are identified in 63–87% of cases [3, 10, 24, 32, 38]. Table I lists the frequency of causes of convulsive status epilepticus.

When convulsive status epilepticus is the initial manifestation of epilepsy, an acute structural lesion of the central nervous system should be considered. Idiopathic epilepsy has never been reported to present with convulsive status epilepticus as the initial symptom in the adult. *Janz* [25] and *Oxbury and Whitty* [33] reported that 20–25% of cases were associated with neoplasms. They emphasized that 50–74% of neoplasms associated with convulsive status epilepticus were localized to the frontal lobe.

Although better substantiated in children, clinical studies on prolonged status epilepticus have demonstrated neurologic sequelae secondary to extensive neuronal damage [1–3]. Rapid and sustained termination of status epilepticus must be the goal of therapy to prevent neurologic sequelae or death.

Table I. Causes of status epilepticus in adults (%)

	Study			
	Janz, 1964 [25] (n = 138)	*Oxbury and Whitty,* 1971 [32] (n = 96)	*Rowan and Scott,* 1970 [38] (n = 42)	*Celesia* 1976 [10] (n = 60)
Idiopathic	21	22	21	25
Cerebrovascular	14	7	7	15
Craniocerebral trauma	17	21	26	12
Infection	9	7	16	2
Metabolic-toxic	2	0	2	13
Neoplasm	20	25	5	5
Other causes	4	9	23	16
Unknown	13	9	0	13

Medical Management of Convulsive Status epilepticus

While the prognosis is influenced by the cause of status epilepticus, rapid and sustained termination reduces the risk of neurologic sequelae and death. Diagnostic and therapeutic protocols have been proposed to achieve these goals in the management of status epilepticus (table II) [19, 47]. Man-

Table II. Medical management of status epilepticus [19, 47]

Time, min	Diagnostic protocol	Therapeutic protocol
0	assess cardiopulmonary status; monitor blood pressure, pulse, ECG, respiration	establish oral airway and nasal O_2 (assisted ventilation may be indicated); establish intravenous line
5	assess electrolytes, calcium, magnesium, phosphorus, blood urea nitrogen, drug screen; complete blood count, arterial blood gas, anticonvulsant levels	glucose i.v.: 50 ml of 50%, thiamine 100 mg i.m.
10	monitor ECG continuously, and blood pressure, pulse, respiration every 2 min throughout intravenous administration of all drugs	diazepam 10–20 mg i.v. at 2 mg/min and phenytoin 15–18 mg/kg at 50 mg/min (reduce rate of administration of anticonvulsants and institute appropriate medical therapy, if cardiopulmonary status becomes unstable)
45	monitor blood pressure, pulse, and arterial blood gases	intubate to assist ventilation and phenobarbital at 25 mg/min to a total of 20 mg/kg; correct all metabolic disturbances
90	monitor EEG if pentobarbital is used	general anesthesia
At cessation of status epilepticus	monitor anticonvulsant levels and fully investigate cause of status epilepticus: skull X-ray, CT scan, EEG, chest X-ray, spinal fluid	maintain all long-term anticonvulsants at therapeutically effective levels; institute therapy for cause of status epilepticus

agement of status epilepticus is not successful, unless all the following goals are accomplished: (1) insure adequate cardiopulmonary function; (2) arrest clinical and electrical status epilepticus within 30 min; (3) establish long-term anticonvulsant therapy to prevent recurrences; (4) prevent and correct metabolic disturbances, and (5) identify and correct causes.

A variety of anticonvulsants are available for use in status epilepticus. However, diazepam, phenytoin, and phenobarbital are the anticonvulsants of choice. To be effective, all anticonvulsants must be given intravenously and in adequate loading doses to achieve therapeutic concentrations. All anticonvulsants have potential cardiopulmonary depressant effects which may accentuate cardiopulmonary complications if administered too rapidly or in combination with other anticonvulsants. Adequate ventilatory and cardiovascular function must be insured at all times.

Diazepam

Intravenous diazepam was introduced in the treatment of status epilepticus as the drug of choice in 1965 [21]. The overall efficacy of diazepam in treatment of status epilepticus is 70%, with another 17% of cases showing only temporary improvement [7]. Diazepam is more effective for control of status epilepticus associated with static and chronic neurologic disorders [36, 39]. Diazepam, when administered intravenously, is rapidly redistributed with a decline to subtherapeutic brain and plasma concentrations over 45 min [37]. It is a useful drug for arresting status epilepticus, but inadequate to prevent recurrences. Therefore, phenytoin must be given in adequate loading doses to prevent recurrences.

Diazepam must be administered intravenously at a dose of 0.15–0.3 mg/kg to a maximum of 20 mg. It should be given at a rate no greater than 2 mg/min to reduce the risk of complications. Continuous infusion of diazepam has been reported to be effective in 66% of cases of status epilepticus refractory to bolus diazepam [20]. Continuous infusion of diazepam would insure constant therapeutic concentrations; however, tolerance to the drug may develop. For this reason phenytoin should be administered to prevent recurrence of seizures.

Complications include respiratory depression, hypotension, and rarely asystole. The risk of respiratory depression is increased by prior use of sedatives including alcohol or barbiturates [5].

Phenytoin

Phenytoin is an effective anticonvulsant in the treatment of generalized tono-clonic status, focal motor status, and partial complex status. Phenytoin is more effective in the treatment of status epilepticus in patients with preexisting epilepsy than in patients who have status epilepticus from acute central nervous system disorders. *Cranford* et al. [13] reported cessation of status epilepticus in 79% of cases with preexisting epilepsy and 54% of cases presenting with status epilepticus from acute neurologic or metabolic disorders. Similar efficacy has been reported by others [45, 49].

To be effective in the treatment of status epilepticus, phenytoin must be administered intravenously in large loading doses. Oral or intramuscular administration of phenytoin does not produce the rapid therapeutic serum concentration necessary to control status epilepticus [14, 50]. Using the intravenous route, phenytoin enters the brain rapidly; however, adequate loading doses must be administered to achieve clinical efficacy. When loading doses of 15–18 mg/kg are administered intravenously, serum concentrations of 18–24 mg/ml are achieved within 30 min of infusion [12]. Maintenance doses of phenytoin should be started within 6–12 h of loading to insure therapeutic serum concentrations.

Intravenous phenytoin should be administered undiluted through saline-flushed intravenous tubing into an arm vein. Heart rate and blood pressure should be monitored every 2 min. The electrocardiogram should be monitored throughout the infusion. The infusion should be 50 mg/min; a rate of 25 mg/min is preferred in elderly patients.

Serious cardiovascular complications from intravenous phenytoin include hypotension and arrythmias. If the following guidelines are observed, serious complications can be avoided: (1) Contraindications to the use of intravenous phenytoin are severe atherosclerotic heart disease, marked bradycardia, and second- or third-degree heart block. (2) The rate of infusion should be 50 mg/min. (3) If hypotension is observed during the infusion, the rate of infusion should be slowed [12].

Phenobarbital

Phenobarbital is an effective anticonvulsant for treatment of convulsive status epilepticus. Phenobarbital must be given intravenously to achieve rapid therapeutic concentration. It may be used as either the first-line or a second-line drug in the treatment.

Goldberg and McIntyre [23] have recommended the initial administration of 250–300 mg of phenobarbital intravenously. This can be repeated every 20–30 min for a total of three doses. Phenobarbital as the initial drug is very effective for status epilepticus associated with anoxia and metabolic disturbances.

As a second-line drug, *Escueta* et al. [19] have recommended the intravenous administration of phenobarbital, if status epilepticus is refractory to diazepam and phenytoin. These authors recommend a maximum dose of 20 mg/kg. Maintenance doses of phenobarbital should be continued to insure therapeutic concentrations to prevent recurrences.

Intravenously administered phenobarbital can produce sedation which makes its use in neurosurgical disorders less desirable. Respiratory depression is the most serious side effect of phenobarbital. It would be wise to insure adequate ventilation prior to the administration of phenobarbital, particularly if any other respiratory depressants have been used.

Refractory Status epilepticus

24% of the treatment failures are related to unsatisfactory management [11]. Reasons for unsatisfactory management are: (1) delay in recognition of status epilepticus; (2) delay in institution of therapy; (3) inadequate anticonvulsant dosage; (4) oral or intramuscular administration; (5) failure to maintain adequate respiration and blood pressure, and (6) failure to institute maintenance anticonvulsant therapy.

Refractory status epilepticus should be recognized within 2 h of presentation. Since refractory status epilepticus is commonly associated with acute neurologic or systemic disorders, identification and treatment of the cause will enhance the therapeutic efficacy of anticonvulsants. If status epilepticus cannot be controlled with adequate doses of diazepam, phenytoin, and phenobarbital, general anesthesia should be instituted. Barbiturate anesthesia using pentobarbital in conjunction with continuous electroencephalographic monitoring or halothane anesthesia may be used [23, 31]. Neuromuscular junction blockade is indicated, if acidosis or life-threatening systemic complications cannot be managed medically. However, neuromuscular junction blockade is not advocated without general anesthesia to arrest cerebral status epilepticus. Prolonged status epilepticus, even with adequate ventilation, is associated with continuous electrical status epilepticus and brain damage [17, 26, 34, 46]. Refractory status epilepticus has been treated with lidocaine and paraldehyde; however, experience in administration and efficacy is limited [6, 8, 15, 27, 41].

Management of Nonconvulsive Status epilepticus

Complex partial status epilepticus is responsive to phenytoin. The diagnosis should be confirmed prior to the administration of intravenous anticonvulsants. Phenytoin should be administered intravenously as outlined in table II. Phenobarbital may be indicated, if complex partial status epilepticus is not reponsive to phenytoin. Maintenance of long-term anticonvulsants is important to prevent recurrence.

The drug of choice for absence status is ethosuximide. Ethosuximide cannot be administered intravenously and must be given orally. Sodium valproate is a second-line drug in the treatment of absence status. Both drugs are effective in treatment of this disorder.

References

1 Aicardi, J.; Chevrie, J.J.: Convulsive status epilepticus in infants and children. A study of 239 cases. Epilepsia *11:* 187–197 (1970).
2 Aicardi, J.; Barton, J.: A pneumoencephalographic demonstration of brain atrophy following status epilepticus. Devl Med. Child Neur. *13:* 660–667 (1971).
3 Aminoff, M.J.; Simon, R.P.: Status epilepticus: causes, clinical features and consequences in 98 patients. Am. J. Med. *69:* 657–666 (1980).
4 Andermann, F.; Robb, J.P.: Absence status. A reappraisal following review of thirty-eight patients. Epilepsia *13:* 177–187 (1972).
5 Bell, D.S.: Dangers of treatment of status epilepticus with diazepam. Br. med. J. *i:* 159–161 (1969).
6 Bernhard, C.G.; Bohm, E.: Local anaesthetics as anticonvulsants: a study on experimental and clinical epilepsy, pp. 57–90 (Almqvist & Wiksell, Uppsala 1965).
7 Browne, T.R.; Penry, J.K.: Benzodiazepines in the treatment of epilepsy. A review. Epilepsia *14:* 277–310 (1973).
8 Browne, T.R.: Drug therapy reviews: drug therapy of status epilepticus. Am. J. Hosp. Pharm. *35:* 915–922 (1978).
9 Celesia, G.G.; Messert, B.; Murphy, M.J.: Status epilepticus of late adult onset. Neurology *22:* 1047–1055 (1972).
10 Celesia, G.G.: Modern concepts of status epilepticus. J. Am. med. Ass. *235:* 1571–1574 (1976).

11 Celesia, G.G.: Prognosis in convulsive status epilepticus. Adv. Neurol. *34:* 55–60 (1983).

12 Cranford, R.E.; Leppik, I.E.; Patrick, B.; Anderson, C.B.; Kostick, B.: Intravenous phenytoin: clinical and pharmacokinetic aspects. Neurology *28:* 874–880 (1978).

13 Cranford, R.E.; Leppik, I.E.; Patrick, B.; Anderson, C.B.; Kostick, B.: Intravenous phenytoin in acute treatment of seizures. Neurology *29:* 1474–1479 (1979).

14 Dam, M.; Olesen, V.: Intramuscular administration of phenytoin. Neurology *16:* 288–292 (1966).

15 De Elio, F.J.; De Jalon, P.G.; Obrador, S.: Some experimental and clinical observations on the anticonvulsive action of paraldehyde. J. Neurol. Neurosurg. Psychiat. *12:* 19–24 (1949).

16 Engel, J.; Ludwig, B.I.; Fetell, M.: Prolonged partial complex status epilepticus: EEG and behavioural observations. Neurology *28:* 863–869 (1978).

17 Epstein, M.H.; O'Connor, J.S.: Destructive effects of prolonged status epilepticus. J. Neurol. Neurosurg. Psychiat. *29:* 251–254 (1966).

18 Escueta, A.V.; Boxley, J.; Stubbs, N.; Waddell, G.; Wilson, W.A.: Prolonged twilight state and automatisms: a case report. Neurology *24:* 331–339 (1974).

19 Escueta, A.V.; Wasterlain, C.; Treiman, D.M.; Porter, R.J.: Management of status epilepticus. New Engl. J. Med. *306:* 1337–1340 (1982).

20 Escueta, A.V.; Bacsal, F.E.: Combination therapy for status epilepticus: intravenous diazepam and phenytoin. Adv. Neurol. *34:* 477–485 (1983).

21 Gastaut, H.; Naquet, R.; Poire, R.; Tassinari, C.A.: Treatment of status epilepticus with diazepam (Valium). Epilepsia *6:* 167–182 (1965).

22 Gastaut, H.: Clinical and electroencephalographic classification of epileptic seizures. Epilepsia *11:* 102–113 (1970).

23 Goldberg, M.A.; McIntyre, H.B.: Barbiturates in the treatment of status. Adv. Neurol. *34:* 499–503 (1983).

24 Hunter, R.A.: Status epilepticus. History, incidence and problems. Epilepsia *1:* 162–188 (1959).

25 Janz, D.: Status epilepticus and frontal lobe lesions. J. neurol. Sci. *1:* 446–457 (1964).

26 James, J.L.; Whitty, C.W.M.: The electroencephalogram as a monitor of status epilepticus suppressed peripherally by curarisation. Lancet *ii:* 239–241 (1961).

27 Lemmen, L.J.; Klassen, M.; Duiser, B.: Intravenous lidocaine in the treatment of convulsions. J. Am. med. Ass. *239:* 2025 (1978).

28 Markand, O.N.; Wheeler, G.L.; Pollack, S.L.: Complex partial status epilepticus (psychomotor status). Neurology *28:* 189–196 (1978).

29 Meldrum, B.S.; Brierley, J.B.: Prolonged epileptic seizures in primates. Ischemic cell change and its relation to ictal physiological events. Archs Neurol. *28:* 10–17 (1973).

30 Meldrum, B.S.; Horton, R.W.: Physiology of status epilepticus in primates. Archs Neurol. *28:* 1–9 (1973).

31 Opitz, A.; Marschall, M.; Degen, R.; Koch, D.: General anesthesia in patients with epilepsy and status epilepticus. Adv. Neurol. *34:* 531–535 (1983).

32 Oxbury, J.M.; Whitty, C.W.M.: Causes and consequences of status epilepticus in adults. Brain *94:* 733–744 (1971).

33 Oxbury, J.M.; Whitty, C.W.M.: The syndrome of isolated epileptic status. J. Neurol. Neurosurg. Psychiat. *34:* 182–184 (1971).

34 Plum, R.; Howse, D.C.; Duffy, T.E.: Metabolic effects of seizures. Res. Publs Ass. Res. nerv. ment. Dis. *53:* 141–157 (1974).

35 Porter, R.J.; Penry, J.K.: Petit mal status. Adv. Neurol. *34:* 61–67 (1983).

36 Prensky, A.L.; Raff, M.C.; Moore, M.J.; Schwab, R.S.: Intravenous diazepam in the treatment of prolonged seizure activity. New Engl. J. Med. *276:* 779–784 (1967).

37 Ramsay, E.R.; Hammond, E.J.; Perchalski, R.J.; Wilder, B.J.: Brain uptake of phenytoin, phenobarbital and diazepam. Archs Neurol. *36:* 535–539 (1979).

38 Rowan, A.J.; Scott, D.F.: Major status epilepticus. Acta neur. scand. *46:* 573–584 (1970).

39 Sawyer, G.T.; Webster, D.D.; Schut, L.J.: Treatment of uncontrolled seizure activity with diazepam. J. Am. med. Ass. *203:* 913–918 (1968).

40 Shalev, R.S.; Amir, N.: Complex partial status epilepticus. Archs Neurol. *40:* 90–92 (1983).

41 Taverner, D.; Bain, W.A.: Intravenous lignocaine as an anticonvulsant in status epilepticus and serial epilepsy. Lancet *ii:* 1145–1147 (1958).

42 Thompson, S.W.; Greenhouse, A.H.: Petit mal status in adults. Ann. intern. Med. *68:* 1271–1279 (1968).

43 Treiman, D.M.; Escueta, A.V.: Status epilepticus; in Thompson, Green, Critical care of neurologic and neurosurgical emergencies, pp. 53–99 (Raven Press, New York 1980).

44 Treiman, D.M.; Escueta, A.V.: Complex partial status epilepticus. Adv. Neurol. *34:* 69–81 (1983).

45 Wallis, W.; Kutt, H.; McDowell, F.: Intravenous diphenylhydantoin in treatment of acute repetitive seizures. Neurology *18:* 513–525 (1968).

46 Wasterlain, C.G.: Mortality and morbidity from serial seizures. Epilepsia *15:* 155–176 (1974).

47 Wasterlain, C.G.: Status epilepticus. Semin. Neurol. *1:* 87–94 (1981).

48 Wieser, H.G.: Temporal lobe or psychomotor status epilepticus. A case report. Electroenceph. clin. Neurophysiol. *48:* 558–572 (1980).

49 Wilder, B.J.; Ramsay, R.E.; Willmore, L.J.; Feussner, G.F.; Perchalski, R.J.; Shumate, J.B.: Efficacy of intravenous phenytoin in the treatment of status epilepticus: kinetics of central nervous system penetration. Ann. Neurol. *1:* 511–518 (1977).

50 Wilensky, A.J.; Lowden, J.A.: Inadequate serum levels after intramuscular administration of diphenylhydantoin. Neurology *23:* 318–324 (1973).

Peggy J. Wisdom, MD,
Department of Neurology, University of Oklahoma Health Sciences Center,
Oklahoma City, OK 73190 (USA)

Prog. crit. Care Med., vol. 2, pp. 36–43 (Karger, Basel 1985)

Mechanisms of Acute Lung Injury

Sami I. Said

Department of Medicine, University of Oklahoma Health Sciences Center and Veterans Administration Medical Center, Oklahoma City, Okla., USA

Major Responses in Acute Lung Injury

Acute lung injury, culminating in the clinical entity of respiratory distress, with diffuse pulmonary infiltrates, falling arterial blood oxygenation, and a stiffening lung (adult respiratory distress syndrome, ARDS), is associated with several pulmonary and extrapulmonary responses [36]:

(1) *Increased pulmonary microvascular permeability,* the key pathophysiologic alteration, is responsible for the major abnormalities in pulmonary gas exchange and pulmonary mechanics and is the most difficult to correct.

(2) *Pulmonary vasoconstriction and bronchoconstriction,* which are frequently present, add to the respiratory distress and may be more amenable to treatment than the increased permeability.

(3) *Systemic hypotension,* a common complication of severe ARDS (as well as a predisposing cause of it), is usually aggravated by certain therapeutic measures, especially the use of positive end-expiratory pressure.

(4) *Coronary vasoconstriction and impaired myocardial function* are associated with experimental lung injury and may result from the action of certain mediators, notably the leukotrienes [11, 27] (see below).

Potential Mediators of Acute Lung Injury

The search for the mediators of acute lung injury is an important area of investigation, and one that is likely to yield information that could reduce the high mortality of ARDS. At present, the identities of these mediators remain only partially known, but new advances toward this goal are rapidly being gained [36]. The potential mediators of lung injury belong to one or more of three groups: humoral substances, cells, and oxygen free radicals. Evidence for the participation of each potential mediator is summarized below.

Humoral Substances

Among humoral substances which have been associated with the pathogenesis of acute lung injury are the biogenic amines histamine and serotonin. Neither of them is believed capable of increasing the permeability of pulmonary microvessels, although they can both contribute to the associated bronchoconstriction and pulmonary vasoconstriction.

The bulk of the work on mediators of lung injury has centered on the possible role of bioactive lipids. These are either arachidonic acid metabolites or platelet-activating factor.

Arachidonic acid metabolites include cyclo-oxygenase products and leukotrienes. The most important representatives of the first group are thromboxane A_2, prostaglandins and prostacyclin. Thromboxane A_2 synthesis is stimulated during acute lung injury induced by a variety of experimental procedures. It is doubtful, however, that thromboxane mediates high-permeability edema in man since inhibition of its synthesis does not protect against pulmonary edema of acute lung injury, with the possible exception of lung injury induced by thrombin [25]. On the other hand, there is ample evidence that thromboxane A_2 contributes to the pulmonary hypertension and decreased compliance induced by *Escherichia coli* endotoxin in sheep and similar changes in other experimental models of acute lung injury [13, 18, 43, 45].

Likewise, the prostaglandins PGE_2, D_2 and $F_{2\alpha}$, which are released with the increased availability of free arachidonic acid, probably are not among the mediators of increased pulmonary microvascular permeability. These compounds could help mediate some of the other responses to injury, such as vasoconstriction and bronchoconstriction [8, 34].

There is little evidence to support a mediator role for prostacyclin in acute lung injury. In fact, some evidence suggests that prostacyclin may serve to modulate certain features of this condition, including pulmonary vasoconstriction and increased vascular permeability.

Leukotrienes C_4 and D_4 (LTC_4 and LTD_4) are lipoxygenase products and are capable of inducing high-permeability edema, as well as bronchoconstriction and pulmonary vasoconstriction in experimental animals [2, 7, 10, 38]. One of the leukotrienes, LTB_4, is particularly potent in attracting and aggregating granulocytes [12, 26], which in turn play a critical role in bringing about the increased permeability of acute lung injury (see below). The effects of selective inhibition of leukotriene synthesis or action are currently being examined to assess the contribution of these compounds in experimental models of the human ARDS.

Platelet-activating factor (PAF) is capable of causing increased pulmonary microvascular permeability in dogs and sheep in vivo [28] and in isolated guinea pig and rabbit lungs in vitro [19]. To what extent PAF actually mediates high-permeability pulmonary edema is still unknown.

Peptides

Of the different biologically active peptides present in the lung, only complement has been demonstrated unequivocally to participate in the mediation of increased pulmonary microvascular permeability [9, 22, 42]. This conclusion is based on the evidence that complement activation (C5a) leads to acute pulmonary edema, related to neutrophil aggregation and activation and the production of toxic oxygen metabolites.

Another peptide, bradykinin, is capable of increasing vascular permeability of systemic, but not pulmonary, vessels. When combined with hypoxia, however, bradykinin may be able to induce pulmonary edema [29].

Enkephalins and endorphins may participate in mediating the hypotension of endotoxin shock, and opiate antagonists may attenuate this hypotension [4, 30]. The possible mediator role of other, newly identified lung peptides [30] has not been investigated.

Enzymes

Proteolytic enzymes, released by granulocytes and alveolar macrophages, can be expected to contribute to acute lung injury. Although the contribution of proteolytic enzymes to acute pulmonary edema remains poorly defined, it is likely that they contribute in particular to the acute lung injury complicating acute pancreatitis.

Role of Cells

It is now clear that certain cells play a key role in mediating the increased vascular permeability of acute lung injury. The most important of these cells are granulocytes, but platelets, mast cells and alveolar macrophages can be major contributors.

There is convincing evidence that granulocytes may be essential for the occurrence of pulmonary edema in acute lung injury due to endotoxin, complement activation and other agents. Depletion of granulocytes protects against acute pulmonary edema in these experimental models [39, 40]. Granulocytes mediate pulmonary edema by releasing upon stimulation free radicals, proteolytic enzymes and arachidonic acid metabolites.

Platelet aggregation in pulmonary microvessels, leading to pulmonary microembolism, is a recognized cause of ARDS. Upon activation and aggregation, platelets release their content of serotonin and other active compounds.

Mast cell degranulation is, of course, responsible for the acute inflammatory responses of anaphylaxis and extrinsic asthma [25]. The contribution of mast cells to the pathogenesis of acute lung injury has not been adequately delineated.

Like granulocytes, alveolar macrophages may release free radicals, proteases and arachidonic acid products, and thus may serve an important mediator role.

Oxygen Free Radicals

Oxygen free radicals, including superoxide anion, hydrogen peroxide, hydroxyl radical and other unstable, but highly toxic compounds are among the most potent mediators of acute lung injury in a variety of conditions [39, 40, 42]. The importance of these radicals is underscored by the demonstration that granulocytes from patients with chronic granulomatous disease, which lack the ability to generate free radicals, do not produce acute pulmonary edema under conditions where normal granulocytes do [39]. Free radical scavengers, including superoxide dismutase, catalase, and various antioxidants, can reduce or prevent experimental lung injury, and offer promise for protection against pulmonary edema [41].

Interactions between Mediators

There is evidence of close interactions between the various mediators of acute lung injury. These interactions occur at several different levels: among different lipid compounds, between lipid and peptide mediators, as well as between humoral mediators, free radicals, and cellular mediators. The following may serve as examples of such interactions:

(1) Some of the actions of leukotrienes are mediated by the stimulation of thromboxane release.

(2) The release of arachidonic acid metabolites and of free radicals is closely associated with the presence and activation of granulocytes.

(3) Complement-induced lung injury depends on the influx of granulocytes and their production of toxic radicals and lipid mediators.

Modulators of Lung Injury

In contrast to the large number and variety of potential mediators of lung injury, few endogenous compounds are known to have the potential to modulate this process. Such modulator ability could derive from the ability to oppose one or more of the responses of acute lung injury (see above). Two naturally occurring compounds, one a lipid and the other a peptide, qualify for such a role. Their biological effects include: vasodilation of pulmonary (as well as coronary and other systemic) vessels, relaxation of bronchial smooth muscle, stimulation of cyclic AMP production, and inhibition of platelet aggregation.

Prostacyclin has been reported to have a protective effect in *E. coli* endotoxemia [24] and in pulmonary microembolism [21]. Vasoactive intestinal peptide, an endogenous bronchodilator and pulmonary vasodilator [15, 33, 37] which counteracts the effects of leukotrienes [16], may have similar protective activity.

Markers of Lung Injury

Because of the high morbidity and mortality of acute lung injury (ARDS), there is a strong and urgent need to identify one or more markers of early lung injury. Such markers or indicators could permit earlier diagnosis and more effective treatment of ARDS. Recent research suggests that certain arachidonic acid metabolites and products of lipid peroxidation may be detectable in blood and bronchoalveolar lavage even with minimal lung injury [1].

Acknowledgment

My thanks to *Neshia Brown, Carrie Winningham* and *Tommie Akard* for help with the manuscript. This research was supported in part by the Medical Research Service of the Veterans Administration and by National Heart, Lung, and Blood Institute Grant HL 30450.

References

1 Attiah, A.; Yoshii, K.; Mojarad, M.; Misra, H.; Kramer, K.; Said, S.I.: Detection of markers of early lung injury induced by small dose of phorbol myristate acetate (PMA) in dogs. Am. Rev. resp. Dis. *129:* A113 (1984).
2 Bach, M.K.: The leukotrienes: their structure, actions, and role in diseases. Current concepts (Upjohn, Kalamazoo 1983).
3 Bizios, R.; Minnear, F.L.; Van der Zee, H.; Malik, A.B.: Effects of cyclooxygenase and lipoxygenase inhibition on lung fluid balance after thrombin. J. appl. Physiol. *55:* 462–471 (1983).
4 Bone, R.C.; Jacobs, E.R.; Potter, D.M.; Hiller, F.C.; Wilson, F.J., Jr.: Endorphins in endotoxin shock. Microcirculation *1:* 285 (1981).
5 Cook, J.A.; Wise, W.C.; Halushka, P.V.: Elevated thromboxane levels in the rat during endotoxic shock. J. clin. Invest. *65:* 227–230 (1980).
6 Crutchley, D.J.; Boyd, J.A.; Eling, T.E.: Enhanced thromboxane B_2 release from challenged guinea pig lung after oxygen exposure. Am. Rev. resp. Dis. *121:* 685–699 (1980).
7 Dahlen, S.-E.; Hedqvist, P.; Hammarström, S.; Samuelsson, B.: Leukotrienes are potent constrictors of human bronchi. Nature, Lond. *288:* 484–486 (1980).
8 Demling, R.; Smith, M.; Gunther, R.; Flunn, J.; Gee, M.: Pulmonary injury and prostaglandin production during endotoxemia in conscious sheep. Am. J. Physiol. *240:* H348 (1981).
9 Desai, U.; Kruetzer, D.L.; Showell, H.; Arroyave, C.V.; Ward, P.A.: Acute inflammatory pulmonary reactions induced by chemotactic factors. Am. J. Path. *96:* 71 (1979).
10 Drazen, J.M.; Venugopalan, C.S.; Austen, K.F.; Brion, F.; Corey, E.J.: Effects of leukotriene E on pulmonary mechanics in the guinea pig. Am. Rev. resp. Dis. *125:* 290–294 (1982).
11 Ezra, D.; Boyd, L.M.; Feuerstein, G.; Goldstein, R.E.: Coronary constriction by leukotriene C_4, D_4, and E_4 in the intact pig heart. Am. J. Cardiol. *51:* 1451–1454 (1983).
12 Ford-Hutchinson, A.W.: Neutrophil aggregating properties of PAF-acether and leukotriene B_4. Int. J. Immunopharmacol. *5:* 17–21 (1983).

13 Frolich, J.; Ogletree, M.; Brigham, K.: Gram-negative endotoxemia in sheep: pulmonary hypertension correlated to pulmonary thromboxane synthesis. Adv. Prostaglandin Thromboxane Res. *7:* 745 (1980).
14 Garcia-Szabo, R.R.; Malik, A.B.: Pancreatitis-induced increase in lung vascular permeability. Am. Rev. resp. Dis. *129:* 580 (1984).
15 Hamasaki, Y.; Mojarad, M.; Said, S.I.: Relaxant action of VIP on cat pulmonary artery: comparison with acetylcholine, isoproterenol, and PGE_1. J. appl. Physiol. *54:* 1607–1611 (1983).
16 Hamasaki, Y.; Saga, T.; Mojarad, M.; Said, S.I.: VIP counteracts leukotriene D_4-induced contractions of guinea pig trachea, lung and pulmonary artery. Trans. Ass. Am. Physns *96:* 406–411 (1983).
17 Hamasaki, Y.; Mojarad, M.; Saga, T.; Tai, H.-H.; Said, S.I.: Platelet activating factor raises airway and vascular pressures and induces edema in lungs perfused with platelet-free solution. Am. Rev. resp. Dis. (in press, 1984).
18 Harlan, R.W.J.; Nadir, B.; Harker, L.; Hildebrandt, J.: Thromboxane A_2 mediates lung vasoconstriction but not permeability after endotoxin. J. clin. Invest. *72:* 911–918 (1983).
19 Heffner, J.E.; Shoemaker, S.A.; Canham, E.M.; Patel, M.; McMurtry, I.F.; Morris, H.G.; Repine, J.E.: Acetyl glyceryl ether phosphorylcholine-stimulated human platelets cause pulmonary hypertension and edema in isolated rabbit lungs: role in thromboxane A_2. J. clin. Invest. *71:* 351–357 (1983).
20 Hinson, J.H., Jr.; Hutchison, A.; Ogletree, M.L.; Brigham, K.L.; Snapper, J.R.: Effect of granulocyte depletion on altered lung mechanics after endotoxemia in sheep. J. appl. Physiol. *55:* 92–99 (1983).
21 Hirose, T.: Prostacyclin as a modulator of acute lung injury; in Said, Pulmonary circulation and pulmonary vascular injury (Futura, Mount Kisco, in press, 1984).
22 Hosea, S.; Brown, E.; Hammer, C.; Frank, M.: Role of complement activation in a model of adult respiratory distress syndrome. J. clin. Invest. *66:* 375–382 (1980).
23 Hüttemeier, P.C.; Watkins, W.D.; Peterson, M.B.; Zapol, W.M.: Acute pulmonary hypertension and lung thromboxane release after endotoxin infusion in normal and leukopenic sheep. Circulation Res. *50:* 688–694 (1982).
24 Krausz, M.M.; Utsunomiya, T.; Feuerstein, G.; Wolf, J.H.N.; Shepro, D.; Hechtman, H.B.: Prostacyclin reversal of lethal endotoxemia in dogs. J. clin. Invest. *67:* 1118–1125 (1981).
25 Lewis, R.A.; Austen, K.F.: Non-respiratory functions of pulmonary cells. Fed. Proc. *36:* 2676 (1977).
26 Lindbom, L.; Hedqvist, P.; Dahlen, S.-E.; Lindgren, J.A.; Årfors, K.-E.: Leukotriene B_4 induces extravasation and migration of polymorphonuclear leukocytes in vivo. Acta physiol. scand. *116:* 105–108 (1982).
27 Michelassi, F.; Landa, L.; Hill, R.F.; Lowenstein, E.; Watkins, W.D.; Petkau, A.J.; Zapol, W.M.: Leukotriene D_4: a potent coronary artery vasoconstrictor associated with impaired ventricular contraction. Science *217:* 841–843 (1982).
28 Mojarad, M.; Hamasaki, Y.; Said, S.I.: Platelet-activating factor increases pulmonary microvascular permeability and induces pulmonary edema. Bull. eur. Physiopathol. resp. (Clin. resp. Physiol.) *19:* 253–256 (1983).

29 O'Brodovich, H.M.; Stalcup, S.A.; Pang, L.M.; Lipset, J.S.; Mellins, R.B.: Bradykinin production and increased pulmonary endothelial permeability during acute respiratory failure in unanesthetized sheep. J. clin. Invest. *67:* 514 (1981).

30 Peters, W.P.; Johnson, M.W.; Friedman, P.A.; Mitch, W.E.: Pressor effect of naloxone in septic shock. Lancet *i:* 529 (1980).

31 Saga, T.; Yoshii, K.; Said, S.I.: Protection by FPL 55712 or indomethacin of leukotriene D4-induced pulmonary edema and airway constriction in guinea pig lungs. Am. Rev. resp. Dis. *129:* A33 (1984).

32 Said, S.I.: Vasoactive peptides and the pulmonary circulation. Ann. N.Y. Acad. Sci. *384:* 207–211 (1982).

33 Said, S.I.: Vasoactive intestinal peptide (Raven Press, New York 1982).

34 Said, S.I.: Pulmonary metabolism of prostaglandins and vasoactive peptides. A. Rev. Physiol. *44:* 257–268 (1982).

35 Said, S.I.: Peptides and lipids as mediators of acute lung injury; in Zapol, Acute respiratory failure. Lung biology in health and disease (Dekker, New York, in press, 1984).

36 Said, S.I.; Guemei, A.; Hara, N.: Bronchodilator effect of VIP in vivo: protection against bronchoconstriction induced by histamine or prostaglandin $F_{2\alpha}$; in Said, Vasoactive intestinal peptide, pp. 185–191 (Raven Press, New York 1982).

37 Samuelsson, B.: Leukotrienes: mediators of immediate hypersensitivity reactions and inflammation. Science *220:* 568–575 (1983).

38 Shasby, D.M.; Vanbenthuysen, K.M.; Tate, R.M.; Shasby, S.; McMurtry, I.; Repine, J.E.: Granulocytes mediate acute edematous lung injury in rabbits and in isolated rabbit lungs perfused with phorbol myristate acetate: role of oxygen radicals. Am. Rev. resp. Dis. *125:* 443–447 (1982).

39 Tate, R.M.; Repine, J.E.: Neutrophils and the adult respiratory distress syndrome. Am. Rev. resp. Dis. *128:* 552–559 (1983).

40 Till, G.O.; Johnson, K.J.; Kunkel, R.; Ward, P.A.: Intravascular activation of complement and acute lung injury. J. clin. Invest. *69:* 1126–1135 (1982).

41 Turrens, J.F.; Crapo, J.D.; Freeman, B.A.: Protection against oxygen toxicity by intravenous injection of liposome-entrapped catalase and superoxide dismutase. J. clin. Invest. *73:* 87 (1984).

42 Utsunomiya, T.; Krausz, M.M.; Levine, L.; Sherpo, D.; Hechtman, H.B.: Thromboxane mediation of cardiopulmonary effects of embolism. J. clin. Invest. *70:* 361–368 (1982).

43 Ward, P.A.; Till, G.O.; Kunkel, R.; Beauchamp, C.: Evidence for role of hydroxyl radical in complement and neutrophil-dependent tissue injury. J. clin. Invest. *72:* 789–801 (1983).

44 Watkins, W.D.; Hüttemeier, P.C.; Kong, D.; Peterson, M.B.: Thromboxane and pulmonary hypertension following *E. coli* endotoxin infusion in sheep: effects of an imidazole derivative. Prostaglandins *23:* 273–285 (1982).

45 Weiss, J.W.; Drazen, J.M.; Coles, N.; McFadden, E.R., Jr.; Weller, P.F.; Corey, E.J.; Lewis, R.A.; Austen, K.F.: Bronchoconstrictor effects of leukotriene C in humans. Science *216:* 196–198 (1982).

S.I. Said, MD, Department of Medicine,
University of Oklahoma Health Sciences Center, Oklahoma City, OK 73190 (USA)

Prog. crit. Care Med., vol. 2, pp. 44–55 (Karger, Basel 1985)

Mechanical Ventilation

Alan T. Aquilina, Robert A. Klocke

Department of Medicine, State University of New York at Buffalo,
Buffalo, N.Y., USA

Mechanical ventilators are devices used to augment or replace ventilatory effort. They can increase alveolar ventilation and deliver higher levels of inspired oxygen, thereby enhancing CO_2 elimination and improving arterial blood oxygenation.

The earliest reference to administering ventilatory support appeared in the Bible [1]. *Vesalius* (1542) and *Hooke* (1700) successfully accomplished artificial ventilation of animals [1]. Following numerous attempts at mechanical ventilation of humans, *O'Dwyer* and *Fell* (1892) successfully developed a J-shaped tube for laryngeal intubation and a bellow-type foot-operated apparatus to treat a patient with edema of the lungs [1, 2].

In 1929 *Drinker and Shaw* [3] described a tank-type respirator which came to be known as the iron lung. It used the principle of alternating externally applied pressures. During poliomyelitis epidemics, this device gained enormous popularity.

The deficiencies of the tank respirators were recognized during World War II and also documented during a polio epidemic in Scandinavia. In Copenhagen (1952) the mortality of bulbar cases of polio was reduced from 80–90% to 47% by the use of a method recommended by the anesthetist *Ibsen;* this was reported by *Lassen* [4] in 1953. The procedure was tracheostomy with manually controlled positive pressure ventilation. This provided the necessary impetus for the development of mechanical ventilators such as the Engstrom and Bang ventilators.

In the United States mechanical ventilators were designed in the 1950s. Specialized intensive care units were developed in the 1960s and positive end-expiratory pressure (PEEP) reintroduced for the treatment of severe hypoxemia [5].

Mechanical ventilators exist in many sizes and shapes and with many functions [6]. Positive pressure ventilators are most commonly divided into two types: pressure-cycled and volume-cycled. In a pressure-cycled machine, the flow of gas from the respirator stops when a pre-set airway pressure is reached. With a volume-cycled machine, flow continues until a specific pre-set volume has been obtained. The pressure required to reach this volume will depend upon the resistance to flow and compliance of the patient's lungs. Either type of ventilator can be used, but a volume-cycled machine is preferred because it delivers a constant tidal volume. The tidal volume of a pressure-cycled machine varies with the resistance and compliance of the lung. The ideal ventilator should have a periodic sigh mechanism, a controlled oxygen concentration setting, variable pressure, flow, and respiratory rate settings, and appropriate alarms. However, constant surveillance must always be maintained and cannot be replaced by an alarm system. Recently, new mechanical devices called high frequency positive pressure ventilators (HFPPV) have been developed. These machines are still experimental and are the subject of ongoing research [7].

Indications

The decision to institute mechanical ventilation cannot be taken lightly. In assessing the need for mechanical ventilation, careful physical examination and determination of arterial blood gas composition are essential. When mechanical ventilation becomes necessary, endotracheal intubation should be carried out using a tube with a highly compliant, large volume cuff, i.e. the so-called 'soft-cuff' [8]. Tracheal damage is much less severe with these new cuffs.

The indications for intubation and mechanical ventilation are summarized in table I. Respiratory failure which does not primarily affect the lung is usually associated with alveolar hypoventilation and acute CO_2 retention. Examples include disorders affecting the central nervous system (sedative overdose, coma, CVA, head trauma), spinal cord disease (Guillain-Barré syndrome, spinal cord trauma), chest wall disease (rib fractures, flail chest), neuromuscular disease (myasthenia gravis, muscular dystrophy), and upper

Table I. Intubation and mechanical ventilation

Indications	*Contraindications*
Hypoventilation – apnea	Patient who is ventilating well with supplemental O_2
Acute respiratory failure with acidemia	Stable chronic respiratory acidosis
Inability to control progressive hypoxemia	Desire to add dead space
Protection of airway in a comatose patient	
Obstruction of the upper airway	
Inability to mobilize secretions	

Table II. Guidelines for ventilatory support in adults with acute respiratory failure

Mechanics	Normal range	Tracheal intubation and ventilation indicated
Respiratory rate	12–20	>35
Vital capacity, ml/kg body weight	65–75	<10–15
Inspiratory force, cm H_2O	75–100	<25

airway obstruction (laryngospasm). Some physiologic guidelines for intubation and ventilation are included in table II [9]. With the exception of central nervous system (CNS) diseases, failure of respiratory function is usually heralded by a decrease in vital capacity, increase in respiratory rate, ineffective cough, and eventually hypercapnia. Respiratory acidosis is an indication of advanced ventilatory failure. Less common indications, usually involving the upper airway, are also listed in table I.

Mechanical ventilation is also indicated for patients with chronic obstructive lung disease and asthma in whom there is progressive respiratory acidosis and failure of conservative measures including low-flow oxygen therapy. These patients can often be identified early by the presence of asynchronous breathing [10]. Normally the chest and abdomen move synchronously during breathing, i.e., both outward during inspiration and inward during expiration. By placing the hands on the chest and abdomen, the physician can evaluate this movement. In patients with obstructive lung disease and progressive respiratory failure, the chest and abdomen move asynchronously during respirations. This breathing pattern and progressive hypercapnia should alert the physician to monitor the patient carefully and institute intubation and mechanical ventilation early.

Inability to provide adequate arterial oxygenation in patients with progressive hypoxemia is an indication for mechanical ventilation. This is seen in patients with severe pneumonia, pulmonary fibrosis and pulmonary edema.

Contraindications to intubation and mechanical ventilation include patients with stable chronic respiratory acidosis, patients with adequate ventilation with supplemental O_2 and those patients in need of added dead space to increase arterial PCO_2.

Practical Considerations

Once the patient is intubated, the next step is to choose the appropriate settings on the ventilator. Important settings include mode of operation, tidal volume, flow rate, respiratory rate, oxygen percentage, pressure limit, sigh volume, and PEEP setting.

There are two basic modes of operation in ventilators: (1) assist/control, and (2) intermittent mandatory ventilation (IMV). These modes describe the means of initiating inspiration from the ventilator.

In the assist/control mode, a minimal respiratory rate is set, and the inspiratory cycle is initiated by a timer in the ventilator (controlled ventilation). In addition, the patient can trigger an inspiratory cycle from the ventilator by an inspiratory effort which is sensed by the machine as negative inspiratory airway pressure (assisted ventilation). The patient, however, cannot breathe spontaneously without ventilator assistance. With this mode, the patient can determine the respiratory rate. It is employed most often when decreased ventilatory drive is present or possible, such as when the patient is sedated.

IMV was designed to wean the patient from the ventilator [11]. It utilizes both the spontaneous breathing of the patient and tidal volumes delivered by positive-pressure ventilation. The patient shares the work of breathing with the ventilator by spontaneous breathing from an oxygen source. At pre-set intervals he receives a supplemental positive-pressure breath from the ventilator (fig. 1). IMV is now the more frequently used mode of ventilation in the awake patient in some hospitals. IMV is preferable in patients who cannot be brought into synchronization with the ventilator and in

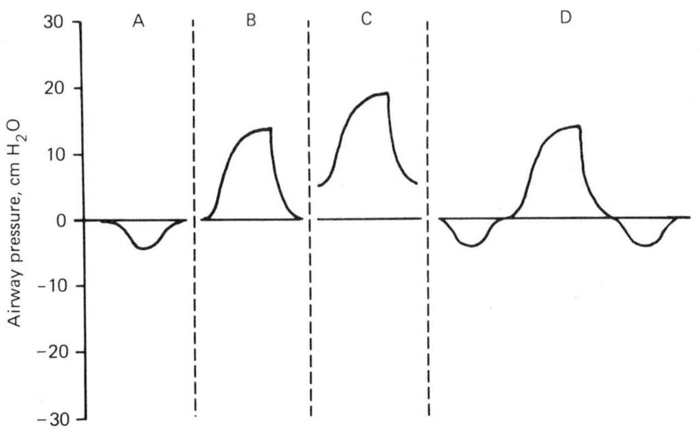

Fig. 1. Airway pressure during ventilation. A = Spontaneous ventilation; B = assist/control positive pressure ventilation; C = assist/control positive pressure ventilation with PEEP; D = intermittent mandatory ventilation. During spontaneous ventilation the airway pressure is below zero. During positive pressure ventilation the airway pressure is above zero. With intermittent mandatory ventilation (D) there is both spontaneous breathing and positive pressure ventilation.

whom sedation is contraindicated. However, it is less desirable than assist/control ventilation for unstable patients with changing neurologic status, shock or other conditions in which the oxygen consumption and the work of breathing should be minimized [12].

Initial ventilator settings require an approximation of the appropriate alveolar ventilation. If the patient has normal lungs, anatomic dead space can be estimated in milliliters equal to ideal body weight (i.e. 2 ml/kg). However, in the presence of obstructive lung disease, 30–50% of delivered tidal volume is dead space volume. Under these circumstances treatment is usually started with a tidal volume of 10–15 ml/kg and a respiratory rate of 10–12/min. This usually corresponds to a minute ventilation (tidal volume × respiratory rate) of 7–12 liters/min. After 20 min arterial blood gases should be analyzed. If the arterial PCO_2 is elevated and the pH is low, the alveolar ventilation is inadequate and should be increased. If the arterial pH is high, the alveolar ventilation is too high, and should be reduced. Blood gas analysis should be repeated until the arterial PCO_2 and arterial pH have reached the desired level. It must be emphasized that the desired PCO_2 is not always 'normal' (35–45 mm Hg). In patients with metabolic acidosis, it may be necessary to hyperventilate the patient to a low PCO_2 in order to maintain blood pH, while the underlying abnormality is identified and corrected. Likewise, in patients with respiratory failure superimposed on chronic respiratory acidosis, a higher than 'normal' PCO_2 is desirable, again maintaining a blood pH in the normal range.

The flow rate is the volume of gas delivered per unit time, usually expressed as liters per minute. Adequate flow rates are necessary for adequate ventilation. Use of the flow control with tidal volume and respiratory rate will establish inspiratory/expiratory time ratios. At the same tidal volume, increasing the flow rate will decrease inspiratory time; a shorter inspiratory time than expiratory time is desirable (i.e. ratio 1:2) and is especially important in obstructive disease.

It is advisable to initiate mechanical ventilation with a high inspired oxygen concentration (40–60%) and maintain this level until blood gas analysis is obtained; the concentration of oxygen can then be reduced if the arterial PO_2 allows this. In a clinical emergency the initial concentration of oxygen should be 100%.

To protect the patient against harmful effects from high pressure, excess pressures are prevented by a pressure limit valve. When the pressure limit is reached, the inspiratory cycle ends and no further volume is delivered. One sets the pressure limit at an acceptable level usually 5–10 cm H_2O higher than peak pressure. The sigh volume is an intermittent deep breathing that is incorporated into the ventilatory pattern; it is used to prevent atelectasis and is usually 2–3 times tidal volume and cycles 3–4 times per hour. However, with large tidal volumes currently used, the need for a sigh volume has decreased.

If severe hypoxemia persists despite mechanical ventilation and high inspired oxygen concentrations, the hypoxemia is likely due to shunting. This frequently occurs in the so-called adult respiratory distress syndrome (ARDS) [13], which is characterized by severe respiratory distress, reduced lung compliance, decreased lung volume, hypoxemia due to shunting of blood through collapsed, nonventilated alveoli, and diffuse parenchymal infiltrates on chest roentgenograms. Any further increase in inspired oxygen concentration will not likely correct this problem. In this situation PEEP is used (fig. 1) [14]. There are valves built into the exhalation limb of the ventilator which allow maintenance of positive airway pressure at the end of expiration. PEEP is effective in ARDS in part because it results in an increase in functional residual capacity (FRC), the volume of gas present in the lungs at end-expiration resulting in an opening of collapsed alveoli, a decrease in intrapulmonary shunting of blood and a rise in arterial PO_2. PEEP is used to avoid O_2 toxicity caused by breathing excessively high O_2 mixtures. PEEP levels from 5 to 20 cm H_2O pressure are usually used; however, as the PEEP increases so does the risk of adverse physiologic effects.

Monitoring

Once ventilatory support is started, monitoring of both the machine and patient is essential to ensure respiratory function. Neither blood gases nor invasive monitoring can substitute for attention to vital signs, intake and output and clinical evaluation of neurologic and cardiopulmonary status.

A frequent 'physical examination' of the ventilator is recommended. A check list should include respiratory rate, tidal volume chosen and delivered, pressure settings, sigh volume and pressure, oxygen concentration of inspired air, control modes, inspired air temperature, water level, PEEP pressure, and inspection of the respiratory tubing. In addition, most ventilators are built with alarms and indicators of these parameters. Most alarm systems provide for early detection of unexpected events such as disconnection of the patient from the ventilators, air leaks, or increase in airway obstruction. The respiratory therapist generally evaluates the function of the ventilator. The physician should assess the need for mechanical ventilation and the ventilatory parameters at least on a daily basis.

Bedside measurements of pulmonary mechanics are noninvasive and can provide valuable information about the patient's status. Delivery of a tidal volume requires application of positive airway pressure to overcome (a) the elasticity of the lung and chest wall, and (b) the resistance to airflow provided by ventilator tubing, the endotracheal tube and the patient's tracheobronchial tree. If only elasticity impeded inflation of the lungs, the change in pressure needed to deliver the tidal volume would be represented by the heavy arrow in figure 2a. The slope of this line, $\Delta V/\Delta P$, reflects the respiratory system compliance and is the inverse of elasticity, i.e., as elasticity increases and the lungs become more 'stiff', compliance falls. The

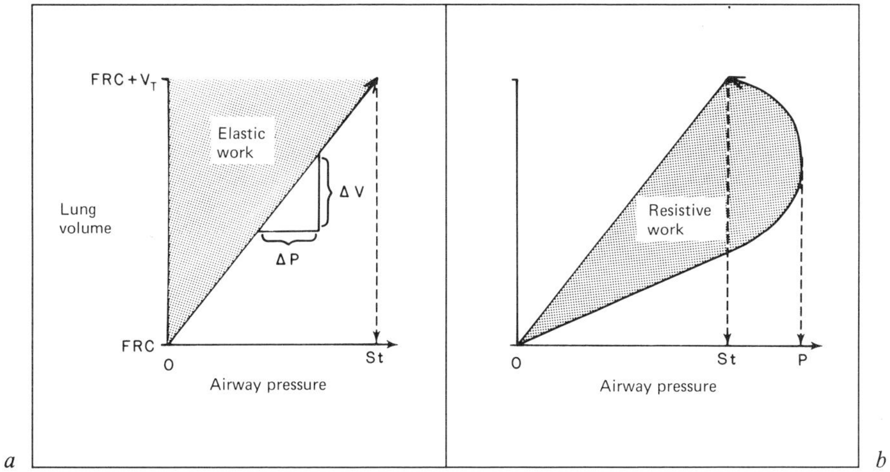

Fig. 2. Pressure volume relationship. *a* The shaded area indicates the work needed to overcome the elastic forces. St = Static pressure; FRC = functional residual capacity. *b* The shaded area represents the work needed to overcome the resistance to airflow during positive pressure ventilation. P = Peak pressure.

shaded area in figure 2a indicates the work needed to overcome elastic forces. However, frictional losses secondary to resistance to airflow also impose a workload during inspiration and in reality the volume-pressure relationship during delivery of the tidal volume resembles the heavy arrow in figure 2b. The shaded area in this panel represents the work required to overcome resistance to airflow. As noted in the figure, there are two airway pressures of interest – static and peak. The static pressure is measured at the end of inspiration and is used to calculate the total compliance of the respiratory system

$$C_{St} = \frac{\Delta V \text{ (tidal volume)}}{\Delta P \text{ (static pressure)}}.$$

When PEEP is used, this pressure must be subtracted from the static pressure before C_{St} is calculated. The normal value in a ventilated patient is greater than 50 ml/cm H_2O. Static pressure is measured at end-inspiration, in the absence of flow, by occluding the expiratory tubing or setting the ventilator for a short period of inspiratory hold. After peak airway pressure is reached, airway pressure falls and reaches a plateau at the static pressure.

'Effective' or 'dynamic' compliance can be measured using peak, rather than static, airway pressure. However, peak pressure reflects the work required to overcome both the elastic properties of the respiratory system and flow-resistive characteristics of the airway. The latter is better estimated by comparing peak and static airway pressures. The difference between peak and static pressures will depend on the flow rate used to deliver the tidal volume and the endotracheal tube size but, in usual circumstances, is no more than 10 cm H_2O. Changes in the peak-static pressure difference at a constant flow rate usually indicate an increase in airway resistance.

Respiratory system compliance is reduced with loss of aerated lung tissue which often occurs in pneumonia, ARDS or lung collapse secondary to pneumothorax. Serial measurements of compliance can be helpful in monitoring the patient's clinical course. Decrements in the peak-static pressure difference (at constant flow rate) reflect improvement in status asthmaticus, acute respiratory failure superimposed on COPD and other airway diseases. The most common cause of a sharp increase in this pressure difference is the presence of secretions obstructing the endotracheal tube or large bronchi.

Complications

Complications of mechanical ventilation are divided into two groups: those associated with failure of the ventilator and others that are due to adverse responses of the patient to mechanical ventilation [15].

Difficulties associated with mechanical failure of the ventilator include power failure, interruption of O_2 supply, gas leaks or tubing obstruction, accidental disconnection of the patient from the ventilator, inadequate humidification, and damaged gas pumping mechanisms.

Among the adverse physiological responses of the patient to mechanical ventilation are: depression of cardiovascular function; abnormalities in electrolytes and acid-base balance; infection and atelectasis, and pulmonary barotrauma.

Any mechanism which increases intrathoracic pressure may reduce venous return and cardiac output. Two factors determine the effect of positive-pressure ventilation on venous return. One is the magnitude and duration of the inspiratory pressure; the higher and longer mean intrathoracic pressure is applied, the more likely it is that venous return will be compromised. The ideal pattern of positive-pressure ventilation was described by *Cournand* et al. [16] as a short inspiratory cycle of low pressure with a longer expiratory phase. Increased airway pressure during mechanical ventilation with PEEP may not only affect venous return but also pulmonary circulation and cardiac output [17]. The other important determinant of venous return is circulating blood volume. If the volume is reduced, the effects of positive-pressure ventilation and PEEP arle likely to be greatly increased. Correction of volume depletion is important when mechanical ventilation is used.

Acid-base and electrolyte disturbances are commonly caused by mechanical ventilation. Respiratory alkalosis, accompanied by electrolyte disturbances, arrhythmias and death have occurred [18]. This most often occurs in patients with chronic respiratory acidosis in whom renal retention of bicarbonate has occurred. In these patients, mechanical ventilation should be adjusted to keep arterial pH normal by avoiding excess changes in arterial PCO_2. Fluid retention often occurs after 48–72 h of mechanical ventilation [19]. This may be partly attributable to increased levels of antidiuretic hormone, decreased glomerular filtration rate or changes in distribution of intrarenal blood flow. The disorder can be detected by careful monitoring of the patient's weight and recording of intake and output.

Atelectasis and pulmonary infection are common complications. The risk of infection can be minimized by meticulous airway care, adequate humidification and aggressive bronchial hygiene. If there is evidence of infection (fever, leukocytosis, physical signs and radiographic evidence), the patient should be treated with antibiotics. The use of antibiotics is guided by regular examination of the sputum and culture.

Among the significant complications of mechanical ventilation is pulmonary barotrauma: pneumothorax, pneumomediastinum, pulmonary interstitial emphysema and subcutaneous emphysema [20]. These are directly related to high airway pressures used to maintain tidal volume. The result is overdistention of alveoli with a resultant rupture and leak of air into the extraparenchymal structures. The risk is increased in patients with stiff, noncompliant lungs where high inflation pressures are needed to maintain adequate alveolar ventilation. PEEP therapy of 10 cm H_2O or greater is associated with an increased incidence of barotrauma.

Other adverse effects associated with mechanical ventilation are gastric distention and gastrointestinal bleeding; these do not appear to be a complication of mechanical ventilation per se but occur frequently in patients with respiratory failure on mechanical ventilators.

With proper monitoring and careful use, mechanical ventilation has improved survival in patients with respiratory failure.

References

1 Eisenberg, L.: History of inhalation therapy equipment; in Dobkin, Ventilators and inhalation therapy, 1st ed., pp. 67–81 (Little, Brown, Boston 1972).

2 Rattenborg, C.C.: Mechanical ventilation; 1st ed., pp. 209–240 (Year Book, Chicago 1981).

3 Drinker, P.; Shaw, L.A.: An apparatus for the prolonged administration of artificial respirations. I. A design for adults and children. J. clin. Invest. *7:* 229–247 (1929).

4 Lassen, H.C.: A preliminary report on the 1952 epidemic of poliomyelitis in Copenhagen with special reference to the treatment of acute respiratory insufficiency. Lancet *i:* 37–41 (1953).

5 Ashbaugh, D.G.; Bigelow, D.B.; Petty, T.C.: Acute respiratory distress in adults. Lancet *ii:* 319–323 (1967).

6 Shapiro, B.A.; Harrison, R.A.; Tront, C.A.: Clinical application of respiratory care; 2nd ed., pp. 311–337 (Year Book, Chicago 1979).

7 Sjöstrand, J.: High-frequency positive-pressure ventilation (HFPPV): a review. Crit. Care *8:* 345–364 (1980).

8 Colice, G.; Matthay, R.A.: Current guidelines for doing tracheal intubation. J. Respir. Dis. *3:* 43–60 (1982).

9 Pontoppidan, H.; Geffin, B.; Lowenstein, E.: Acute respiratory failure in the adult. New Engl. J. Med. *287:* 690–698, 743–752, 799–806 (1972).

10 Gilbert, R.; Ashutosh, K.; Auchincloss, J.H., Jr.; Rana, S.; Peppi, D.: Prospective study of controlled oxygen therapy. Poor prognosis of patients with asynchronous breathing. Chest *71:* 456–462 (1977).

11 Downs, J.G.; Klein, E.F., Jr.; Desautels, D.; Modell, J.H.; Kirby, R.R.: Intermittent mandatory ventilation: a new approach to weaning patients from mechanical ventilators. Chest *64:* 331–335 (1973).

12 Luce, J.M.; Pierson, D.J.; Hudson, L.D.: Intermittent mandatory ventilation. Chest *79:* 678–685 (1981).

13 Connors, A.F.; McCaffree, D.R.; Rogers, R.M.: Adult respiratory distress syndrome. Disease a Month *27:* 1–79 (1981).

14 Weisman, I.M.; Rinaldo, J.E.; Rogers, R.M.: Positive end-expiratory pressure in respiratory failure. New Engl. J. Med. *307:* 1381–1384 (1982).

15 Zwillich, C.W.; Pierson, D.J.; Creagh, C.E.; Sutton, F.D.; Schlatz, E.; Petty, T.L.: Complications of assisted ventilation: a prospective study of 354 consecutive episodes. Am. J. Med. *57:* 161–170 (1974).

16 Cournand, A.; Motley, H.L.; Werko, L.; Richards, D.W.: Physiologic studies of effects of intermittent positive-pressure breathing on cardiac output in man. Am. J. Physiol. *152:* 162–174 (1948).
17 Dorinsky, P.M.; Whitcomb, M.E.: The effect of PEEP on cardiac output. Chest *84:* 210–216 (1983).
18 Kilburn, K.H.: Shock, seizures, and coma with alkalosis during mechanical ventilation. Ann. intern. Med. *65:* 977–984 (1966).
19 Sladen, A.; Laver, M.B.; Pontoppidan, H.: Pulmonary complications and water retention in prolonged mechanical ventilation. New Engl. J. Med. *279:* 448–452 (1968).
20 Cullen, D.J.; Caldera, D.L.: The incidence of ventilator-induced pulmonary barotrauma in critically ill patients. Anesthesiology *50:* 185–190 (1979).

A.T. Aquilina, MD, Department of Medicine,
State University of New York at Buffalo, Buffalo, NY 14214 (USA)

Cardiovascular System

Prog. crit. Care Med., vol. 2, pp. 56–68 (Karger, Basel 1985)

Hypertensive Emergencies

Ronald D. Brown

University of Oklahoma Health Sciences Center, Oklahoma City, Okla., USA

Overview

A marked increase in systemic arterial blood pressure is a threat to life. A hypertensive emergency exists when such an increase in blood pressure causes a sudden deterioration of cerebral function, cardiovascular decompensation, uncontrollable bleeding or an acute decrease in renal function. The blood pressure of patients with a hypertensive emergency should be lowered to safe levels within minutes to an hour by the parenteral administration of antihypertensive drugs. Less severe, but still alarming increases in blood pressure, when not accompanied by signs or symptoms of target organ malfunction, constitute a hypertensive urgency. These patients can be treated effectively with oral antihypertensive drugs to lower their blood pressure over a period of hours to a few days. There is excellent evidence that a judicious reduction of blood pressure markedly improves the dismal prognosis of untreated malignant hypertension [12, 15].

Etiology and Pathophysiology

Hypertension of any etiology may become severe and enter into a malignant phase. Untreated essential hypertension is the most frequent condition that precedes malignant hypertension, especially in young black males. In a recent series, renovascular hypertension was the cause of accelerated or malignant hypertension in 43% of 56 white patients and in 7% of 29 black patients [7]. Patients with glomerulonephritis, pyelonephritis, sclerodermal renal disease, a pheochromocytoma, oral contraceptive hypertension and even primary aldosteronism [3] may enter an accelerated phase of hypertension. Therefore, once the patient has been treated for severe hypertension and blood pressure is controlled, diagnostic procedures for secondary forms of hypertension should be performed. Digital subtraction angiography or renal arteriography to diagnose renal artery stenosis should be delayed 7–14 days to minimize the risk of exacerbating any renal insufficiency.

In the accelerated phase, a vicious circle develops in which the severely elevated levels of blood pressure cause vascular damage, further impairing renal blood flow, which decreases renal function and in most cases causes an increase in circulating angiotensin II. The decline in renal function and the increase in angiotensin II worsen the hypertension. The arteriolopathy produced by severe hypertension consists of severe luminal narrowing due mainly to intimal thickening. Some patients have fibrinoid necrosis. Glomerular obsolescence of varying degrees is widespread [23]. Reduction of blood pressure reverses the vascular changes and, with time, healing occurs and organ function improves.

Hypertensive Emergencies

Hypertensive crises that require immediate treatment are listed in table I and are discussed in this section.

Malignant Hypertension

Malignant hypertension is characterized by a marked increase in blood pressure, with diastolic blood pressures usually greater than 140 mm Hg, retinal flame-shaped hemorrhages and cotton-wool exudates, and papilledema. Renal insufficiency with microscopic hematuria, cylindruria and proteinuria is common. Some patients develop left ventricular failure. The term 'accelerated hypertension' is applied to patients who have severe hypertension with retinal hemorrhages and exudates, but no papilledema.

Hypertensive Encephalopathy

Hypertensive encephalopathy is characterized by the insidious onset of increasingly severe global headaches, blurred vision, alterations in consciousness to varying degrees and a diastolic blood pressure which is generally higher than 140 mm Hg [5, 11]. Occasionally, patients may present with predominantly gastrointestinal symptoms and have projectile vomiting. Patients with a very recent onset of hypertension, especially young patients with acute glomerulonephritis and women with toxemia of pregnancy, may develop hypertensive encephalopathy at considerably lower diastolic blood pressure levels. It is thought that the cerebral circulation of patients with long-standing hypertension adapts to elevated blood pressures and such patients are able to autoregulate cerebral blood flow at higher pressure levels than patients with an acute onset of hypertension. If not treated, patients with encephalopathy develop progressive deterioration of cerebral function with the appearance of somnolence, stupor, convulsions and death. There may be focal neurological deficits which suggest the presence of a mass lesion or a stroke and confuse the diagnosis. Computerized tomography of the head, lumbar puncture and digital subtraction angiography are useful methods to differentiate these conditions.

Conditions That Mimic Malignant Hypertension and Hypertensive Encephalopathy

Acute pulmonary edema may cause severe hypertension secondary to acute increases in circulating catecholamines and angiotensin II which cause intense vasoconstriction and an acute increase in peripheral vascular resistance. When the pulmonary edema resolves, the patient becomes normotensive. Uremia is often associated with hypertension and a metabolic encephalopathy which may be confused with hypertensive encephalopathy. Cerebral vascular accidents, subarachnoid hemorrhages, brain tumors and head injuries may present with mental status changes, seizures and secondary hypertension. Other conditions to consider are post-ictal hypertension, cerebral vasculitis such as occurs in patients with lupus erythematosus, and acute anxiety states with hyperventilation. The key to differentiating these conditions from malignant hypertension is the absence of the characteristic neuroretinopathy of malignant hypertension.

Other Hypertensive Emergencies

Moderate or severe hypertension complicated by acute left ventricular failure, dissecting aortic aneurysm or arterial bleeding are hypertensive emergencies. Examples of arterial bleeding which require prompt reduction

Table I. Hypertensive emergencies

Malignant hypertension
Hypertensive encephalopathy
Conditions caused or complicated by moderate to severe hypertension
Acute left ventricular failure
Dissecting aortic aneurysm
Severe or dangerous arterial bleeding
Intracranial hemorrhage
Leaking abdominal aortic aneurysm
Bleeding at vascular suture lines
Uncontrolled epistaxis
Acute coronary insufficiency

in blood pressure are an intracranial hemorrhage, a leaking abdominal aortic aneurysm, bleeding at vascular suture lines after cardiovascular surgery, and severe uncontrolled nose bleeds.

Treatment of Hypertensive Emergencies

Patients with any of the hypertensive emergencies listed in table I should be admitted to the hospital, preferably to an intensive-care unit, placed at bed rest, and undergo an initial evaluation. This evaluation should include a brief history and physical examination to assess the status of the cerebrovascular and cardiovascular systems, a serum creatinine, blood area nitrogen, serum electrolytes, urinalysis, complete blood count, chest X-ray and an electrocardiogram. Plasma or urinary catecholamines should also be obtained. Dietary sodium should be limited to 90 mEq daily and close attention paid to fluid and electrolyte balance.

Drug therapy to lower the blood pressure should be started before the results of all the admission laboratory tests are available.

Drug Treatment

A wide assortment of antihypertensive drugs (table II) can be administered parenterally to treat patients who have a hypertensive emergency. There are parenteral drugs that reduce blood pressure by direct vasodila-

Table II. Parenteral drugs for hypertensive emergencies

Drug	Mechanism	Packaging	Dose	Route	Time of onset	Duration	Contraindications
Sodium nitroprusside (Nipride®)	vasodilator	50 mg/vial	0.5–10 μg/kg/min	i.v.	< 1 min	3–5 min	hepatic and renal insufficiency
Diazoxide (Hyperstat®)	vasodilator	300 mg/ 20 ml ampule	75–300 mg	i.v. bolus	1–2 min	4–24 h	acute left ventricular failure, aortic dissection, acute coronary insufficiency
Hydralazine (Apresoline®)	vasodilator	20 mg/ 1 ml ampule	10–40 mg	i.v. bolus	10–20 min	3–8 h	acute left ventricular failure, aortic dissection, acute coronary insufficiency
Nitroglycerin	vasodilator	variable	5–500 μg/min	i.v.	1–2 min	minutes	none
Trimethaphan camsylate (Arfonad®)	ganglionic blocker	500 mg/ 10 ml ampule	0.3–6 mg/min	i.v.	1–2 min	10 min	after abdominal surgery

tion, e.g., sodium nitroprusside, nitroglycerin, diazoxide and hydralazine, or by interfering with functions of the sympathetic nervous system, e.g., trimethaphan. Parenteral methyldopa, reserpine and pentolinium are not included since their use has declined in recent years, as more effective and easier to use drugs have become available.

Oral antihypertensive drugs should be started as soon as it is feasible, thereby eliminating protracted parenteral therapy.

Sodium Nitroprusside

Sodium nitroprusside has become the drug used most often to treat hypertensive emergencies because of its predictable rapid onset of action, its brief duration of effect, the lack of any absolute contraindications, and relative freedom from toxicity [20, 25]. Sodium nitroprusside is a direct vasodilator which decreases peripheral vascular resistance. It also dilates capacitance vessels. Thus, nitroprusside decreases both preload and afterload. Nitroprusside is packaged as a powder, 50 mg/vial, which is dissolved in 500 ml 5% dextrose and water. The contents should be shielded from light by wrapping the bottle with aluminum foil to prevent deterioration of the drug. Begin the infusion at the rate of 0.5 μg/kg/min using an infusion pump, such as an IVAC or Harvard pump or a minidrip infusion set. The rate is doubled every 2 min until the blood pressure falls and then the dose is titrated to maintain the diastolic pressure at the desired level, usually between 100 and 120 mm Hg during the initial few hours of treatment. The dose required varies from 0.5 to 10 μg/kg/min. A more concentrated solution of nitroprusside (up to 200 mg/500 ml) can be used for patients requiring the larger doses, thereby avoiding the infusion of large fluid volumes. The hypotensive effect ends within minutes after the infusion is discontinued.

The advantages of nitroprusside are many and its disadvantages are few. It is the most predictably effective parenteral antihypertensive agent available. Its onset and offset of action are very rapid so blood pressure can readily be titrated. It reduces both preload and afterload which is an advantage when treating patients with acute cardiac decompensation. It does not have any direct central sedative effects which is an advantage in patients being treated for hypertensive encephalopathy or central nervous dysfunction due to a stroke. In these patients, drugs with sedative properties confuse the clinical evaluation of the response to treatment and should not be used.

The major disadvantage of nitroprusside is the need to closely titrate the dose which necessitates constant observation in an intensive-care unit. Sodium nitroprusside is metabolized to cyanide in a number of tissues which in turn is converted to thiocyanate by the liver. The thiocyanate is excreted by the kidneys. Therefore, severe liver or renal impairment are relative contraindications to the use of this agent. Cyanide poisoning is rare and only occurs when extremely high doses are used. Thiocyanate toxicity can be minimized by administering orally effective antihypertensives as soon as possible and weaning the patient off nitroprusside within 24–48 h as the oral agents take effect. If thiocyanate blood levels exceed 10–12 mg/dl, the dose needs to be reduced.

Diazoxide

Diazoxide is a direct vasodilator which decreases peripheral vascular resistance, but unlike sodium nitroprusside does not dilate capacitance vessels nor decrease preload [13]. Diazoxide is packaged ready to use in a 300 mg/20 ml ampule. A 75 mg (5 ml) test dose should be injected intravenously and 5–10 min later the remainder of the vial injected if the blood pressure has not responded. The use of such a test dose will prevent severe hypotensive responses. Minibolus administration (doses of 1–3 mg/kg) at intervals of 5–15 min are as effective as injecting the entire vial while offering improved safety.

Diazoxide causes sodium and water retention, impairs glucose tolerance, induces a reflex tachycardia and increases myocardial contractility and left ventricular work. It should not be used in patients with an acute dissection of the aorta or acute coronary insufficiency and should be used with caution in patients with left ventricular failure.

Hydralazine

Hydralazine is a direct vasodilator. Since it causes a reflex tachycardia and increased myocardial contractility and left ventricular work, it should not be used in patients with an aortic dissection, acute coronary insufficiency or acute left ventricular failure due to acute severe hypertension. It is packaged ready to use in a 20 mg/1.0 ml ampule. The usual dose is 10–40 mg. It has an advantage over the other vasodilators in that it can be administered intramuscularly. Hydralazine is useful for the treatment of blood pressure increases that are not life-threatening and as an adjunct to other therapy to control sudden increases in blood pressure.

Nitroglycerin

Nitroglycerin is a direct vasodilator which like nitroprusside dilates both arterioles and capacitance vessels [1]. There is an extensive experience with its use in the perioperative period to control hypertension associated with intratracheal intubation, anesthesia, skin incision, sternotomy, cardiac bypass and in the immediate postsurgical period [8]. Recently, its use in treating medical hypertensive emergencies has increased but to date there are no large series of patients reported. The drug is diluted to 100 μg/ml in 5% dextrose and water and infused intravenously using an infusion set made of tubing that does not absorb the nitroglycerin. The initial dose is 5 μg/min which is titrated in 5 μg/min increments every 3–5 min until blood pressure control is attained. Additional measures to lower blood pressure should be started since the duration of action of intravenous nitroglycerin is very short. There are no known contraindications to its use, but our experience is limited. A case of methemoglobinemia due to high-dose intravenous nitroglycerin (30 μg/kg/min) has been reported [9].

Trimethaphan Camsylate

Trimethaphan camsylate is primarily a ganglionic blocking agent but it may also exert a direct vasodilator effect. It is packaged 50 mg/ml in 10-ml ampules. The contents of the ampule should be diluted to 500 ml (1 mg/ml) with 5% dextrose and water and infused intravenously at an initial rate of 3–4 mg/min. The rate should be doubled every 5 min until there is a decrease in blood pressure and then titrated to maintain the blood pressure at the desired level. Trimethaphan does not increase myocardial contractility, cardiac output or left ventricular work, therefore it can be used to treat hypertensive emergencies that are complicated by aortic dissection, coronary insufficiency or acute left ventricular failure. Due to its lack of effects on the central nervous system, it is also useful for the treatment of hypertensive encephalopathy.

Because it causes bowel and bladder atony, trimethaphan should not be used in the postoperative period to treat patients who have undergone abdominal surgery.

Diuretics

As a rule, diuretics are not needed during the initial phase of therapy unless there is evidence of volume overload. However, they generally should be used if the patients require prolonged vasodilator therapy since fluid retention is a common complication of such therapy.

Special Therapeutic Situations

Dissections of Aortic Aneurysms

One of the most serious complications of hypertension is an acute dissection of an aortic aneurysm. One should reduce the blood pressure of these patients to normal or subnormal levels as rapidly as possible. Reserpine was used commonly in the past, but currently trimethaphan and sodium nitroprusside are the drugs of choice. The addition of a β-blocker to sodium nitroprusside therapy is recommended to reduce further myocardial contractility and cardiac output. Drugs that increase cardiac output, such as hydralazine and diazoxide, should not be used since the increase in cardiac contractile force may accelerate the rate of dissection.

Acute Left Ventricular Failure

When the left ventricle fails as a direct consequence of severe hypertension, the failure and consequent pulmonary edema respond dramatically to rapid lowering of blood pressure. In such patients, reduction of blood pressure is a more effective method to treat the pulmonary edema than the use of digitalis and morphine. A rapidly acting diuretic, either furasemide or ethacrynic acid, and an antihypertensive drug, such as sodium nitroprusside, that rapidly reduces both preload and afterload should be administered intravenously. During therapy, it may be necessary to monitor pulmonary wedge pressure with a Swan-Ganz catheter to decide at what rate to infuse the sodium nitroprusside. Drugs that tend to augment venous return, such as diazoxide or hydralazine, should not be used to treat patients with hypertension-induced pulmonary edema.

Intracranial Hemorrhage

Patients who have an intracranial hemorrhage associated with severe hypertension present difficult diagnostic and therapeutic problems. Often it is impossible to determine whether the hemorrhage itself increased the patient's blood pressure or the patient had pre-existing severe hypertension which led to the bleeding episode. There is a divergence of opinion on how to treat these patients, but most physicians recommend that the diastolic blood pressure be lowered to approximately 100–110 mm Hg if the patient was known to be hypertensive prior to the hemorrhage and to 90 mm Hg if there is no prior history of high blood pressure. Sodium nitroprusside is recommended and the blood pressure should be reduced gradually over a period of 30 min. If there is no deterioration of neurologic function when the blood pressure is reduced, the blood pressure should be maintained at the lower level. If the neurologic status of the patient worsens, the rate of infusion should be reduced and the blood pressure allowed to increase to a level that provides better cerebral perfusion and an improvement of neurological function. This same rule applies to any patient who has deterioration of cerebral function while being vigorously treated for hypertension [14].

Angina pectoris

When severe hypertension is complicated by coronary insufficiency, the blood pressure should be lowered gradually over 15–20 min to reduce the work load and oxygen demands of the myocardium which will relieve the ventricular ischemia. Sodium nitroprusside favorably affects left ventricular function during acute ischemia. This property of sodium nitroprusside and its rapid and controllable action make it the drug of choice for treating such patients. Diazoxide and hydralazine are not good choices since both may cause a reflex tachycardia and increased cardiac output, thereby increasing left ventricular work and myocardial oxygen demands.

Postoperative Hypertension

Acute increases in blood pressure in the immediate postoperative period are most likely to occur after open heart surgical procedures requiring cross-clamping of the aorta or after an operation on the carotid artery. Because vascular suture lines may be endangered, prompt reduction of blood pressure is indicated. Sodium nitroprusside was commonly used but intravenous nitroglycerin is now being administered with increasing frequency. Severe pain and anxiety contribute to postoperative hypertension. Judicious use of narcotics and thorazine to relieve pain and anxiety will often reduce blood pressure. Thorazine also inhibits α-adrenoreceptor function, thereby decreasing peripheral vascular resistance and blood pressure.

Treatment of Hypertensive Urgencies

Hypertensive urgencies can be treated with oral antihypertensive drugs since blood pressure need not be reduced as rapidly as in a hypertensive emergency. Several regimens have been recommended. We have found that clonidine loading is effective in most patients. The initial dose is 0.2 mg orally, followed by 0.1 mg orally every hour up to four to five doses as needed to lower the blood pressure to safer levels [2, 6, 24]. The patient should then be continued on clonidine 0.1–0.2 mg twice or three times a day and the dose subsequently adjusted. A diuretic may have to be added to this regimen.

Captopril administered orally using an initial dose of 10–50 mg has also been reported to be effective in hypertensive urgencies and in some patients with hypertensive emergencies, including a few with early signs of hypertensive encephalopathy [4, 10, 16, 18, 19, 22]. The maximal blood pressure response occurs within 45–90 min. With additional experience, it is likely that we will find captopril is useful to treat patients with severe hypertension complicated by left ventricular failure or angina since it reduces both preload and afterload and decreases cardiac work and myocardial oxygen needs. We recommend that patients receive a 6.25 mg test dose of captopril since some patients respond with a marked reduction in blood pressure to higher doses, especially if they have received diuretics or other antihypertensive drugs prior to receiving captopril, or have high-renin type hypertension.

Parenteral preparations of captopril and new angiotensin-converting enzyme inhibitors, such as MK-422, or enalapril, should be available in the future which will make it easier to titrate the initial dose and may make these drugs more useful to treat hypertensive emergencies.

Other drugs used successfully to treat hypertensive urgencies include minoxidil [17, 21], hydralazine with propranolol and prazosin. The addition of a rapidly acting loop diuretic to these drugs is often used but is probably not necessary during initial therapy unless there is evidence of volume overload.

References

1 Abrams, J.: Nitroglycerin and long-acting nitrates. New Engl. J. Med. *302:* 1234–1237 (1980).

2 Anderson, R.J.; Hart, G.R.; Crumpler, C.P.; Reed, W.G.; Matthews, C.A.: Oral clonidine loading in hypertensive urgencies. J. Am. med. Ass. *246:* 848–850 (1981).

3 Beevers, D.G.; Brown, J.J.; Ferriss, J.B.; Fraser, R.; Lever, A.F.; Robertson, J.I.S.; Tree, M.: Renal abnormalities and vascular complications in primary hyperaldosteronism. Evidence on tertiary hyperaldosteronism. Q. Jl Med. *45:* 401–410 (1976).

4 Case, D.B.; Atlas, S.A.; Sullivan, P.A.; Laragh, J.H.: Acute and chronic treatment of severe and malignant hypertension with the oral angiotensin-converting enzyme inhibitor captopril. Circulation *64:* 765–771 (1981).
5 Chester, E.M.; Agamanolis, D.P.; Banker, B.Q.; Victor, M.: Hypertensive encephalopathy: A clinicopathologic study of 20 cases. Neurology *28:* 928–939 (1978).
6 Cohen, I.M.; Katz, M.A.: Oral clonidine loading for rapid control of hypertension. Clin. Pharmacol. Ther. *24:* 11–15 (1978).
7 Davis, B.A.; Crook, J.E.; Vestal, R.E.; Oates, J.A.: Prevalence of renovascular hypertension in patients with grade III or IV hypertensive retinopathy. New Engl. J. Med. *301:* 1273–1276 (1979).
8 Flaherty, J.T.; Magee, P.A.; Gardner, T.L.; Potter, A.; MacAllister, N.P.: Comparison of intravenous nitroglycerin and sodium nitroprusside for treatment of acute hypertension developing after coronary artery bypass surgery. Circulation *65:* 1072–1077 (1982).
9 Gibson, G.R.; Hunter, J.B.; Raabe, D.S., Jr.; Manjoney, D.L.; Ittleman, F.P.: Methemoglobinemia produced by high-dose intravenous nitroglycerin. Ann. intern. Med. *96:* 615–616 (1982).
10 Griswold, W.; McNeal, R.; O'Connor, D.; Reznik, V.; Mendoza, S.: Oral converting enzyme inhibitor in malignant hypertension. Archs Dis. Childh. *57:* 235–237 (1982).
11 Healton, E.B.; Brust, J.C.; Feinfeld, D.A.; Thomson, G.E.: Hypertensive encephalopathy and the neurologic manifestations of malignant hypertension. Neurology *32:* 127–132 (1982).
12 Kaplan, N.M.: Hypertensive crisis; in Clinical hypertension; 2nd ed., p. 166 (Williams & Wilkins, Baltimore 1978).
13 Koch-Weser, J.: Diazoxide. New Engl. J. Med. *294:* 1271–1274 (1976).
14 Ledingham, J.G.G.; Rajagopalan, B.: Cerebral complications in the treatment of accelerated hypertension. Q. Jl Med. *48:* 25–41 (1979).
15 Lee, T.H.; Alderman, M.H.: Malignant hypertension. N.Y. State J. Med. *78:* 1389–1391 (1978).
16 Levin, L.; Logan, K.: Response of malignant hypertension with refractory cardiac failure to captopril. S. Afr. med. J. *58:* 217–218 (1980).
17 Linas, S.L.; Nies, A.S.: Minoxidil. Ann. intern. Med. *94:* 61–65 (1981).
18 Monnens, L.; Drayer, J.; De Jong, M.: Malignant hypertension in a child with hemolytic-uremic syndrome treated with captopril. Acta paediat. scand. *70:* 583–585 (1981).
19 Oberfield, S.E.; Case, D.B.; Levine, L.S.; Rapaport, R.; Rauh, W.; New, M.I.: Brief clinical and laboratory observations: Use of oral angiotensin I-converting enzyme inhibitor (captopril) in childhood malignant hypertension. J. Pediat. *95:* 641–644 (1979).
20 Palmer, R.F.; Lasseter, K.C.: Sodium nitroprusside. New Engl. J. Med. *292:* 294–297 (1975).
21 Pettinger, W.A.: Minoxidil and the treatment of severe hypertension. New Engl. J. Med. *303:* 922–926 (1980).
22 Saragoca, M.A.; Homsi, E.; Ribeiro, A.B.; Filho, S.R.F.; Ramos, O.L.: Hemodynamic mechanism of blood pressure response to captopril in human malignant hypertension. Hypertension *5:* suppl. 1, pp. I-53–I-58 (1983).

23 Sinclair, R.A.; Antonovych, T.T.; Mostofi, F.K.: Renal proliferative arteriopathies and associated glomerular changes: a light and electron microscopic study. Human Pathol. *7:* 565–588 (1976).

24 Spitalewitz, S.; Porush, J.G.; Oguagha, C.: Use of oral clonidine for rapid titration of blood pressure in severe hypertension. Chest *83:* suppl., pp. 404–407 (1983).

25 Tuzel, I.; Limjuco, R.; Kahn, D.: Sodium nitroprusside in hypertensive emergencies. Curr. ther. Res. *17:* 95–106 (1975).

R.D. Brown, MD, Professor of Medicine,
University of Oklahoma Health Sciences Center,
Oklahoma City, OK 73106 (USA)

Prog. crit. Care Med., vol. 2, pp. 69–86 (Karger, Basel 1985)

Pitfalls in the Interpretation of Hemodynamic Data

Paul V. Carlile

University of Oklahoma Health Sciences Center and Veterans Administration Medical Center, Oklahoma City, Okla., USA

Since the introduction of the flow-directed, right heart (Swan-Ganz) catheter in 1970, continuous hemodynamic monitoring of critically ill patients with circulatory and/or respiratory failure has gained widespread acceptance. Measurements of flow, intravascular pressures, and the oxygen tension or saturation in mixed venous blood provide information not readily available from clinical or radiographic evaluation, and sequential measurements enable the physician to assess changes over time and the outcome of therapeutic interventions. However, the use of hemodynamic monitoring depends not only on a properly calibrated system that yields reliable measurements but also on an understanding of how altered physiology or therapeutic interventions may affect the validity and interpretation of these measurements. The purpose of this chapter is to examine: (1) factors affecting the interpretation of intravascular pressure measurements, especially the pulmonary wedge pressure, and (2) hemodynamic alterations during positive end-expiratory pressure (PEEP).

Interpretation of Intravascular Pressure Measurements

Bedside measurement of left ventricular pressure with the right heart catheter provides information about the state of left ventricular filling and the potential for fluid accumulation in the lung. The left ventricular end-diastolic volume (LVEDV) is an important determinant of ventricular performance (Frank-Starling relationship) but is difficult to measure clinically. Since LVEDV is related to the distending pressure by the diastolic pressure-volume relationship of the ventricle, pressure and volume are considered

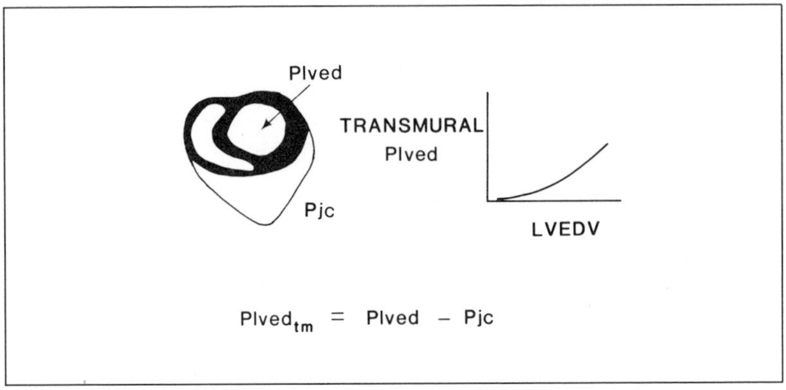

Fig. 1. The distending or *transmural* pressure of the left ventricle is the difference between the intracavitary pressure of the ventricle, Plved, and the juxtacardiac pressure, Pjc. There is a curvilinear relationship between the left ventricular end-diastolic volume, LVEDV, and the transmural left ventricular end-diastolic pressure, $Plved_{tm}$.

interchangeable, and it is this pressure that is estimated at the bedside. The distending or transmural pressure of the left ventricle ($Plved_{tm}$) is the difference between the pressure inside the ventricle at end-diastole, left ventricular end-diastolic pressure or Plved, and the pressure around the heart, juxtacardiac pressure or Pjc, which is assumed to equal pleural pressure (fig. 1 and equation 1).

$$Plved_{tm} = Plved - Pjc. \qquad (1)$$

In normal subjects there is no significant pressure gradient between the pulmonary artery and left ventricle at end-diastole because of the low resistance of the pulmonary circulation, and, as a result, Plved agrees closely with the pulmonary wedge pressure (Ppw) [59] or pulmonary artery end-diastolic pressure (Ppaed) [3, 22]. Since juxtacardiac pressure is slightly subatmospheric, left ventricular end-diastolic pressure, Ppw, and Ppaed, measured with atmospheric pressure as a zero reference, will underestimate $Plved_{tm}$. (Throughout this chapter all vascular pressures are measured with atmosphere as a zero reference unless otherwise indicated to be a transmural pressure or identified by the subscript 'tm'.) If Pjc is relatively constant, the error would be minimal, and changes in the pulmonary artery end-diastolic pressure or wedge pressure should reflect changes in transmural left ventricular end-diastolic pressure. Therefore, the use of pressures obtained with the right heart catheter (Ppaed or Ppw) to reflect left ventricular end-diastolic volume depends upon several assumptions: (1) close agreement between right heart pressures and the left ventricular end-diastolic pressure; (2) a fixed relationship between Plved and $Plved_{tm}$ (i.e., minimal or no change in pleural pressure and Pjc); (3) a constant left ventricular diastolic pressure-volume relationship.

Relationship between Right Heart Pressures and the Plved

The low resistance of the pulmonary circulation in normal subjects results in equalization of the end-diastolic pressures in the pulmonary artery and the left ventricle [3, 22]. However, in the presence of pulmonary vascular disease and elevated pulmonary vascular resistance, Ppaed overestimates left ventricular end-diastolic pressure [22, 37], left atrial pressure (Pla) [36, 68], and Ppw [53, 57, 58] (fig. 2). A discrepancy between end-diastolic pressures in the pulmonary artery and left ventricle also occurs with moderately increased heart rates in the range of 125 beats/min [3, 22]. Since elevated pulmonary vascular resistance is a common finding in patients with acute respiratory failure [73], chronic obstructive lung disease [8], or acute myocardial infarction [53], the pulmonary artery end-diastolic pressure cannot be used to reflect left ventricular preload in most critically ill patients. Furthermore, the assumption that the Ppaed – Ppw difference will remain fixed in a given patient is also not justified since this difference will be only as constant as those factors (heart rate and pulmonary vascular resistance) which cause it.

In the presence of left ventricular disease, pulmonary wedge pressure may underestimate left ventricular end-diastolic pressure [27, 53]. *Braunwald and Frahm* [4], investigating the hemodynamic function of the left atrium, found that the difference between left ventricular end-diastolic pressure and mean left atrial pressure averages 0.2 Torr in normal subjects and 9.0 Torr (range 1–18) in patients with left ventricular disease characterized by increased volume or decreased compliance. In normal subjects left atrial contraction results in an elevation of both Plved and mean atrial pressure, but in the presence of left ventricular disease and high atrial pressures, atrial contraction raises the left ventricular end-diastolic pressure *without* a concomitant increase in mean left atrial pressure. The result is improved ventricular performance because the ventricle moves to a higher end-diastolic volume but without the cost of increased left atrial pressure, which would increase the hydrostatic pressure in pulmonary vessels [4]. Since agreement between pulmonary wedge and left atrial pressure is not

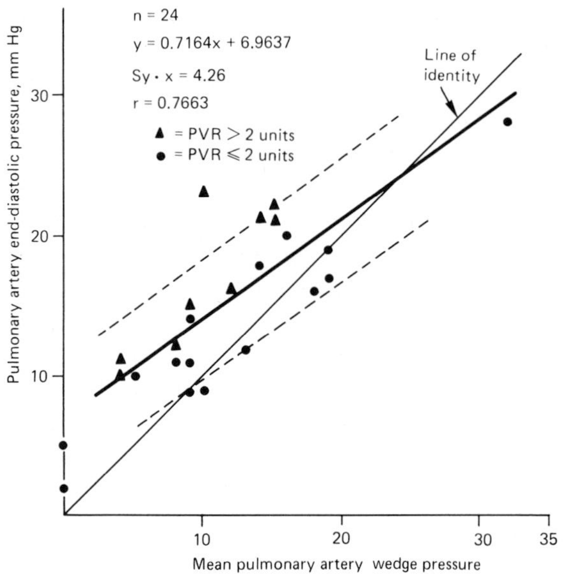

Fig. 2. The relationship between pulmonary artery end-diastolic pressure and mean pulmonary artery wedge pressure for 24 paired determinations in patients with acute myocardial infarction. Measurements in patients with elevated pulmonary vascular resistance (PVR) are identified by triangles and those from patients with low PVR by circles. The average difference (± SEM) between the two measurements was 1.3 ± 0.7 Torr for the 15 paired measurements when PVR was low and 6.7 ± 0.8 ($p < 0.001$) for the 9 measurements with elevated PVR [from 53, with permission].

affected by impaired LV performance [39, 41], Ppw reflects the pressure which promotes fluid transudation in the lung but underestimates Plved in patients with left ventricular disease. This discrepancy is tolerable in most clinical situations since it is the risk of pulmonary congestion and edema that necessarily limits manipulations of LV filling pressure. However, when precise quantification of left ventricular function is desired, direct measurements of Plved may be required, although it has been suggested that the 'a' wave of the pulmonary wedge pressure could be used [27, 53].

Measurement of pressure in the left heart with a wedged pulmonary artery catheter requires the presence of a continuous column of fluid between the left heart and the tip of the catheter, but this condition may not

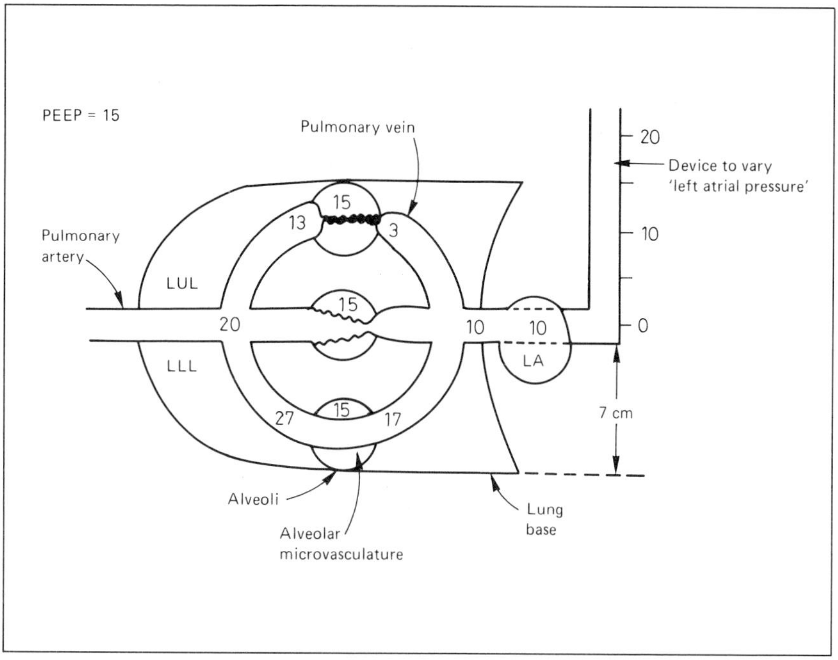

Fig. 3. Schematic representation of a lung in a supine animal with vascular and alveolar pressures illustrating the vertical gradient of hydrostatic pressures in the lung and the effect of increased alveolar pressure (due to PEEP) on the patency of the pulmonary microvasculature (all pressures in cm H_2O). The top of the lung would be in zone I, and the center in zone II. A catheter wedged in zone III at the bottom of the lung would be expected to reflect left atrial pressure. LUL = Left upper lobe; LLL = left lower lobe; LA = left atrium [from 67, with permission].

be met in some lung regions with reduced blood flow. Pulmonary capillaries are collapsible vessels, and their patency is determined by the pressure difference across the vessel wall [70]. The pressure around the capillary is alveolar pressure. Since the pulmonary circulation is a low pressure system under the influence of gravity, there is a vertical gradient of hydrostatic pressures throughout the lung, and the pressure inside pulmonary capillaries is not uniform (fig. 3). In nondependent or 'zone I' lung regions, capillaries are compressed because the surrounding alveolar pressure exceeds capillary inflow pressure, which is pulmonary artery pressure less the pressure drop determined by the vertical height of the region above the heart. In 'zone II' regions alveolar pressure is less than inflow but greater than the outflow pressure of the capillary, and flow through this region is described as a vascular waterfall or Starling resistor, since the driving pressure for flow is inflow minus the surrounding (alveolar) pressure. In zones I and II a continuous fluid column between the left atrium and the pulmonary artery catheter tip is not present, but in 'zone III' (inflow pressure > outflow pressure > alveolar pressure) this condition is satisfied. If a catheter does not enter zone III, left atrial pressure is overestimated because the pressure recorded by the transducer is a function of the vertical height of the catheter tip above the level of the transducer as well as the alveolar pressure transmitted to the catheter [56, 64, 67]. Animal studies indicate that wedging of the catheter outside zone III and overestimation of left atrial pressure are more likely if: (1) the catheter tip is located at a level vertically above the left atrium [67]; (2) alveolar pressure is elevated by PEEP [56, 67]; or (3) left atrial pressure is low [66, 74].

Few studies have evaluated the effect of these conditions on the relationship between Pla and Ppw in the human. *Lappas* et al. [39] found good agreement between left atrial and pulmonary wedge pressures over the range of 6–35 Torr in 18 patients following cardiac or major vascular surgery, but vertical position of the Swan-Ganz catheter and amount (if any) of positive end-expiratory pressure were not reported. *Shasby* et al. [64] found good agreement between the Pla and Ppw in patients on mechanical ventilation without PEEP regardless of the vertical height of the catheter tip but poor agreement during PEEP ventilation when the tip was above the left atrium or Pla was low. *Jardin* et al. [35] found close agreement between Ppw and Plved during mechanical ventilation with PEEP $\leqslant$ 10 cm H_2O but overestimation of Plved at PEEP greater than 10 cm H_2O (vertical height of the catheter not reported). Since catheters below the left atrial level appear to be accurate even at high levels of PEEP [64, 67], lateral chest radiographs may be useful to assess the reliability of a high pulmonary wedge pressure, especially in the presence of PEEP > 10 cm H_2O.

Effect of Altered Pleural Pressure on Hemodynamic Measurements

Since the transmural pressure of the left ventricle or any cardiac chamber is the difference between the intracavitary pressure, i.e., the pressure inside the chamber, and the juxtacardiac pressure, Plved and Ppw will not change in the same direction as $Plved_{tm}$ when alterations in pleural and juxtacardiac pressure occur. Rearrangement of equation 1 indicates that left ventricular end-diastolic pressure (measured relative to atmosphere) may be thought of as the sum of the $Plved_{tm}$ and Pjc (equation 2).

$$Plved = Plved_{tm} + Pjc \quad (2)$$

$$\Delta Plved = \Delta Plved_{tm} + \Delta Pjc \quad (3)$$

Therefore, a change in the Plved (or Ppw) could reflect a change in left ventricular filling (i.e., $Plved_{tm}$) and/or a change in pleural and juxtacardiac pressure (equation 3). During a spontaneous inspiratory effort juxtacardiac pressure falls and transmural pressure rises as venous return increases, but the net result is a decrease in intracavitary pressure measured relative to atmosphere. During positive pressure inspiration pleural pressure and Pjc increase, and transmural pressure declines, but the net result is an increase in intracavitary pressure. Clearly the Ppw or any other intrathoracic vascular pressure should be measured at end-expiration so that changes in juxtacardiac pressure and the disparity between intracavitary and transmural pressures are minimized. This underscores the importance of recording pressure tracings on calibrated paper to determine the end-expiration point, since it is difficult to determine from an oscilloscope or digital meter. However, changes in Pjc may *not* be minimized at the point of end-expiration under some conditions.

Pleural pressure is subatmospheric during passive exhalation in quietly breathing subjects, but when exhalation requires active muscular effort in patients with respiratory failure, pleural and juxtacardiac pressures may be elevated at the point chosen as 'end-expiration'. End-expiratory pleural pressure may be in the range of +20 to 30 Torr in patients with chronic airway obstruction [54] and +5 Torr in asthmatic subjects [48], and may also be elevated in subjects with diffuse lung disease during intermittent mandatory ventilation [63]. One approach to this problem would be to use an esophageal balloon to estimate pleural pressure and calculate transmural filling pressures. Since use of the esophageal balloon is complex and impractical in the usual clinical setting, alternative solutions have been sought, but none has proven ideal. *Rice* et al. [54], studying patients during exacerbations of chronic obstructive pulmonary disease, found that end-expiratory Ppw reflected pleural pressure (measured as esophageal pressure) but that the electronically averaged Ppw agreed with the transmural wedge pressure (the difference of Ppw and esophageal pressure) within $\pm$ 3 Torr (fig. 4). However, in patients with very large pleural pressure swings ($>$20 Torr) mean pressures overestimated the transmural Ppw by as much as 17 Torr [54]. Another shortcoming of the electronically averaged pressure is the difficulty of deciding whether a change in average filling pressure represents

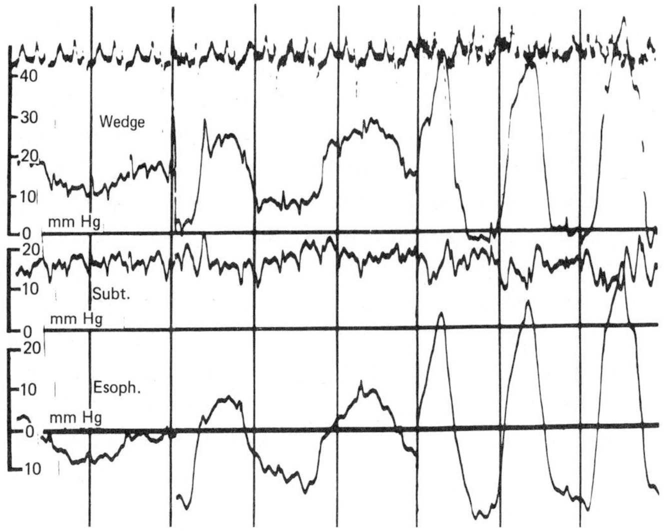

Fig. 4. Recording of pulmonary wedge pressure (Wedge), esophageal pressure (Esoph), and the difference between the two (Subt) as an estimate of transmural left ventricular filling pressure during quiet breathing followed by hyperventilation. The pulmonary wedge pressure reflects pleural pressure rather than transmural filling pressure, even at 'end-expiration' [from 54, with permission].

altered circulatory function or a change in pleural pressure due to altered respiratory mechanics or ventilatory pattern. *Schuster and Seeman* [63] advocate measuring the Ppw during a brief period of muscle paralysis in mechanically ventilated patients when elevation of end-expiratory vascular pressures by active exhalation is suspected. This aproach is obviously not applicable in spontaneously breathing patients and carries some risk of hypoxemia during paralysis even in patients on mechanical ventilation.

When positive end-expiratory pressure is used in the treatment of respiratory failure, juxtacardiac pressure increases due to transmission of airway pressure to the pleural space and compression of the heart by the expanding lungs [26, 44]. The increase in Pjc is determined by lung and chest wall compliance [12] and the amount of PEEP applied, and the effect on the Ppw is a function of the increase in juxtacardiac pressure and the attendant reduction in venous return (equation 3). Application of PEEP in experimental animals increases cardiac filling pressures measured relative to atmosphere [11, 40, 52, 61], whereas in human subjects it may increase the Ppw by as much as 12 Torr or have no effect [16, 20, 73]. The variable effect of PEEP on the Ppw in human subjects may reflect variability in the state of left ventricular filling when PEEP is applied [19] or, in some instances, minimal increases in pleural and juxtacardiac pressure in the presence of extremely stiff lungs.

Clearly, interpretation of the pulmonary wedge pressure during ventilation with positive end-expiratory pressure is difficult since PEEP: (1) increases pleural pressure, (2) decreases venous return, and (3) may create areas of zone I or II lung. Since the effect of PEEP is to increase the pulmonary wedge pressure relative to the $Plved_{tm}$, a low Ppw measured during PEEP ventilation with a properly calibrated system should be accepted as valid. A high filling pressure may represent the true state of the circulation or an artifact, and in this situation it is common to repeat the measurement while PEEP is briefly discontinued. This practice has been criticized because of the risk of hypoxemia and the doubtful value of the measurements [69]. Although the risk of hypoxemia is acceptable in selected patients ventilated with 100% oxygen beforehand [17, 38], the measurements are difficult to interpret because of the hemodynamic changes accompanying the removal of PEEP. If Ppw falls when PEEP is discontinued, the lower value more closely approximates $Plved_{tm}$ than the PEEP value. More commonly Ppw does not change when PEEP is removed, probably due to offsetting effects of the decrease in airway pressure on venous return and juxtacardiac pressure.

More precise estimates could be made if the change in pressure around the heart could be predicted from the level of PEEP applied. Observations in humans with adult respiratory distress syndrome indicate that 10–35% of the amount of PEEP applied is transmitted to the heart [35], but the methods used to measure pleural pressure in this study may underestimate juxtacardiac pressure [26, 45]. Data from animal studies indicate that the change in juxtacardiac pressure is approximately one-half of the amount of PEEP applied [26, 45]. For example, 15 cm H_2O of PEEP would elevate the Ppw by 5.3 Torr (15 cm $H_2O \times 0.5 \times 0.7$ Torr/cm H_2O = 5.3 Torr), and 10 cm H_2O by 3.5 Torr. However, this relationship holds only if lung and chest wall compliance are approximately equal [12], and it is unclear whether it can be applied in human subjects.

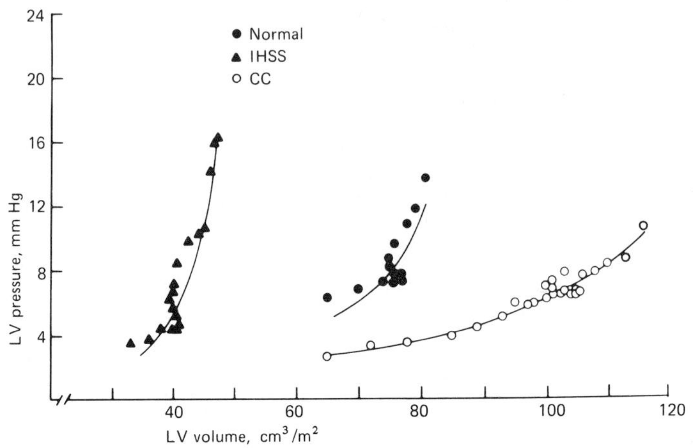

Fig. 5. Left ventricular diastolic pressure-volume curves from one normal subject and patients with a chronic pressure overload condition (idiopathic hypertrophic subaortic stenosis, IHSS) and a chronic volume overload condition (congestive cardiomyopathy, CC) [from 28, with permission].

Left Ventricular Diastolic Pressure-Volume Relationship

The curvilinear relationship between left ventricular pressure and volume during diastole reflects the interaction of factors both intrinsic to the ventricular chamber and external to it. Principal among these factors are ventricular relaxation, passive elastic properties of the ventricle, viscous properties, the pericardium, and interaction with the right ventricle [31]. Since these factors may be altered by disease, the LV diastolic pressure-volume (P-V) relationship is not fixed, and alterations of curve shape or position may occur. Chronic conditions characterized by an increase in ventricular wall thickness (hypertension, aortic stenosis, IHSS) or altered composition of the ventricular wall (amyloidosis, hemochromatosis, fibrosis) shift the diastolic pressure-volume curve so that normal or low diastolic volumes require high diastolic pressures [28, 29, 31, 32]. Chronic volume overload conditions such as congestive cardiomyopathy and aortic or mitral regurgitation may displace the curve such that high diastolic volumes are associated with normal or only mildly increased filling pressures [28, 31, 32] (fig. 5). Both acute and chronic coronary artery disease increase diastolic

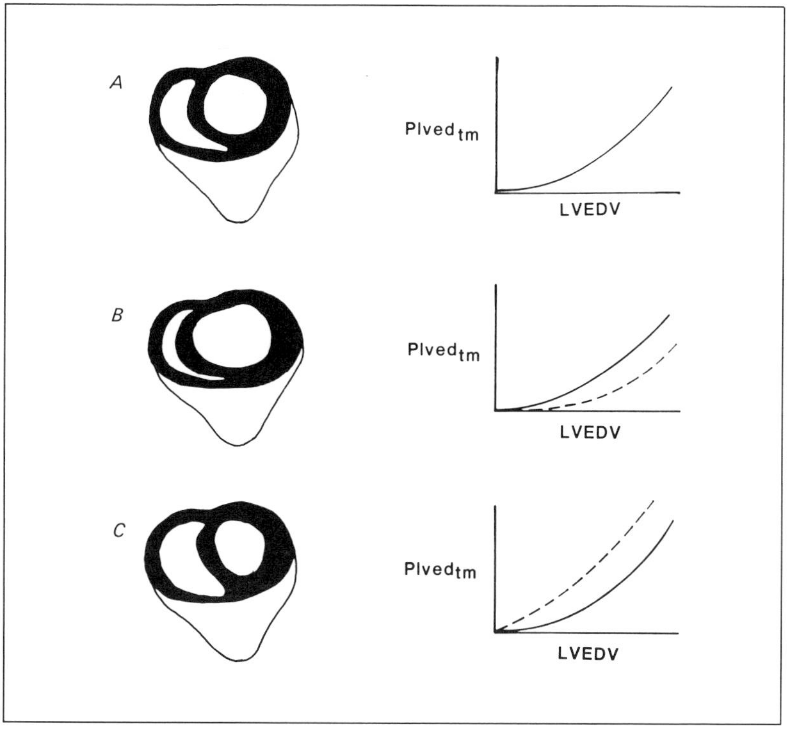

Fig. 6. Ventricular interdependence. *A* Normal. *B* Unloading of the right ventricle and rightward shift of the interventricular septum decrease the stiffness of the left ventricle, resulting in a new diastolic pressure-volume relationship (dashed line). *C* Pressure loading of the right ventricle and leftward shift of the septum increase the stiffness of the left ventricle, resulting in a new diastolic pressure-volume relationship (dashed line).

stiffness [5, 18, 21, 29, 30], as do pericardial constriction and tamponade. Administration of nitroprusside [1, 6] or nitroglycerin [42] shifts the LV pressure-volume curve in the direction of lower filling pressures, presumably by reducing right ventricular pressures and altering the position of the interventricular septum [42] (fig. 6B). The clinical implications of altered LV diastolic function are clear: (1) it cannot be assumed that the relationship between Plved or Ppw and the left ventricular end-diastolic volume is the same from one patient to the next; (2) the relationship is not necessarily constant in the same patient and can be altered acutely by therapeutic interventions or disease; (3) disparity between the radiographic assessment of ventricular size and measured filling pressure may be explained by an altered P-V relationship; and (4) hydrostatic pulmonary edema may occur with minimal or no abnormalities of contractile function if diastolic stiffness is increased [21].

Influence of PEEP on Ventricular Function

Ventilation with positive end-expiratory pressure reduces cardiac output in most patients with acute respiratory failure [23, 38]. The magnitude of the reduction in cardiac output is a function of several factors including the level of PEEP applied, intravascular volume status, cardiac function, and lung and chest wall compliance. While it seems reasonable to assume that positive airway pressure and the attendant increase in pleural pressure impede venous return, thereby reducing cardiac output [2, 13, 40, 52], confusing observations made in several laboratories have called this explanation into question.

If PEEP reduces cardiac output solely by decreasing venous return, then both transmural right and left ventricular filling pressures should fall. However, several groups of investigators have found that when PEEP is applied in experimental animals, transmural right and left ventricular pressures do not fall commensurately with stroke volume, or larger transmural pressures are required to maintain cardiac output and stroke volume constant, indicating impaired performance of both ventricles [10, 11, 51, 55, 61, 62]. While some investigators have suggested that PEEP impairs ventricular function by humoral or reflex mechanisms [9, 43, 47], indices of contractile function are unchanged or even increased during PEEP [24, 35, 55, 60]. Observations from several different laboratories in both experimental animals and human subjects have indicated that the hemodynamic effects of PEEP are explained by mechanical interdependence of the ventricles. When the lungs are hyperinflated by PEEP, the rise in pulmonary vascular resistance associated with increased lung volume [71] increases right ventricular afterload. Right ventricular loading results in a shift of the interventricular septum toward the left ventricle with the result that the LV is stiffer during diastole and left ventricular filling is reduced at the same filling pressure (fig. 6C) [34, 35, 60].

However, recent careful observations in animals indicate that the reduction in cardiac output during PEEP is explainable by a reduction in preload due to mechanical interaction of the heart and lungs. These studies demonstrate that pleural and esophageal pressure underestimate the pressure exerted on the outside of the heart by PEEP-expanded lungs, and, as a result, transmural ventricular pressures measured relative to pleural or esophageal pressure overestimate true distending pressure [15, 26, 45]. *Wise* et al. [72] examined ventricular function during PEEP in open chest animals on right heart bypass. Although any right ventricular influence on the left ventricular diastolic pressure-volume relationship was excluded, PEEP still produced a rightward shift in the Frank-Starling relationship. Direct measurements of pressure in the pericardial space indicated that juxtacardiac pressure exceeds atmospheric pressure during 15 cm H_2O PEEP and that this increased pressure around the heart explains the apparent right shift of the ventricular function curve during PEEP [72]. *Fewell* et al. [26] found that cardiac output, LVEDV, and Plved are unchanged during PEEP when the lungs are held away from the heart in open chest animals. When direct measurements of juxtacardiac pressure are used to calculate transmural ventricular pressures, PEEP does not alter the diastolic pressure-volume relationship [25] or the ventricular function curve [44] of either ventricle in closed chest animals. In summary, the best evidence from animal studies leads to the conclusion that PEEP decreases cardiac output by a reduction in the end-diastolic volumes of the right and left ventricles without impaired contractility or altered LV diastolic function.

The relationship of PEEP and ventricular function is further complicated by the finding that cardiac output may actually rise during PEEP in some subjects [33, 46]. The most likely explanation for this observation is the effect of PEEP on left ventricular afterload. Afterload, the wall tension or stress developed by ventricular muscle during systole, is a function of ventricular geometry, radius, and systolic pressure. For clinical purposes afterload is usually represented by systolic intraventricular pressure, but when intrathoracic pressure is altered, afterload is better represented by the transmural ventricular systolic pressure. This is more easily understood if one considers a hypothetical situation in which juxtacardiac pressure were raised to the level of aortic pressure; the ventricle would be compressed mechanically by the surrounding pressure, and ejection of blood could occur passively in the absence of any tension development by the ventricle. Alternatively, if intrathoracic pressure is markedly reduced, the pressure difference between the thorax and the extrathoracic arterial bed is increased, and additional tension is required to move blood out of the thorax. Consistent with this reasoning are the observations that: (1) frequent coughing maintains aortic pressure and consciousness in the presence of ventricular fibrillation [14]; (2) a Mueller maneuver (inspiration against a closed glottis) impairs ventricular performance in the presence of an unchanged or increased LVEDV [7, 65]; (3) increasing intrathoracic pressure with abdominal and chest binders improves cardiac function [49, 50]. Thus, PEEP may improve left ventricular performance by decreasing transmural ventricular systolic pressure and afterload. Augmentation of cardiac output during PEEP is more likely in patients with underlying ventricular dysfunction [33, 46], and this may reflect the fact that afterload reduction has a greater effect on LV function than decreased venous return in a volume-unresponsive failing heart.

References

1 Alderman, E.L.; Glantz, S.A.: Acute hemodynamic interventions shift the diastolic pressure-volume curve in man. Circulation *54:* 662–671 (1976).

2 Ashbaugh, D.G.; Petty, T.L.: Positive end-expiratory pressure. Physiology, indications, and contraindications. J. thorac. cardiovasc. Surg. *65:* 165–170 (1973).

3 Bouchard, R.J.; Gault, J.H.; Ross, J.: Evaluation of pulmonary arterial end-diastolic pressure as an estimate of left ventricular end-diastolic pressure in patients with normal and abnormal left ventricular performance. Circulation *44:* 1072–1079 (1971).

4 Braunwald, E.; Frahm, C.J.: Studies on Starling's law of the heart. IV. Observations on the hemodynamic functions of the left atrium in man. Circulation *24:* 633–642 (1961).

5 Bristow, J.D.; Van Zee, B.E.; Judkins, M.P.: Systolic and diastolic abnormalities of the left ventricle in coronary artery disease. Studies in patients with little or no enlargement of ventricular volume. Circulation *42:* 219–228 (1970).

6 Brodie, B.R.; Grossman, W.; Mann, T.; McLaurin, L.P.: Effects of sodium nitroprusside on left ventricular diastolic pressure-volume relations. J. clin. Invest. *59:* 59–68 (1977).

7 Buda, A.J.; Pinsky, M.R.; Ingels, N.B.; Daughters, G.T.; Stinson, E.B.; Alderman, E.L.: Effect of intrathoracic pressure on left ventricular performance. New Engl. J. Med. *301:* 453–459 (1979).

8 Burrows, B.; Kettel, L.J.; Niden, A.H.; Rabinowitz, M.; Diener, C.F.: Patterns of cardiovascular dysfunction in chronic obstructive lung disease. New Engl. J. Med. *286:* 912–918 (1972).

9 Cassidy, S.S.; Eschenbacher, W.L.; Johnson, R.L.: Reflex cardiovascular depression during unilateral lung hyperinflation in the dog. J. clin. Invest. *64:* 620–626 (1979).

10 Cassidy, S.S.; Eschenbacher, W.L.; Robertson, C.H.; Nixon, J.V.; Blomqvist, G.; Johnson, R.L.: Cardiovascular effects of positive-pressure ventilation in normal subjects. J. appl. Physiol. *47:* 453–461 (1979).

11 Cassidy, S.S.; Robertson, C.H.; Pierce, A.K.; Johnson, R.L.: Cardiovascular effects of positive end-expiratory pressure in dogs. J. appl. Physiol. *44:* 743–750 (1978).

12 Chapin, J.C.; Downs, J.B.; Douglas, M.E.; Murphy, E.J.; Ruiz, B.C.: Lung expansion, airway pressure transmission, and positive end-expiratory pressure. Archs Surg. *114:* 1193–1197 (1979).
13 Cournand, A.; Motley, H.L.; Werko, L.; Richards, D.W.: Physiological studies of the effects of intermittent positive pressure breathing on cardiac output in man. Am. J. Physiol. *152:* 162–174 (1948).
14 Criley, J.M.; Blaufuss, A.H.; Kissel, G.L.: Cough-induced cardiac compression. Self-administered form of cardiopulmonary resuscitation. J. Am. med. Ass. *236:* 1246–1250 (1976).
15 Culver, B.H.; Marini, J.J.; Butler, J.: Lung volume and pleural pressure effects on ventricular function. J. appl. Physiol. *50:* 630–635 (1981).
16 Davison, R.; Parker, M.; Harrison, R.A.: The validity of determinations of pulmonary wedge pressure during mechanical ventilation. Chest *73:* 352–355 (1978).
17 DeCampo, T.; Civetta, J.M.: The effect of short-term discontinuation of high-level PEEP in patients with acute respiratory failure. Crit. Care Med. *7:* 47–49 (1979).
18 Diamond, G.; Forrester, J.S.: Effect of coronary artery disease and acute myocardial infarction on left ventricular compliance in man. Circulation *45:* 11–19 (1972).
19 Ditchey, R.V.: Volume-dependent effects of positive airway pressure on intracavitary left ventricular end-diastolic pressure. Circulation *69:* 815–821 (1984).
20 Divertie, M.B.; McMichan, J.C.; Michel, L.; Offord, K.P.; Ness, A.B.: Avoidance of aggravated hypoxemia during measurement of mean pulmonary artery wedge pressure in ARDS. Chest *83:* 70–74 (1983).
21 Dodek, A.; Kassebaum, D.G.; Bristow, J.D.: Pulmonary edema in coronary-artery disease without cardiomegaly. Paradox of the stiff heart. New Engl. J. Med. *286:* 1347–1350 (1972).
22 Falicov, R.E.; Resnekov, L.: Relationship of the pulmonary artery end-diastolic pressure to the left ventricular end-diastolic and mean filling pressures in patients with and without left ventricular dysfunction. Circulation *42:* 65–73 (1970).
23 Falke, K.J.; Pontoppidan, H.; Kumar, A.; Leith, D.E.; Geffin, B.; Laver, M.B.: Ventilation with end-expiratory pressure in acute lung disease. J. clin. Invest. *51:* 2315–2323 (1972).
24 Fewell, J.E.; Abendschein, D.R.; Carlson, C.J.; Murray, J.F.; Rapaport, E.: Continuous positive-pressure ventilation decreases right and left ventricular end-diastolic volumes in the dog. Circulation Res. *46:* 125–132 (1980).
25 Fewell, J.E.; Abendschein, D.R.; Carlson, C.J.; Rapaport, E.; Murray, J.F.: Continuous positive-pressure ventilation does not alter ventricular pressure-volume relationship. Am. J. Physiol. *240:* H821–H826 (1981).
26 Fewell, J.E.; Abendschein, D.R.; Carlson, C.J.; Rapaport, E.; Murray, J.F.: Mechanism of decreased right and left ventricular end-diastolic volumes during continuous positive-pressure ventilation in dogs. Circulation Res. *47:* 467–472 (1980).
27 Fisher, M.L.; DeFelice, C.E.; Parisi, A.F.: Assessing left ventricular filling pressure with flow-directed (Swan-Ganz) catheters. Chest *68:* 542–547 (1975).
28 Gaasch, W.H.; Cole, J.S.; Quinones, M.A.; Alexander, J.K.: Dynamic determinants of left ventricular diastolic pressure-volume relations in man. Circulation *51:* 317–323 (1975).
29 Gaasch, W.H.; Levine, H.J.; Quinones, M.A.; Alexander, J.K.: Left ventricular compliance: mechanisms and clinical implications. Am J. Cardiol. *38:* 645–653 (1976).

30 Glantz, S.A.; Parmley, W.W.: Factors which affect the diastolic pressure-volume curve. Circulation Res. *42:* 171–180 (1978).

31 Grossman, W.; McLaurin, L.P.: Diastolic properties of the left ventricle. Ann. intern. Med. *84:* 316–326 (1976).

32 Grossman, W.; McLaurin, K.P.; Stefadouros, M.A.: Left ventricular stiffness associated with chronic pressure and volume overloads in man. Circulation Res. *35:* 793–800 (1974).

33 Harken, A.H.; Brennan, M.F.; Smith, B.; Barsmian, E.M.: The hemodynamic response to positive end-expiratory ventilation in hypovolemic patients. Surgery *76:* 786–793 (1974).

34 Haynes, J.B.; Carson, S.D.; Whitney, W.P.; Zerbe, G.O.; Hyers, T.M.; Steele, P.: Positive end-expiratory pressure shifts left ventricular diastolic pressure-area curves. J. appl. Physiol. *48:* 670–676 (1980).

35 Jardin, F.; Farcot, J.C.; Boisante, L.; Curien, N.; Margairaz, A.; Bourdarias, J.P.: Influence of positive end-expiratory pressure on left ventricular performance. New Engl. J. Med. *304:* 387–392 (1981).

36 Jenkins, B.S.; Bradley, R.D.; Branthwaite, M.A.: Evaluation of pulmonary arterial end-diastolic pressure as an indirect estimate of left atrial mean pressure. Circulation *42:* 75–78 (1970).

37 Kaltman, A.J.; Herbert, W.H.; Conroy, R.J.; Kossmann, C.E.: The gradient in pressure across the pulmonary vascular bed during diastole. Circulation *34:* 377–384 (1966).

38 Kumar, A.; Flake, K.J.; Geffin, B.; Aldredge, C.F.; Laver, M.B.; Lowenstein, E.; Pontoppidan, H.: Continuous positive-pressure ventilation in acute respiratory failure. New Engl. J. Med. *283:* 1430–1436 (1970).

39 Lappas, D.; Lell, W.A.; Gabel, J.C.; Civetta, J.M.; Lowenstein, E.: Indirect measurement of left-atrial pressure in surgical patients – pulmonary-capillary wedge and pulmonary-artery diastolic pressures compared with left-atrial pressure. Anesthesiology *38:* 394–397 (1973).

40 Lenfant, C.; Howell, B.J.: Cardiovascular adjustments in dogs during continuous pressure breathing. J. appl. Physiol. *15:* 425–428 (1960).

41 Luchsinger, P.C.; Seipp, H.W.; Patel, D.J.: Relationship of pulmonary artery-wedge pressure to left atrial pressure in man. Circulation Res. *11:* 315–318 (1962).

42 Ludbrook, P.A.; Byrne, J.D.; McKnight, R.C.: Influence of right ventricular hemodynamics on left ventricular diastolic pressure-volume relations in man. Circulation *59:* 21–31 (1979).

43 Manny, J.; Grindlinger, G.; Mathe, A.A.; Hechtman, H.B.: Positive end-expiratory pressure, lung stretch, and decreased myocardial contractility. Surgery *84:* 127–132 (1978).

44 Marini, J.J.; Culver, B.H.; Butler, J.: Effect of positive end-expiratory pressure on canine ventricular function curves. J. appl. Physiol. *51:* 1367–1374 (1981).

45 Marini, J.J.; O'Quin, R.; Culver, B.H.; Butler, J.: Estimation of transmural cardiac pressures during ventilation with PEEP. J. appl. Physiol. *53:* 384–391 (1982).

46 Mathru, M.; Rao, T.L.K.; El-Etr, A.A.; Pifarre, R.: Hemodynamic response to changes in ventilatory patterns in patients with normal and poor left ventricular reserve. Crit. Care Med. *10:* 423–426 (1982).

47 Patten, M.T.; Liebman, P.R.; Hechtman, H.B.: Humorally mediated decreases in cardiac output associated with positive end expiratory pressure. Microvasc. Res. *13:* 137–139 (1977).
48 Permutt, S.: Relation between pulmonary arterial pressure and pleural pressure during the acute asthmatic attack. Chest *63:* suppl., pp. 25S–27S (1973).
49 Pinsky, M.R.; Summer, W.R.: Cardiac augmentation by phasic high intrathoracic pressure support in man. Chest *84:* 370–375 (1983).
50 Pinsky, M.R.; Summer, W.R.; Wise, R.A.; Permutt, S.; Bromberger-Barnea, B.: Augmentation of cardiac function by elevation of intrathoracic pressure. J. appl. Physiol. *54:* 950–955 (1983).
51 Prewitt, R.M.; Wood, L.D.H.: Effect of positive end-expiratory pressure on ventricular function in dogs. Am. J. Physiol. *236:* H534–H544 (1979).
52 Qvist, J.; Pontoppidan, H.; Wilson, R.S.; Lowenstein, E.; Laver, M.B.: Hemodynamic responses to mechanical ventilation with PEEP. Anesthesiology *42:* 45–55 (1975).
53 Rahimtoola, S.H.; Loeb, H.S.; Ehsani, A.; Sinno, M.Z.; Chuquimia, R.; Lal, R.; Rosen, K.M.; Gunnar, R.M.: Relationship of pulmonary artery to left ventricular diastolic pressures in acute myocardial infarction. Circulation *46:* 283–290 (1972).
54 Rice, D.L.; Awe, R.J.; Gaasch, W.H.; Alexander, J.K.; Jenkins, D.E.: Wedge pressure measurement in obstructive pulmonary disease. Chest *66:* 628–632 (1974).
55 Robotham, J.L.; Lixfeld, W.; Holland, L.; MacGregor, D.; Bromberger-Barnea, B.; Permutt, S.; Rabson, J.L.: The effects of positive end-expiratory pressure on right and left ventricular performance. Am. Rev. resp. Dis. *121:* 677–683 (1980).
56 Roy, R.; Powers, S.R.; Feustel, P.J.; Dutton, R.E.: Pulmonary wedge catheterization during positive end-expiratory pressure ventilation in the dog. Anesthesiology *46:* 385–390 (1977).
57 Rubin, L.J.; Peter, R.H.: Hemodynamics at rest and during exercise after oral hydralazine in patients with cor pulmonale. Am. J. Cardiol. *47:* 116–122 (1981).
58 Rubin, L.J.; Peter, R.H.: Oral hydralazine therapy for primary pulmonary hypertension. New Engl. J. Med. *302:* 69–73 (1980).
59 Sapru, R.P.; Taylor, S.H.; Donald, K.W.: Comparison of the pulmonary wedge pressure with the left ventricular end-diastolic pressure in man. Clin. Sci. *34:* 125–140 (1968).
60 Scharf, S.M.; Brown, R.; Saunders, N.; Green, L.H.; Ingram, R.H.: Changes in canine left ventricular size and configuration with positive end-expiratory pressure. Circulation Res. *44:* 672–678 (1979).
61 Scharf, S.M.; Caldini, P.; Ingram, R.H.: Cardiovascular effects of increasing airway pressure in the dog. Am. J. Physiol. *232:* H35–H43 (1977).
62 Scharf, S.M.; Ingram, R.H.: Influence of abdominal pressure and sympathetic vasoconstriction on the cardiovascular response to positive end-expiratory pressure. Am. Rev. resp. Dis. *116:* 661–670 (1977).
63 Schuster, D.P.; Seeman, M.D.: Temporary muscle paralysis for accurate measurement of pulmonary artery occlusion pressure. Chest *84:* 593–597 (1983).
64 Shasby, D.M.; Dauber, I.M.; Pfister, S.; Anderson, J.T.; Carson, S.B.; Manart, F.; Hyers, T.M.: Swan-Ganz cathetrer location and left atrial pressure determine the accuracy of the wedge pressure when positive end-expiratory pressure is used. Chest *80:* 666–670 (1981).

65 Summer, W.R.; Permutt, S.; Sagawa, K.; Shoukas, A.A.; Bromberger-Barnea, B.: Effects of spontaneous respiration on canine left ventricular function. Circulation Res. *45:* 719–728 (1979).
66 Todd, T.R.J.; Baile, E.M.; Hogg, J.C.: Pulmonary arterial wedge pressure in hemorrhagic shock. Am. Rev. resp. Dis. *118:* 613–616 (1978).
67 Tooker, J.; Huseby, J.; Butler, J.: The effect of Swan-Ganz catheter height on the wedge pressure-left atrial pressure relationship in edema during positive-pressure ventilation. Am. Rev. resp. Dis. *117:* 721–725 (1978).
68 Trichet, B.; Falke, K.; Togut, A.; Laver, M.B.: The effect of pre-existing pulmonary vascular disease on the response to mechanical ventilation with PEEP following open-heart surgery. Anesthesiology *42:* 56–67 (1975).
69 Weisman, I.M.; Rinaldo, J.E.; Rogers, R.M.: Positive end-expiratory pressure in adult respiratory failure. New Engl. J. Med. *307:* 1381–1384 (1982).
70 West, J.B.; Dollery, C.T.; Naimark, A.: Distribution of blood flow in isolated lung; relation to vascular and alveolar pressures. J. appl. Physiol. *19:* 713–724 (1964).
71 Whittenberger, J.L.; McGregor, M.; Berglund, E.; Borst, H.G.: Influence of state of inflation of the lung on pulmonary vascular resistance. J. appl. Physiol. *15:* 878–882 (1960).

Paul V. Carlile, MD, University of Oklahoma Health Sciences Center,
Oklahoma City, OK 73190 (USA)

Prog. crit. Care Med., vol. 2, pp. 87–98 (Karger, Basel 1985)

Pulmonary Thromboembolism

D. Robert McCaffree

University of Oklahoma Health Sciences Center, Veterans Administration Medical Center, Oklahoma City, Okla., USA

Pulmonary thromboembolic disease continues to be a major contributor to mortality and morbidity as well as a diagnostic and therapeutic challenge to clinicians. The exact incidence of symptomatic and significant pulmonary emboli remains an area of controversy. *Dalen and Alpert* [8] have estimated over 600,000 occurrences per year in the United States. *Robin* [21], on the other hand, argues that pulmonary embolism is overdiagnosed, giving as evidence findings in two studies that only 17 and 40% of patients strongly suspected of having a pulmonary embolus on the basis of the clinical picture and perfusion lung scan actually had emboli confirmed by angiography [3, 19]. One recent retrospective review of final autopsy diagnoses at Peter Bent Brigham Hospital between 1973 and 1977, a period during which 61% of deaths (1,455 of 2,372) were autopsied, found pulmonary emboli reported in 14% (or 216) of the autopsies [10]. These were further divided into 'major' or 'minor' emboli on the basis of anatomic location and clinical impact. One quarter (or 54) of the emboli were judged to be 'major'. Only 16 of these 54 (30%) were correctly diagnosed premortem, a percentage very close to the estimation of correct premortem diagnoses of *Dalen and Alpert* [8]. The above studies tend to support the view that pulmonary embolism is both over- and underdiagnosed, depending upon the clinical situation, and suggest that accurate diagnosis is difficult.

Diagnosis

The same autopsy study by *Goldhaber* et al. [10] also evaluated factors associated with correct antemortem diagnoses. The factors associated with a correct antemortem diagnosis – proven venous thrombosis, postsurgical

Table I. Clinical risk factors for pulmonary thromboembolism

Prior history of pulmonary thromboembolism	Thrombotic disorders
Recent surgery (particularly pelvic and hip surgery)	Advanced disorders
Immobilization	Advanced age
Congestive heart failure	Estrogens

Table II. Presenting symptoms and signs in the UPET

Symptoms	%	Signs	%
Dyspnea	81	Respiration > 16/min	87
Pleural pain	72	Rales	53
Apprehension	59	Increased P_2	53
Cough	54	Pulse > 100/min	44
Hemoptysis	34	Temperature 37.8 °C	42
Sweats	26	S_3, S_4	34
Syncope	14	Sweating	34
		Phlebitis	33
		Cyanosis	18

state, and the obtaining of lung scans and pulmonary angiograms – suggest, not surprisingly, that one must first consider the possibility. Pneumonia, congestive heart failure, and old age (greater than 70 years) were all associated with failure to make the correct premortem diagnosis, and all three might mimic or mask the effects of a pulmonary embolus.

The clinical settings in which the presence of thromboembolic disease should be more strongly suspected are listed in table I. Most of these conditions are associated with stasis of blood flow (bed rest, congestive heart failure) or altered coagulation (estrogens, release of tissue thromboplastin during surgery).

The signs and symptoms of pulmonary embolism are well known and nonspecific. The most frequent findings from the Urokinase Pulmonary Embolism Trial (UPET) [23] are listed in table II. However, the presence of these signs and symptoms in an appropriate clinical setting should arouse one's suspicion for the presence of a pulmonary embolus and lead to more definitive evaluation.

There are several laboratory adjuncts in making a diagnosis, but all have their shortcomings. Therefore, it is common to employ multiple tests in arriving at a diagnosis. The two most sensitive screening tests are the arterial blood gas determinations and the radioisotopic perfusion lung scan. One must remember, however, that a normal Pa_{O_2} does not rule out the possibility of a pulmonary embolus as proven in the UPET in which 12% of patients with proven pulmonary emboli had normal Pa_{O_2} values. On the other hand, a normal perfusion lung scan does, for all practical purposes, rule out that possibility. An abnormal perfusion lung scan cannot be used to prove the diagnosis, however, since the lung scan is sensitive to a great many diseases affecting the lungs, including chronic airflow obstruction and pneumonia.

Attempts have been made to increase the specificity of the perfusion lung scan by assessing the likelihood that the perfusion defects found on the scan are associated with a pulmonary embolus. In these schemes, a 'high-probability' scan exhibits peripheral, concave, segmental, or larger defects which do not correspond with any alterations on the chest radiograph. On the other hand, a 'low-probability' scan exhibits patchy, subsegmental defects or defects associated with abnormalities on the chest radiograph. Others have proposed the use of ventilation scans in conjunction with perfusion scans to improve the diagnostic yield. The principle underlying the use of ventilation scans is that in chronic diseases, decreases in blood flow will be accompanied by decreases in ventilation. Thus, one will find 'matching' defects of both ventilation and perfusion. On the other hand, acute decreases in perfusion will not be accompanied immediately by a decrease in ventilation, and one will find ventilation maintained in areas where perfusion is absent, i.e., a ventilation-perfusion 'mismatch'. The exact role of ventilation scans has remained somewhat controversial. Recently, however, two studies seem to corroborate that the ventilation scans can be useful in specific situations [6, 15]. *Cheely* et al. [6] found angiographically proven emboli in 23 of 25 patients with ventilation-perfusion mismatching involving lobes or multiple segments. They did not find that subsegmental defects were useful. Similarly, *Hull* et al. [15] found angiographically proven pulmonary emboli in 30 of 35 patients with segmental or greater defects and ventilation-perfusion mismatching. Moreover, these authors also combined venography with angiography and found evidence of deep venous thrombosis or pulmonary emboli in 32 of these same 35 patients. These studies support the view that segmental or greater perfusion defects with maintained ventilation (a ventilation-perfusion 'mismatch') lends strong support to the diagnosis of pulmonary embolism. On the other hand, a ventilation-perfusion 'match' cannot be used to rule out the possibility, nor can scans with subsegmental defects be used to establish or rule out the diagnosis.

The most specific test is pulmonary angiography. This should be utilized when one needs to be as certain as possible of the diagnosis, which is most of the time. However, it is an invasive procedure with a low but definite incidence of morbidity and mortality and requires technical expertise and equipment which may not be available at all hospitals. Even when such capabilities are present, it may not be possible or advisable to utilize angiography in all patients suspected of having a pulmonary embolus. One must, therefore, rely on the other less specific tests such as the ventilation and perfusion lung scans in some circumstances.

Since the majority of patients with pulmonary embolism will have evidence of deep venous thrombosis, there may be circumstances in which the simple demonstration of deep venous thrombosis associated with the clinical picture of pulmonary embolism would be strong enough support to establish the diagnosis. In fact, in the above-mentioned study by *Hull* et al. [15] 29 of 41 patients with angiographically proven pulmonary emboli had venographically proven deep venous thrombosis. However, venograms are also technically demanding and invasive procedures and thus other less invasive diagnostic tests which can be employed at the bedside have been suggested. Some of these include Doppler flow determinations, impedance plethysmography, ^{125}I-labeled fibrinogen scanning, and phleborheography. All but the ^{125}I-fibrinogen scans depend upon the demonstration of decreased flow through the venous system. The ^{125}I-fibrinogen is incorporated into the actively forming clots so that external counting will find increased radioactivity over areas with clots. Each of these techniques has its uses and limitations, but *Hull* et al. [14] have found a high correlation between venography and the combined use of ^{125}I-fibrinogen scanning and impedance plethysmography. Based upon their experience, they have recommended replacing venography in hospitalized patients with the above two noninvasive tests.

Other laboratory tests may help in the differential diagnosis or serve as adjuncts to the above tests. The chest radiograph usually has nonspecific changes, but is necessary in interpreting the perfusion and ventilation lung scans. In the UPET, the two most common findings on chest radiograph were consolidation and elevation of a hemidiaphragm. The electrocardiogram likewise was frequently abnormal, but the most common abnormalities were nonspecific ST and T wave changes. However, since acute myocardial infarction is frequently part of the differential diagnosis, the electrocardiogram can be extremely useful. Other tests such as the determination of fibrin and fibrinogen degradation products may be useful, but are not widely used [4]. Other chemical tests such as the determination of lactate dehydrogenase, serum glutamic-oxaloacetic transaminase and bilirubin are of no value.

Newer diagnostic tests such as digital subtraction angiography and the use of indium-labeled platelets in a perfusion lung scan are being evaluated, but their usefulness has not yet been determined.

Prophylaxis

With all the difficulties in trying to diagnose the disease, its prevention is by far preferable wherever possible. There are two different clinical settings for prophylaxis: (1) prevention of pulmonary emboli in the first place (primary prophylaxis) and (2) prevention of recurrence once the disease is diagnosed (secondary prophylaxis). Primary prophylaxis includes: (1) using mechanical means to decrease stasis or (2) altering the coagulability of the blood. The mechanical means which have been evaluated include elevation of the legs, exercising the calf muscles by pushing against a footboard, early ambulation following surgery, elastic stockings, electrical stimulation of the calf muscles, and pneumatic compression of the calf. These have all enjoyed varying degrees of success, but the ones that appear to be most useful and successful are early ambulation, electrical stimulation of the calf, and the use of the pneumatic boot. However, awake patients do not tolerate the electrical stimulation of the calf well, and pneumatic compression has not gained wide acceptance.

Therefore, in most situations primary prophylaxis is directed at altering blood coagulation. Warfarin has long been shown to be an effective anticoagulant and prophylactic, but has a high incidence of complications and is contraindicated in the surgical patient in the intraoperative and immediate postoperative period. Low-dose heparin (5,000 U s.c. every 12 h) has been shown to be effective in a wide variety of medical and surgical patients and has a low incidence of complications [17]. Recent trials administering dihydroergotamine (to induce venous constriction) along with low-dose heparin have shown promise for this approach as well. The original investigations with low-dose heparin alone found no increase in postoperative bleeding, but recent reports in the United States indicate that this nevertheless may occur [20]. Therefore, at present, it should be used only for those surgical patients at greatest risk for developing deep venous thrombosis.

There are some patients in whom low-dose heparin is not an effective prophylaxis: (1) those undergoing a suprapubic prostatectomy and (2) those undergoing hip surgery. Because of these limitations other agents have been tried. Low molecular weight dextran has been used, primarily in patients undergoing orthopedic procedures, with varying success rates. Aspirin has been proven to be useful in males undergoing total hip replacement [11]. *Harris* et al. [11], using 600 mg of aspirin twice daily, starting 24 h prior to surgery, demonstrated in men a decrease in the incidence of deep venous thrombosis from 56 to 17% when compared with placebo. This same effect was not noted in females. Other antiplatelet agents, such as sulfinpyrazone, dihydroxychloroquine, and dipyridamole, have been evaluated. At the present time, the only definitive statement that can be made is that dipyridamole (Persantine) is not effective.

Once a pulmonary embolus has occurred, attention must be focused on prevention of recurrent emboli which are associated with increased morbidity and mortality. There are two primary ways of approaching this: (1) mechanical interruption of the flow in the inferior vena cava and (2) anticoagulation.

Mechanical 'sieving' of clots used to be done primarily by surgical ligation or plication, but is now most commonly done by the transvenous placement of a filtering device, such as the Greenfield filter. This is most commonly utilized in the face of recurrent emboli despite adequate anticoagulation or in patients in whom the risk of anticoagulation is unacceptable. Its use should also be considered in patients with significant hemodynamic compromise in whom a second embolus may prove fatal, since anticoagulants will not remove the source for recurrent emboli. The complications of these devices include perforation of the vessel wall, spontaneous migration of the filter, downstream propagation of a clot, renal vein thrombosis, and infection.

Since the early study by *Coon and Willis* [7] demonstrating decreased recurrences in people taking warfarin, this agent has remained the anticoagulant of widest use in secondary prophylaxis. However, warfarin has a high incidence of bleeding complications, and in recent years investigators have evaluated the efficacy of fixed low-dose heparin regimens [5, 13], adjusted-dose heparin [12], and lower dose warfarin regimens [16]. *Bynum and Wilson* [5] and *Hull* et al. [13] reported the results of their studies using a fixed low-dose heparin regimen, each reaching a different conclusion as to the efficacy. However, the designs of the studies were somewhat different. In the study by *Bynum and Wilson* [5] the patients were fully anticoagulated for 4 weeks and then received 6 months of prophylaxis, whereas in the study of *Hull* et al. [13] the patients were fully anticoagulated for 2 weeks and then received 45–90 days of prophylaxis. In the former study there was a high incidence of recurrence with either heparin or warfarin (29 and 38%, respectively), but a much higher incidence of major bleeding with warfarin (17 compared with 0%). Thus they concluded that low-dose heparin was the better prophylaxis. *Hull* et al. [13] also found a major difference between warfarin and heparin in major bleeding (12 vs. 0%), had a similarly high rate of recurrence with the heparin regimen (26%), but had no recurrences with warfarin. Therefore, their conclusion was that low-dose heparin was not effective as a prophylaxis against recurrence. Subsequently, *Hull* et al. [12] have evaluated adjusting the dose of subcutaneous heparin given every 12 h to keep the partial thromboplastin time (PTT) obtained 6 h after heparin at 1.5 times the control value and have found a low incidence both of bleeding (2 vs. 17% of those taking warfarin) and recurrence (4%) and thus feel that this regimen is effective. *Hull* et al. [16] have evaluated adjusting warfarin dosage by using a prothrombin time determination more sensitive than the method most widely employed in the United States. The Manchester comparative reagent is more sensitive than Simplastin to changes in the vitamin K dependent coagulation factors and allows for a lower dose of warfarin being given; this resulted in fewer bleeding complications (4 vs 22% in the more intensely anticoagulated group) while maintaining a low rate of recurrences (2% in both groups) [16]. They concluded that this also is an effective method of prophylaxis without incurring the high risk of bleeding complications using higher doses of warfarin.

Therapy

There are three major therapeutic approaches: (1) mechanical removal of clots; (2) stopping of the clotting process through the use of anticoagulants, and (3) dissolution of clots through the use of fibrinolytic agents.

The mechanical removal of clots will not be discussed in any detail, in part because the role and efficacy of open surgical removal remains unclear. One technique that does offer some promise is the use of a suction catheter to remove the clots [24], but this technique is not widely available.

Heparin Therapy

Anticoagulation with heparin has been the mainstay of therapy, but interestingly, its efficacy has only been demonstrated in one prospective study of 20 patients [1]. Heparin anticoagulation will stop or slow thrombus formation, will prevent platelets from adhering to the emboli and releasing numerous potent vasoactive substances, and has been shown to reduce recurrent emboli. However, heparin will not eliminate potential sources for recurrent emboli, alter the hemodynamic disturbances in the immediate postembolic period, or prevent permanent impairment to the pulmonary vascular bed.

At the present time two of the major controversies surrounding the use of heparin are whether to infuse it intermittently or continuously and how to monitor the heparin therapy. Some prospective studies [9, 22] have demonstrated increased bleeding with intermittent versus continuous infusion. On the other hand, at least one retrospective study [26] demonstrated no overall increase in bleeding between continuous and intermittent infusion, but in a retrospectively identified 'high-risk' group, there was a significant increase in bleeding with intermittent therapy. However, intermittent therapy was also associated with a much lower recurrence rate. The factor used to identify the 'high-risk' group for bleeding included: age greater than 60 years, uremia, diastolic blood pressure greater than 115 mm Hg, recent surgery, trauma or gastrointestinal bleeding, massive pulmonary emboli, and any documented hemostatic defect. The authors' review of initial data in this study indicated that intermittent therapy resulted in more heparin being given per 24 h and might explain both the increased bleeding and the lower recurrence rate. However, when the daily heparin dose was equalized between the two methods of administration, continuous infusion still resulted in more recurrences. Thus, the physician continues to face the dilemma of the best method of administration of heparin. From the currently available evidence, it appears that continuous infusion will, in general, be associated with less bleeding and that intermittent infusion will, in general, be associated with less recurrences. By either method, patients generally will require 25,000–40,000 U/24 h.

The question of how to monitor the effects of heparin therapy on the coagulation system also reflects the risk of bleeding and recurrence. Some authors argue that a high PTT, i.e., greater than 1.5–2 times the control value, cannot reliably be associated with bleeding complications. However, in one of the above studies [26], those patients who bled tended to have a higher PTT than those who did not. Moreover, one investigation has shown that recurrences were reduced by keeping the PTT at least 1.5 times the control value [2]. From the present information it appears that a PTT should be obtained to demonstrate the therapeutic effects of heparin, and then the PTT may need to be periodically checked to document continued therapeutic efficacy. Particularly in patients with high risk of bleeding complications, it would also be advisable to periodically monitor the PTT to assure that it is not greatly above twice the control value.

Thrombolytic Therapy

The other major mode of therapy, used in conjunction with heparin, is the use of thrombolytic agents. Their use has been the subject of several excellent recent reviews [18, 25]. At the present time, the two agents available and of proven efficacy are urokinase, a human protein derived from cultured human fetal kidney cells, and streptokinase, a protein derived from streptococci. Human tissue plasminogen activator is currently being evaluated, but is not yet available for clinical use. When it is, it might well replace streptokinase.

The advantages of thrombolytic therapy are: (1) it will remove the source of recurrent emboli; (2) it will protect venous valves and prevent further damage; (3) it will help return the acutely altered hemodynamics to their normal state, and (4) it may prevent permanent damage to the pulmonary vascular bed. However, thrombolytic therapy has never been shown to reduce mortality in massive pulmonary embolus.

There are also several disadvantages of thrombolytic therapy: (1) it will reliably dissolve any recently formed clots and will create bleeding in recent wounds including vascular puncture sites; (2) streptokinase, being a foreign protein, will commonly cause fever and, less commonly, allergic reactions, and (3) this therapy is expensive.

There are several contraindications to the use of thrombolytic agents, all of them related to bleeding or the possibility of emboli to the brain. The absolute contraindications include: active internal bleeding, evidence of a cerebral vascular accident in the last 2 months, or any other active intracranial process. Relative contraindications include: any recent surgery, trauma, childbirth or gastrointestinal bleeding, severe hypertension, a left-heart thrombus (because of the danger of emboli), hemorrhagic diabetic retinopathy, an age greater than 75 years, preexisting coagulation defects, and pregnancy.

When these agents first became available some clinicians were hesitant to use them because of the rather complicated recommendations for dosage determination and adjustment. However, it has been demonstrated now that a simplified fixed dose regimen is very effective. At the present time the following approach appears to be simple and effective. Once pulmonary embolism is proven by angiography, the patient is first started on high-dose heparin therapy, while the specified thrombolytic agent is obtained. Once the agent is available, the heparin therapy is discontinued. One may either monitor the PTT until the effect of the heparin is gone or, more practically, wait for about 2 h, at which time there should be little or no anticoagulant effect from the heparin. During this time a baseline thrombin time (or other appropriate laboratory monitor, such as the euglobulin lysis time) is obtained. Once this is obtained, urokinase, 2,000 CTA U/pound body weight, is infused over 10 min and then 2,000 CTA U/pound body weight hourly for 12–24 h. If one is using streptokinase, then 250,000 U is infused over 20–30 min initially, then followed by 100,000 U/h for the next 24–72 h. 3–4 h after starting the infusion, the thrombin time (or other test used to demonstrate a 'lytic state') is obtained to document a therapeutic effect. The thrombin time should be five times the patient's control value. If there is no therapeutic effect, then the infusion rate can either be increased by 50% or can be decreased. If neither maneuver is effective, the thrombolytic therapy is stopped and heparin restarted.

With the use of thrombolytic therapy, one can anticipate minor superficial bleeding from puncture sites in all patients. This can usualy be handled by local care with pressure dressings and other means. Most patients receiving streptokinase will develop fever which can be controlled by antipyretics or a cooling blanket. Serious internal bleeding in patients without any known predisposing factors occurs in only 5–10% of the patients.

Once the thrombolytic therapy is completed and the infusion stopped, the thrombin time is followed until it is normal. Then the heparin therapy is once again instituted, so that the patient receives a full 7- to 10-day thrombolytic and anticoagulant therapy prior to the institution of any secondary prophylaxis.

In summary, the diagnosis of pulmonary embolism remains a clinical challenge, requiring the synthesis of information from multiple sources. Once the diagnosis is established, the selection of therapy must be tailored to each individual patient's requirements. While heparin remains the mainstay of therapy in many settings, the combined use of thrombolytic agents and heparin may often prove to be more advantageous without increasing the risks.

References

1 Barrett, D.W.; Jordan, J.C.: Anticoagulant drugs in the treatment of pulmonary embolism: a controlled clinical trial. Lancet *i:* 1309–1312 (1960).

2 Basu, D.; Gallus, A.; Hirsh, J.; Cade, J.: A prospective study of the value of monitoring heparin treatment with the activated partial thromboplastin time. New Engl. J. Med. *287:* 324–327 (1972).

3 Bell, W.R.; Simon, T.L.: A comparative analysis of pulmonary perfusion scans with pulmonary angiograms. From a National Cooperative Study. Am. Heart J. *92:* 700–706 (1976).

4 Bynum, L.T.; Crotty, C.M.; Wilson, J.E., III: Diagnosis value of tests of fibrin metabolism in patients predisposed to pulmonary embolism. Archs intern. Med. *139:* 283–285 (1979).

5 Bynum, L.J.; Wilson, J.E.: Low-dose heparin therapy in the long-term treatment of venous thrombosis. New Engl. J. Med. *306:* 189–234 (1982).

6 Cheely, E.; McCartney, W.H.; Perry, J.R.; Delany, D.J.; Bustak, L.; Wynia, V.H.; Griggs, T.P.: The role of noninvasive tests versus pulmonary angiography in the diagnosis of pulmonary embolism. Am. J. Med. *70:* 17–22 (1981).

7 Coon, W.W.; Willis, P.W.: Recurrence of venous thromboembolism. Surgery *73:* 823–827 (1973).

8 Dalen, J.E.; Alpert, J.S.: Natural history of pulmonary embolism. Prog. cardiovasc. Dis. *17:* 259–269 (1975).

9 Glazier, R.L.; Crowell, E.B.: Randomized prospective trial of continuous versus intermittent heparin therapy. J. Am. med. Ass. *236:* 1365–1367 (1976).

10 Goldhaber, S.Z.; Hennekens, C.H.; Evans, D.A.; Newton, E.C.; Godleski, J.J.: Factors associated with correct antemortem diagnosis of major pulmonary embolism. Am. J. Med. *73:* 822–826 (1982).

11 Harris, W.H.; Salzman, E.W.; Athanasoulis, C.A.; Waltman, A.C.; DeSanctis, R.W.: Aspirin prophylaxis of venous thromboembolism after total hip replacement. New engl. J. Med. *297:* 1246–1249 (1977).

12 Hull, R.; Delmore, T.; Carter, C.; Hirsh, J.; Genton, E.; Gent, M.; Turpie, B.; McLoughlin, D.: Adjusted subcutaneous heparin versus warfarin sodium in the long-term treatment of venous thrombosis. New Engl. J. Med. *306:* 189–234 (1982).

13 Hull, R.; Delmore, T.; Genton, E.; Hirsh, J.; Gent, M.; Sackatt, D.; McLoughlin, D.; Armstrong, P.: Warfarin sodium versus low-dose heparin in the long-term treatment of venous thrombosis. New Engl. J. Med. *301:* 855–858 (1979).

14 Hull, R.D.; Hirsh, J.; Sackatt, D.L.; Taylor, D.W.; Carter, C.; Turpie, A.G.G.; Zielinsky, A.; Powers, P.; Gent, M.: Replacement of venography in suspected venous thrombosis by impedance plethysmography and I-fibrinogen leg scanning. Ann. intern. Med. *94:* 12–15 (1981).

15 Hull, R.D.; Hirsh, J.; Carter, C.J.; Jay, R.M.; Dodd, P.E.; Ockelford, P.A.; Coates, G.; Gill, G.J.; Turpie, A.G.G.; Doyle, D.J.; Buller, H.R.: Pulmonary angiography, ventilation lung scanning, and venography for clinically suspected pulmonary embolism with abnormal perfusion lung scans. Ann. intern. Med. *98:* 891–899 (1983).

16 Hull, R.; Hirsh, J.; Jay, R.; Carter, C.; England, C.; Gent, M.; Turpie, A.G.G.; McLoughlin, D.; Dodd, P.; Thomas, M.; Raskob, G.; Ockelford, P.: Different inten-

sities of oral anticoagulant therapy in the treatment of proximal-vein thrombosis. New Engl. J. Med. *307:* 1676–1681 (1982).
17 Kakkar, V.V.; Corrigan, T.P.; Fossard, D.P.: Prevention of fatal post-operative embolism by low-dose heparin: an international multicentre trial. Lancet *ii:* 45 (1975).
18 Marder, V.J.: The use of thrombolytic agents: choice of patient, drug administration, laboratory monitoring. Ann. intern. Med. *90:* 802–808 (1980).
19 McNeil, B.J.: A diagnostic strategy using ventilation-perfusion studies in patients suspect for pulmonary embolism. J. nucl. Med. *17:* 613–616 (1976).
20 Pachter, H.L.; Riles, T.S.: Low-dose heparin: bleeding and wound complications in the surgical patient. Ann. Surg. *186:* 669–673 (1977).
21 Robin, E.D.: Overdiagnosis and overtreatment of pulmonary embolism: the emperor may have no clothes. Ann. intern. Med. *87:* 775–781 (1977).
22 Salzman, E.W.; Deykin, D.; Shapiro, R.M.; Rosenberg, R.: Management of heparin therapy: controlled prospective trial. New Engl. J. Med. *292:* 1046–1050 (1975).
23 Sasahara, A.A.; Hyers, T.M.; Cole, C.M.; Ederer, F.; Murray, J.A.; Wenger, N.D.; Sherry, S.; Stengele, J.M.: Urokinase pulmonary embolism trial. A national comparative study. Circulation *47:* suppl. 2, pp. 1–80 (1973).
24 Scoggins, W.G.; Greenfield, L.J.: Transvenous pulmonary embolectomy for acute massive pulmonary embolism. Chest *71:* 213–216 (1977).
25 Sherry, S.; Bell, W.R.; Duckert, F.H.; Fletcher, A.P.; Gurewich, V.; Long, D.M.; Marder, V.J.; Roberts, H.; Salzman, E.W.; Sasahara, A.; Verstraete, M.: Thrombolytic therapy in thrombosis. National Institutes of Health consensus development conference. Ann. intern. Med. *93:* 141–144 (1980).
26 Wilson, J.E.; Bynum, L.J.; Parkey, R.W.: Heparin therapy in venous thromboembolism. Am. J. Med. *70:* 808–816 (1981).

D. Robert McCaffree, MD, University of Oklahoma Health Sciences Center, Veterans Administration Medical Center, Oklahoma City, OK 73126 (USA)

Prog. crit. Care Med., vol. 2, pp. 99–105 (Karger, Basel 1985)

Selection of Intravenous Fluids for Resuscitation

Charles L. Rice

Intensive Care Unit, Michael Reese Hospital and Medical Center, Chicago, Ill., USA

Introduction

The objectives of fluid administration for resuscitation are the restoration of adequate cardiac output and the replacement, where necessary, of lost interstitial fluid volume. Fluid therapy for correction of electrolyte disturbances and the use of blood and blood products in resuscitation are addressed in other chapters.

In treating a patient in shock, the distinctions drawn between hemorrhagic, cardiogenic, and septic shock are important, but need not delay the administration of fluid. For the patient in hemorrhagic shock, the rationale for fluid administration is self-evident: the patient has lost at least 20% of normal intravascular volume, and that volume must be restored. For victims of septic shock, too, some intravascular volume may have been lost, and, in addition, there is a greater intravascular space to be filled, due to an increase in venous capacitance and a fall in systemic vascular resistance. The administration of fluid to a patient in cardiogenic shock is not as straightforward. Nevertheless, *Russell* et al. [1] demonstrated that many patients in cardiogenic shock are, in fact, volume depleted, and that one can take advantage of Starling's law and obtain an increase in cardiac output by the careful administration of fluid.

Choice of Fluid: Starling's Hypothesis and the 'Colloid-Crystalloid' Debate

In 1895, *Starling* [2] developed a hypothesis to explain fluid movement across capillary membranes (fig. 1). His observations, made in the hindlimb of a dog, were extrapolated to the lung, and were used to explain the devel-

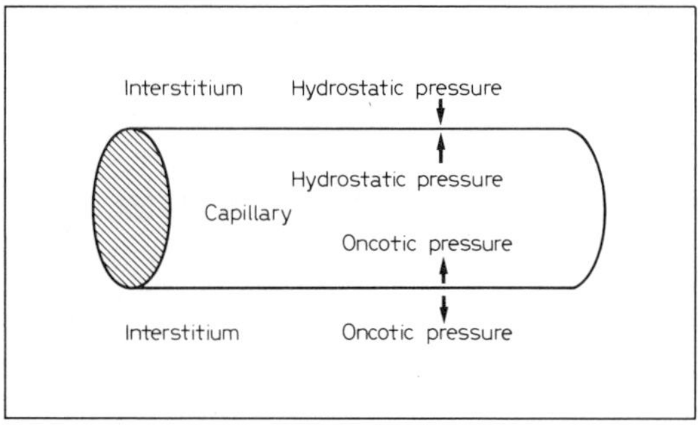

Fig. 1. Starling's hypothesis.

opment of pulmonary edema in combat casualties in Vietnam who had been resuscitated with large quantities of crystalloid. It was postulated that with the administration of large amounts of colloid-free fluid, the oncotic pressure keeping fluid within the pulmonary capillary was exceeded by the hydrostatic pressure, driving fluid into the interstitium. Expressed mathematically, the equation is generally written:

$$Q_f = K_f [(Pmv - Ppmv) - \sigma_f (\pi mv - \pi pmv)],$$

where Q_f = net transvascular flow of fluid; K_f = apparent fluid filtration coefficient; Pmv = microvascular hydrostatic pressure; Ppmv = perimicrovascular interstitial hydrostatic pressure (IP); σ_f = apparent reflection coefficient; πmv = plasma protein oncotic pressure (COP); πpmv = perimicrovascular protein oncotic pressure.

The equation holds that fluid movement across the capillary is equal to the differences in the hydrostatic and oncotic pressures on either side of the capillary membrane, these pressures being modified by two coefficients. The first is K, the filtration coefficient, which represents the rate of fluid movement across the capillary per unit of pressure gradient, per unit time, per unit of tissue mass. The second is σ, the reflection coefficient. Since an oncotic pressure can only be exerted across a semipermeable membrane, σ defines the degree of permeability for a given protein (actually any oncotically active solute). *Starling* assumed that $\sigma = 1$, meaning that all proteins within the capillary remain inside, and all outside remain outside. As σ falls, oncotic pressure becomes less and less important in affecting transvascular flow.

It has been argued that resuscitation with crystalloid solutions decreases πmv, and therefore must result in an increase in lung water. What is the evidence for this?

In 1959, *Guyton and Lindsey* [3] measured lung water in dogs after increasing left atrial pressure (LAP). They found that lung water began to accumulate in normal dogs when LAP exceeded 25 Torr. After plasmapheresis and reduction of albumin to <2 g%, the hydrostatic pressure (LAP) necessary to produce pulmonary edema was decreased to 12 Torr – but at LAP <12, there was no evidence of lung water increase.

Zarins et al. [4], using a jugular venous pouch preparation in baboons for the collection of pulmonary lymph, lowered the colloid oncotic pressures to near zero by plasmapheresis while keeping LAP constant at 8 mm Hg. Although *peripheral* edema occurred, there was no increase in lung water. In addition, the fall in lymph COP exactly paralleled the fall in plasma COP. If lymph COP is taken to represent interstitial COP, no decrease in the term ($\pi mv - \pi pmv$) occurs. This phenomenon is referred to as 'interstitial washout' and is thought to be one of the factors which helps to keep the interstitium (and hence the alveoli) dry.

The obvious conclusion to be drawn from these two studies is that oncotic pressure is important only to the extent that it allows for increases in hydrostatic pressure. If hydrostatic pressure is kept at normal levels, pulmonary edema does not occur even with oncotic pressures of nearly zero.

Resuscitation

Animal Studies

Lung water was measured gravimetrically in rats bled and then resuscitated with either Ringer's lactate or 5% plasma protein fraction (PPF) solution [5]. No evidence was found that there was greater accumulation of lung water when animals were resuscitated without colloid.

Moss et al. [6] studied baboons subjected to hemorrhagic shock and resuscitated either with Ringer's lactate or albumin solutions. The group receiving Ringer's solution required five times the shed volume to restore vital signs, whereas the group receiving albumin required twice the shed volume. There was no evidence of pulmonary edema in either group.

In contrast to these studies, *Holcroft and Trunkey* [7] found that animals resuscitated with PPF had an increase in lung water while there was no increase in those treated with Ringer's solution.

Human Studies

By the mid-1970s, sufficient evidence was available from animal studies indicating that neither albumin nor salt solution resuscitation was inherently harmful. The next step was to address the question in man. As is often the case in clinical trials, the strategies employed made interpretation of the data difficult in some of these studies. What factors should be considered in evaluating such studies?

(1) *Blood replacement:* Red cells must be given to attain some reasonable level of hematocrit. If whole blood is used, however, substantial quantities of albumin will be given the crystalloid-treated group. Blood replacement, therefore, should be in the form of packed cells.

(2) *End points:* The volume of fluid given should be based on physiologic end points, such as heart rate, blood pressure, urine output or cardiac output. There is no arbitrary formula which takes into account physiologic differences between patients.

The first human trial was reported by *Skillman* et al. [8]. 16 patients undergoing elective abdominal aortic surgery were studied. The patients received either 500 ml Ringer's lactate/h or a bolus of albumin followed by 1 liter of 5% albumin. Blood loss was replaced with an average of 3 liters whole blood. The colloid group received an average of 141 g of albumin the day of surgery and 70 g the first postoperative day. The crystalloid group received 31 g of albumin on the day of surgery and 69 g the next day. Both groups received an additional 50 g of albumin contained in the 3 liters whole blood during the operation. The authors reported a significant difference in oncotic pressure between the Ringer's lactate and colloid groups (22 vs. 27 Torr). There was no difference in the alveolar-arterial oxygen gradient (A-aDO_2). They did observe a correlation between the amount of sodium infused and the A-aDO_2.

This study violates both criteria outlined above: whole blood was used and resuscitation was by a formula rather than physiologic end points. Moreover, both groups received substantial quantities of albumin, and no difference in A-aDO_2 could be shown.

Another study in similar patients was reported by *Virgilio* et al. [9]. In this study, 14 patients received Ringer's lactate and 15 received 5% albumin in Ringer's lactate. Hematocrit was maintained at 30% by transfusion of packed cells and fluids in both groups were given to maintain pulmonary capillary wedge pressure, cardiac output, and urine output at acceptable levels. An average of 11 liters was required in the group receiving Ringer's lactate and 6 liters in the group receiving albumin on the day of surgery. No deaths occurred in either group, nor was there any difference in intrapulmonary shunt or other measurements of pulmonary function. 2 patients developed pulmonary edema; both were in the colloid group. These 2 patients underscore the cardinal role of hydrostatic pressure in lung water accumulation. They both developed pulmonary edema after their wedge pressures abruptly rose to approximately 25 Torr. When the colloid oncotic pressure-pulmonary capillary wedge pressure was correlated with intrapulmonary shunt, no relationship was found. This study concluded that resuscitation could be safely accomplished without albumin in patients undergoing elective aortic surgery.

Lowe et al. [10] examined the same issue with a similar protocol in 141 trauma victims. 84 patients received Ringer's lactate and packed cells and 55 received 5% albumin in Ringer's lactate and packed cells. There were 3 deaths in each group. There were no differences in pulmonary function between the groups.

We can summarize these and other studies as follows: (1) There is no evidence that volume resuscitation without colloid leads to an increased incidence of pulmonary edema. (2) The most important factor leading to pulmonary edema is capillary hydrostatic pressure. As long as this is kept at normal levels, pulmonary edema is unlikely to occur, irrespective of colloid oncotic pressure. (3) Some evidence exists that the infusion of albumin, especially in the septic patient, may result in increased amounts of albumin in the pulmonary interstitium. The clinical significance of this observation is unknown.

Crystalloid: The Choices

For reasons not entirely clear, most surgical services tend to use Ringer's lactate solution for volume resuscitation, while most medicine services seem to prefer so-called normal saline (0.9%). While the difference in sodium content is modest (133 vs. 155 mEq/l), the difference in anion concentration is marked: chloride, 105 vs. 155 mEq, lactate, 28 vs. 0 mEq. This difference results in the frequent observation of a nonanion gap (hyperchloremic) metabolic acidosis in patients resuscitated with normal saline. While this acidosis is almost always self-limited, there is no evidence that it is in any way beneficial, and it prevents following metabolic acidosis to gauge adequacy of resuscitation.

The objection to Ringer's lactate is that it would seem paradoxical to infuse lactate into a patient with lactic acidosis. The liver is, however, capable of metabolizing substantial amounts of lactic acid once its perfusion is restored to normal. The only setting in which the infusion of Ringer's lactate should be avoided is the patient with severe hepatocellular dysfunction. In that case, 5% dextrose with 0.45% saline with 100 mEq of sodium bicarbonate added per liter is a very appropriate resuscitative fluid.

Colloids: The Choices

While albumin (first bovine, then human) has been the colloid of choice for several years, other oncotically active fluids are available. The original pooled plasma has been abandoned because of the risk of hepatitis. PPF (Plasmanate, Protenate, Plasmatein) is an aqueous solution consisting of approximately 5% plasma proteins – 85% of which is albumin and 15% globulins. It offers no advantage over albumin. Hydroxy-ethyl starch has received substantial attention because of its somewhat lower cost. Physiologically, it appears to be virtually equivalent to albumin. If a colloid solution is chosen for volume resuscitation, care must be taken to guard against abrupt increases in filling pressure, which may result in pulmonary edema.

References

1 Russell, R.O.; Rackley, C.E.; Pombo, J.; et al.: Effects of increasing left ventricular filling pressures in patients with acute myocardial infarction. J. clin. Invest. *49:* 1539 (1970).
2 Starling, E.H.: On the absorption of fluids from the connective tissue spaces. J. Physiol., Lond. *19:* 312–326 (1895).
3 Guyton, A.C.; Lindsey, A.W.: Effect of left atrial pressure and decreased plasma protein concentration on the development of pulmonary edema. Circulation Res. *7:* 649–657 (1959).
4 Zarins, C.K.; Rice, C.L.; Peters, R.M.; Virgilio, R.W.: Lymph and pulmonary response to isobaric reduction in plasma oncotic pressure in baboons. Circulation Res. *43:* 925–930 (1978).
5 Schloerb, P.R.; Hunt, P.T.; Plummer, H.A.; Cage, G.K.: Pulmonary edema after replacement of blood loss by electrolyte solutions. Surgery Gynec. Obstet. *135:* 893–896 (1972).

6 Moss, G.S.; Siegel, D.C.; Cochin, A.; Fresquez, V.: Effects of saline and colloid solutions on pulmonary function in hemorrhagic shock. Surgery Gynec. Obstet. *133:* 53–58 (1971).

7 Holcroft, J.W.; Trunkey, D.D.: Extravascular lung water following hemorrhagic shock in baboons: comparison between resuscitation with Ringer's lactate and plasmanate. Ann. Surg. *180:* 408–417 (1974).

8 Skillman, J.J.; Restall, S.; Salzman, E.W.: Randomized trial of albumin vs. electrolyte solutions during abdominal aortic operations. Surgery *78:* 219–303 (1975).

9 Virgilio, R.W.; Rice, C.L.; Smith, D.E., et al.: Crystalloid vs. colloid resuscitation: Is one better? Surgery *85:* 129–139 (1979).

10 Lowe, R.J.; Moss, G.S.; Jilek, J.; Levine, H.A.: Crystalloid vs. colloid in the etiology of pulmonary failure after trauma: a randomized trial in man. Surgery *81:* 676–683 (1977).

Charles L. Rice, MD, Director, Intensive Care Unit,
Michael Reese Hospital and Medical Center, 29th Street and Ellis Avenue,
Chicago, IL 60616 (USA)

Prog. crit. Care Med., vol. 2, pp. 106–117 (Karger, Basel 1985)

Use of Pharmacologic Agents in the Hypoperfusion Syndrome

Thomas L. Whitsett

Clinical Pharmacology Program, University of Oklahoma Health Sciences Center, Oklahoma City, Okla., USA

While there are numerous etiologic factors that may cause or contribute to hypoperfusion, most patients begin the syndrome with a state of low cardiac output. In the past, and too often in the present, drugs with strong vasoconstrictive (alpha$_1$-adrenergic) action have dominated pharmacologic therapy. However, raising blood pressure at the expense of constricting flow to vital organs not only reduces perfusion but increases ventricular afterload which may further impair cardiac performance. Thus, efforts directed toward improving cardiac output and lowering ventricular afterload are more likely to improve perfusion than drugs that primarily act on the resistance factor of the blood pressure equation (fig. 1).

It is important to recognize the signs and symptoms of hypoperfusion for making an early diagnosis as well as serving as a general parameter for monitoring therapeutic responsiveness. Depressed sensorium, cool clammy skin, peripheral cyanosis and urine output < 40 ml/h reflect hypoperfusion. Also, understanding the relationship between tissue perfusion, blood pressure, and cardiac output is important in evaluating patients and prescribing appropriate therapy.

Heart Rate

Sinus bradycardia (heart rate < 60) and tachycardia (heart rate > 140) are usually not major factors causing hypoperfusion but may aggravate existing conditions. Atropine, isoproterenol or a pacemaker are considerations for bradycardia. Tachycardia presents more of a challenge since it is a common response to sympathetic stimulation and sympathomimetic ther-

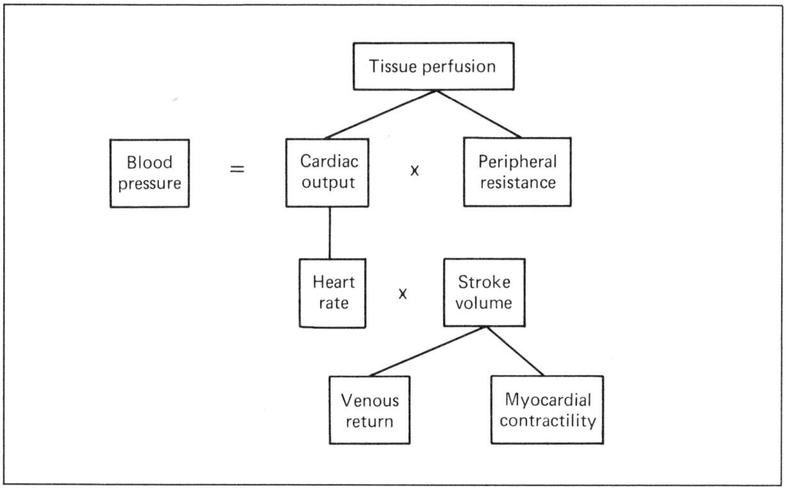

Fig. 1. There is a crucial relationship between tissue perfusion, cardiac output and peripheral resistance. Inadequate cardiac output is the major contributing factor in the hypoperfusion syndrome.

apy. While slowing the heart rate is best accomplished by alleviating such contributing factors as hypoxia, acidosis, fever and hypovolemia, digoxin administration may be helpful.

Stroke Volume

Stroke volume is determined by the adequacy of venous return and myocardial contractility. Pulse pressure roughly correlates with stroke volume and is a helpful clinical measurement for following the results of therapy. A decrease in pulse pressure reflects either a decrease in venous return or depressed myocardial contractility and usually precedes the hypoperfusion syndrome.

Venous Return

Inadequate venous return is common in hypoperfusion, and if it is not present at the beginning, it often emerges with time. The sympathetic activity associated with hypoperfusion and drugs that stimulate alpha$_1$-adrenergic receptors compound the problem since they result in a net loss of fluid to the extravascular space. Venous vasodilators, e.g. nitroglycerin and nitroprusside may aggravate this problem by expanding the capacitance bed, thus lowering ventricular filling pressure. Left ventricular filling pressure < 8–12 mm Hg may significantly decrease cardiac output because of a loss of the Starling forces. Diuretics occasionally contribute to the hypovolemia that complicates the hypoperfusion syndrome.

Myocardial Contractility

If venous return is adequate and hypoperfusion persists, depressed myocardial contractility is likely. Hypoxemia (arterial $PO_2 < 60$ mm Hg) and acidosis (arterial pH < 7.3) are factors that contribute to myocardial depression and their correction may improve ventricular function. Also these factors may interfere with the effects of the sympathomimetic agents. Beta-adrenergic blockers, quinidine-like antiarrhythmic agents and calcium channel antagonists depress cardiac function and constitute a relative contraindication in patients with hypoperfusion. If their use is necessary, the addition of digoxin may lessen this problem.

Approach to Therapy

While alleviating the etiology of the hypoperfusion syndrome is important, it is often either impossible or requires so much time that other therapeutic modalities are required. Prior to instituting pharmacologic therapy, attention should be directed to: (1) maintaining adequate venous return with appropriate fluid replacement, and (2) regulating blood gases and pH with the appropriate use of oxygen, assisted ventilation and sodium bicarbonate.

In many instances this may be adequate to reverse or prevent further progression of the syndrome. If these measures do not correct the hypoperfusion, the use of drugs should be considered.

Pharmacologic Agents

A number of drugs that have been used in treating hypoperfusion are listed in table I. While there may be circumstances in which each of these drugs can be helpful, those deserving major consideration include sympathomimetics, vasodilators and glucocorticoids.

Adrenergic Pharmacology

Effects of the adrenergic nervous system are mediated through the alpha- and beta-adrenergic receptors. While the $beta_1$ and $beta_2$ subdivisions are more commonplace, the $alpha_1$ and $alpha_2$ categories are less well known. The $alpha_1$ receptor (postsynaptic) subserves vasoconstriction,

Table I. Drugs used in treating the hypoperfusion syndrome

Sympathomimetics	Heparin
Vasodilators	Calcium gluconate
Glucocorticoids	Atropine
Glucagon	Naloxone
Insulin-glucose-potassium infusion	PGI_2

Table II. Adrenergic receptor functions

Organ	Receptor	Function	Blocked by
Heart	$beta_1$	rate, contractility, AV conduction	beta blockers
Blood vessels	$beta_2$	arterial dilatation	beta blockers
	$alpha_1$	arterial and venous constriction	alpha blockers (phentolamine, phenoxybenzamine, chlorpromazine, prazosin)
	$alpha_2$	inhibits NE release	blocked by above except prazosin; stimulated by clonidine
Bronchioles	$beta_2$	dilatation	beta blockers
Other			
Renin	$beta_2$	secretion	beta blockers
Insulin	$alpha_1$	secretion	alpha blockers
	$beta_2$	secretion	beta blockers
Liver	$beta_2$	glycogenolysis and gluconeogenesis	beta blockers
Fat cells	$beta_1$	lipolysis	beta blockers

resides in the effector cell and represents the functions historically associated with alpha-adrenergic activity. The $alpha_2$ receptor (presynaptic) mediates a negative feedback on norepinephrine release and resides on the sympathetic nerve ending of both the central and peripheral nervous system. The pertinent aspects of adrenergic receptor function are listed in table II.

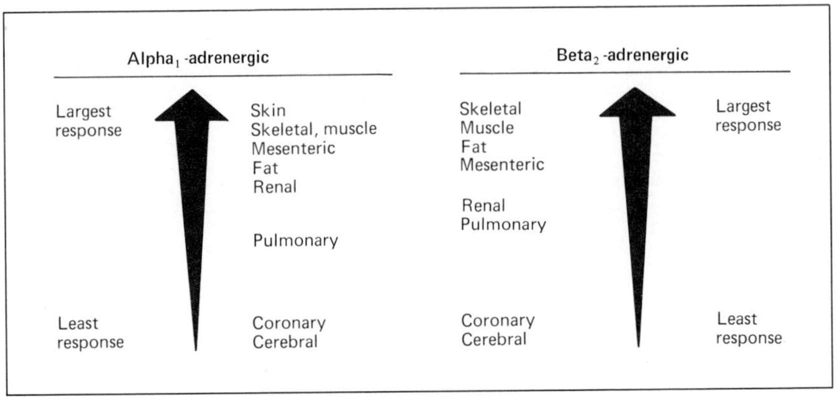

Fig. 2. A hierarchy of adrenergic responsiveness exists among various organs. The higher the sensitivity, the larger the responsiveness.

Also, a hierarchy exists among the various vascular beds, and for a given degree of sympathetic stimulation, there is a variable response; probably related to receptor density as shown in figure 2. Thus, drugs that stimulate these receptors will have a more pronounced effect on the structures that possess increased sensitivity.

One more factor seems particularly relevant concerning adrenergic pharmacology. For any given degree of alpha$_1$-adrenergic stimulation, the postcapillary sphincters respond more than the precapillary sphincters. The result of this is an increase in hydrostatic pressure and a net loss of fluid to the extravascular space. This decreases venous return which may lead to inadequate cardiac output. The resulting increase in interstitial fluid can further interfere with organ and cellular function. Increasing colloid osmotic pressure has an opposite effect.

Sympathomimetic Drugs

The sympathomimetic drugs have either inotropic, pressor or mixed activity. The pharmacologic and hemodynamic effects of these drugs are shown in table III.

The decision when to use a sympathomimetic and which one is not always clear. However, if the hypoperfusion has not been corrected by providing adequate venous return and maintaining normal arterial gases and pH, then a sympathomimetic agent should be considered. While dopamine is often considered the agent of choice in most circumstances, dobutamine

Table III. Drugs used in shock [from ref. 7, with permission]

	Sites of action: heart		Sites of action: blood vessels		Hemodynamic response			
	contractility (inotropic) $beta_1$	SA node rate (chronotropic)[1] $beta_1$	vasoconstriction alpha	vasodilatation $beta_2$	renal perfusion	cardiac output	total peripheral resistance	blood pressure
Inotropic								
Isoproterenol	+++	+++	0	+++	↑ or ↓	↑	↓	↑[2] ↓[3]
Dobutamine	+++	0 to +	0 to +	0 to +	↑	↑	↓	0 to ↑
Dopamine	+++	+	0 to +++[4]	0[5]	↑[4] or ↓	↑	↓[4] or ↑	0 to ↑
Epinephrine	+++	+++	+++	++	↓	↑	↓	↑[2] ↓[3]
Mixed								
Norepinephrine	++	++[1]	+++	0	↓	↑ or ↓	↑	↑
Ephedrine	++	++[1]	+	0 to +	↓	↑	↑ or ↓	↑
Mephentermine	+	+	0 to +	++	↑ or ↓	↑	0 to ↑	↑
Pressors								
Metaraminol	0 to +	0 to +[1]	++	+	↓	↑ or ↓	↑	↑
Methoxamine	0	0[1]	+++	0	↓	0 or ↓	↑	↑
Phenylephrine	0	0[1]	+++	0	↓	↓	↑	↑

+++ = pronounced effect; ++ = moderate effect; + = slight effect; 0 = no effect; ↑ = increase; ↓ = decrease.

1 Decreased heart rate may result from reflex mechanisms.

2 Systolic effect.

3 Diastolic effect.

4 Effects are dose dependent.

5 Dilates renal and splanchnic beds via dopaminergic effect at doses < 10–12 μg/kg/min.

is preferred if there is a cardiogenic component with left ventricular filling pressure. If bradycardia is thought to be a contributing factor, isoproterenol might be preferred. Norepinephrine is advisable in the presence of a neurogenic component or if arterial pressure is critically low (< 60 mm Hg).

It is important to have specific treatment objectives in mind when using a sympathomimetic agent (table IV). If systolic blood pressure is

Table IV. General treatment objectives

Sensorium	oriented
Blood pressure	systolic at least 90 mm Hg
Urine output	larger than 40 ml/h
Central venous pressure	12–15 cm H_2O
Pulmonary capillary wedge pressure	12–18 mm Hg
Skin	warm, no cyanosis
Blood gases	pH 7.35–7.5
	PCO_2 30–35 mm Hg
	PCO_2 80–100 mm Hg
Hemoglobin	12–14 g%

increased to 100 mm Hg and tissue perfusion does not improve, the patient has probably not been helped. A further increase in blood pressure would only be beneficial if it improved perfusion. At this point, administering more intravenous fluid should be considered or the addition of a vasodilator may be indicated to reduce ventricular afterload and filling pressure.

Precaution with the use of sympathomimetics is indicated under certain circumstances. Atrial fibrillation with a rapid ventricular response poses a special situation when isoproterenol, dopamine and dobutamine are used. These compounds facilitate atrioventricular conduction and may result in a pronounced tachycardia. Therefore, a digitalis preparation should be administered prior to the sympathomimetic agent. In general, these compounds should be avoided in patients with idiopathic hypertrophic subaortic stenosis. Also, pressor effects of these drugs may be enhanced in patients receiving tricyclic antidepressants or monoamine oxidase inhibitor agents.

Norepinephrine

The predominant effect of norepinephrine is a direct $alpha_1$-adrenergic mediated vasoconstriction, while the effect of exogenous norepinephrine on $alpha_2$ receptors is inconsequential. The $beta_1$-adrenergic effect on myocardial contractility is increased to a greater degree than heart rate. Norepinephrine may be of value in severe hypotension if there is an inadequate response to fluids, proper ventilation and dopamine or dobutamine. The treatment objectives with norepinephrine are similar to those of other sympathomimetic agents. If systolic pressure is increased to 100 mm Hg and hypoperfusion improves, the effect was beneficial; if perfusion is not improved, other therapeutic modalities should be considered.

Isoproterenol

The cardiac ($beta_1$) and vasodilator ($beta_2$) effects of isoproterenol are equivalent. However, as shown in figure 2, there are disparate responses among various vascular beds. While the positive inotropic effect of isoproterenol may be desirable, the rather pronounced increase in heart rate may be arrhythmogenic and further increase myocardial O_2 consumption. Bradycardia, on the other hand, could be a contributing factor to the hypoperfusion and here isoproterenol might be beneficial. However, there are very few instances when isoproterenol is indicated.

Dopamine

Dopamine acts both directly by stimulation of the receptor and indirectly by release of norepinephrine from sympathetic nerve endings. It exerts the following effects: (1) it is a $beta_1$-adrenergic agonist (not $beta_2$) that increases contractility more than heart rate; (2) there is a dopaminergic (nonbeta-adrenergic) vasodilation of the renal and splanchnic vascular beds; (3) there is an $alpha_1$-adrenergic vasoconstriction at higher doses.

Dopamine is used in hypoperfusion when a positive inotropic effect and an increase in renal blood flow is not achieved by expanding the intravascular volume and correcting the blood gases. Dopamine is administered by continuous intravenous infusion at an initial dose of 2–5 μg/kg/min (the dose should be titrated against the desired effects). At higher doses ($>$ 12 μg/kg/min) $alpha_1$-adrenergic vasoconstrictive components begin to predominate, resulting in a reduction of the enhanced renal and splanchnic blood flow and possibly an elevation of left ventricular filling pressure. At doses larger than 30 μg/kg/min, the effects are comparable to norepinephrine. If a patient has a high degree of vasoconstriction prior to the initiation of dopamine, it is doubtful that the dopaminergic effect will be manifest. In some patients who otherwise would require a large dose of dopamine it is helpful to hold the infusion rate at approximately 5–10 μg/kg/min, to add dobutamine and increase it to the desired endpoint.

Dobutamine

Dobutamine acts directly on the $beta_1$-adrenergic receptors in the heart, resulting in an inotropic effect with minimal chronotropic activity. In patients with congestive heart failure, the increase in contractility has been associated with a reduction in left ventricular filling pressure. This contrasts with the effects of dopamine which may increase left ventricular filling pressure. Dobutamine also has weak $alpha_1$- and $beta_2$-adrenergic effects that are mutually antagonistic and of seemingly little clinical importance.

The usual dose of dobutamine varies from 2 to 15 μg/kg/min given by intravenous infusion. Its major use is to augment myocardial contractility and cardiac output in patients with hypoperfusion. It is also used in combination with a low dose of dopamine as noted above.

Vasodilator Therapy

Extensive experience exists regarding the use of vasodilators in patients with impaired cardiac function. Previously, chlorpromazine, phentolamine or phenoxybenzamine were used. Today, nitroprusside and nitroglycerin are the major vasodilators, and table V lists their cardiovascular effects. Because the effects of these drugs can be dramatic and excessive amounts will produce opposite hemodynamic effects, it is strongly recommended that a Swan-Ganz catheter be used to monitor left ventricular filling pressure, cardiac output and peripheral vascular resistance.

Both nitroprusside and nitroglycerin dilate the venous capacitance bed to a greater degree than the arterial tree; however, nitroglycerin has a relatively larger venous component than nitroprusside, and nitroprusside has a relatively larger arterial component than nitroglycerin. Thus, if the left ventricular filling pressure is thought to predominate the impaired hemodynamics, nitroglycerin is preferred. If afterload is thought to predominate, nitroprusside is preferred.

Table V. Cardiovascular effect of nitroprusside and nitroglycerin

Action	Response	Implications
Venous		
Dilation	↓ central venous pressure (CVP) or wedge pressure	↓ pulmonary congestion ↓ myocardial O_2 consumption
Excessive dilation	↓↓ CVP or wedge pressure (PCW < 8 mm Hg)	↓ cardiac output
Arterial		
Dilation	↓ vascular resistance (± blood pressure)	↓ afterload ↑ cardiac output
Excessive dilation	↓↓ blood pressure	↓ coronary flow

Nitroprusside

Nitroprusside has an immediate onset of action, and must be administered by continuous intravenous infusion because of its brief duration of action. It is converted to cyanomethemoglobin and free cyanide which is converted to thiocyanate in the liver. Thiocyanate is eliminated by the kidneys and has a half-life of approximately 4 days in patients with normal renal function. Approved indications for use of nitroprusside are hypertensive emergencies and controlled hypotension during surgical procedures. In addition, it has been used 'investigationally' to treat lactic acidosis due to impaired peripheral perfusion, and in combination with dopamine or norepinephrine to counteract their vasoconstrictive effects.

An average starting intravenous infusion rate is 1 μg/kg/min. This may be increased every 5–10 min as necessary. In patients with impaired renal function the infusion rate should not exceed 10 μg/kg/min. If obvious tolerance develops, cyanide toxicity should be suspected. The earliest and most reliable evidence of cyanide toxicity is metabolic acidosis. Amyl nitrite inhalation, intravenous sodium thiosulfate or hydroxocobalamin may be used to treat cyanide toxicity. Also, thiocyanate levels may accumulate and cause toxicity with infusions lasting several days and especially in patients with impaired renal function. Symptoms of thiocyanate toxicity, e.g. nausea, muscle spasms, tinnitus, blurred vision, delirium, hyperreflexia and convulsions, emerge at plasma levels around 5–10 μg/ml. Thiocyanate also inhibits the uptake and binding of iodine, therefore it should be used with caution in patients with hypothyroidism.

Nitroglycerin

Intravenous nitroglycerin is used in unstable angina, congestive heart failure associated with acute myocardial infarction, production of controlled hypotension during surgical procedures and control of blood pressure in perioperative hypertension. It has an immediate onset of action but because of a transient duration, intravenous infusion is necessary to maintain drug effect.

The average starting infusion rate is 5–10 μg/min. The rate is increased as necessary every 3–5 min by 5–10 μg/min increments. Final infusion rates usually range from 35 to 60 μg/min. Some physicians like to administer a 50- to 200-μg loading dose prior to the infusion. The dose of nitroglycerin should be titrated against blood pressure, presence of angina or ischemic ECG changes. Further increases in dose should not be made if headache or a 20 mm Hg drop in blood pressure develops.

Some patients with normal or low left ventricular filling pressures may be hypersensitive to nitroglycerin and respond to doses as small as 5 μg/min. These patients require especially careful titration and monitoring.

Glucocorticoids

Increased secretion of adrenocortical hormones is a normal physiologic response to the hypoperfusion syndrome. If a patient is responding poorly to therapy, a relative or true adrenal insufficiency should be considered, and 200 mg hydrocortisone administered intravenously. If the response is favorable, 100 mg should be given every 6 h.

Controversy remains regarding the efficacy of large doses of glucocorticoids in the treatment of hypoperfusion syndromes. Experimentally, improved cell and membrane permeability, stabilization of lysosomes, increased tissue oxygen delivery, improved cardiovascular and cell metabolism have been observed. While this is an impressive list of effects, questions remain whether these can be achieved in patients who are not pretreated with pharmacologic doses of glucocorticoids.

In patients, it has been difficult to demonstrate unequivocal efficacy. This may be partially due to the great difficulty in conducting controlled studies in patients who are critically ill. However, there is some evidence that glucocorticoids are efficacious in patients with septic shock. If they are to be efficacious in other types of hypoperfusion, they must be administered early before the syndrome has become irreversible. The two drugs that are generally used are dexamethasone 3–6 mg/kg, or methylprednisolone 30 mg/kg. These doses may be repeated every 8–12 h for 2 days. Continued efficacy beyond that period is doubtful, and there is little risk of toxicity when therapy is of a short duration.

Naloxone

Beta-endorphin is one of several brain peptides with narcotic-like activity that is released in response to stress. Endorphins have been implicated in shock and may be responsible for the vasodilation occasionally seen in the early phase of septic shock. The narcotic antagonist naloxone has been administered to patients with hypoperfusion with an occasional encouraging response. Doses of 0.4 mg have produced transient reversal of hypotension and the duration of action has been approximately 1 h. An intravenous infusion of 0.03 μg/kg/min has been used successfully after a 0.4 mg intravenous dose. While this therapy is very experimental, it is fortunately quite safe and without overt toxicity.

Suggested Reading

1 Cohn, J.N.; Tristani, E., et al.: Studies in clinical shock and hypotension. Clin. Invest. *48:* 2008–2018 (1969).

2 Goldberg, I.: Dopamine – clinical uses of an endogenous catecholamine. New Engl. J. Med. *291:* 707–710 (1974).

3 Berk, J.L.: Monitoring the patient in shock. Surg. Clins N. Am. *55:* 713 (1975).

4 Moser, K.M.; Spragg, R.G.: Use of the balloon-tipped pulmonary artery catheter in pulmonary disease. Ann. intern. Med. *98:* 53–58 (1983).

5 Higgins, T.L.; Sivak, E.D.; O'Neil, D.M.; Graves, J.W.; Foutch, D.G.: Reversal of hypotension by continuous naloxone infusion in a ventilator-dependent patient. Ann. intern. Med. *98:* 47–49 (1983).

6 Hill, N.S.; Antman, E.M.; Green, L.H.; Alpert, J.S.: Intravenous nitroglycerin: a review of pharmacology, indications, therapeutic effects and complications. Chest *79:* 69–76 (1981).

7 Kostrup, E.K., et al.: Facts and comparisons (a supplemental loose leaf references service), St. Louis, Mo.

8 Sonnenblick, E.H.; Frishman, W.H., et al.: Drug therapy: dobutamine: a new synthetic cardioactive sympathetic amine. New Engl. J. Med. *300:* 17–24 (1979).

9 Flaherty, J.T.; Magee, P.A.; Gardner, T.L.; Potter, A.; MacAllister, N.P.: Comparison of intravenous nitroglycerin and sodium nitroprusside for treatment of acute hypertension developing after coronary artery bypass surgery. Circulation *65:* 1072–1077 (1982).

Thomas L. Whitsett, MD, Professor of Medicine, V.A. Hospital,
921 NE 13th Street, Oklahoma City, OK 73104 (USA)

Prog. crit. Care Med., vol. 2, pp. 118–132 (Karger, Basel 1985)

Blood and Blood Substitutes

E.R. Eichner

University of Oklahoma Health Sciences Center, Oklahoma City, Okla., USA

Overview

The transfusion of blood ranks as a therapeutic milestone in the history of medicine. The first transfusion of sheep blood to humans in 1667 was followed by a gap of 150 years until human blood began to be used sporadically for transfusion to man. In recent decades, however, transfusional therapy has evolved rapidly. More than 10 million blood transfusions are now given yearly in the United States, and the modern blood bank can dispense approximately 20 components of blood. The now widely used anticoagulant-preservative citrate-phosphate-dextrose-adenine allows refrigerated storage of blood for 35 days, and the new variant, with more dextrose and twice as much adenine, promises possible usage of blood stored up to 42–49 days [1]. Blood can be stored frozen for at least 10 years, and frozen blood has found a defined, albeit narrow, clinical role. Modern technology has made blood transfusion generally safe, although, as will be detailed below, fatal hemolytic reactions still occur in the operating room and the intensive care unit. Subclinical infectious hepatitis occurs in 10% of transfusion recipients, and there is great national concern today that our 'newest epidemic', acquired immunodeficiency syndrome, can be spread by blood and blood products [2]. An eloquent history of blood transfusion by *Diamond* [3] is recommended for general reading.

As recent practical reviews have indicated, modern transfusional therapy is component therapy [4, 5]. Most patients need only certain components of blood, and we can make better community use of whole blood by separating it into its components. This chapter will not deal with blood bank procedures for producing the components and will consider only those components most likely to be needed in the intensive care unit. The focus will be on the red blood cell and its possible substitutes with platelet transfusions as an additional consideration. Granulocyte transfusions will be omitted because guidelines for their use are still evolving and apply more to oncology units than to intensive care units. The selection of intravenous fluids for resuscitation, covered in another chapter, will be alluded to as a frame of reference.

Indications and Contraindications

General

Transfusion is supportive, not specific, therapy. In general, if transfusions in an anemic patient can be avoided, they should be avoided; if they are necessary, the fewer given, the better. Most hematologists agree that blood transfusions are overused [4, 5]. Physicians, perhaps, tend to underestimate the ability of the body to compensate for anemia and to underestimate the hazards of transfusion, probably because immediate, serious reactions are now rare and the major infectious complication, hepatitis, is delayed and usually subclinical. One gets the impression that the decision to transfuse is made rather easily, while the decision, for example, to give a drug that causes hepatitis in 10% of the recipients is given more thought.

Specific

The only valid indications for transfusion of blood or blood components are: to restore critical deficits in blood volume, to improve the oxygen-carrying capacity by correcting severe anemia, and to minimize bleeding from coagulation disorders. Transfusions of blood are *not* indicated to provide a tonic, to speed convalescence after an operation, to accelerate wound healing, or to treat hypoalbuminemia.

Single-unit transfusions are often unnecessary. The hazards of transfusion are thought to outweigh the putative benefits of single-unit transfusions in almost all circumstances. Yet, there are rare exceptions. Examples among medical patients include the elderly patient with severe pernicious anemia who needs only one unit of packed red cells to reverse congestive heart failure before the vitamin B_{12} begins to work, and the patient with severe, autoimmune hemolytic anemia who needs one unit per day to survive until specific therapy begins to work [6]. Another example might be the anemic patient in the unit with severe respiratory failure on near-maximal respiratory support with a PO_2 of 40 mm Hg and a hemoglobin of 8 g/dl. A single-unit transfusion here might increase oxygen transport enough to avoid mechanical ventilation, although the in vivo consequence of the increased blood viscosity after transfusion is an imponderable. A rather complex nomogram has recently been offered to facilitate decisions regarding the need for blood transfusions in patients with impaired oxygen delivery [7]. While there may also be rare exceptions among surgical patients, single-unit transfusions are generally to be discouraged, and are especially questionable when the estimated blood loss at surgery is only 500 ml or the preoperative hemoglobin is 9.5 g/dl and a single unit is given to bring the hemoglobin ove the 'magic line' of 10 g/dl for an operation.

Preoperative transfusion is overused. A recent review offers a balanced perspective of the need for preoperative transfusion [8]. It is pointed out that the customary requirement for a hemoglobin of 10 g/dl is unduly rigid, since consideration of the cardiac output and the position of the oxygen dissociation curve should go into the equation for each patient. For certain young persons with chronic anemia, normal blood volume, good cardiac output, and normal circulation, a hemoglobin of 8 g/dl can be acceptable for an operation. In contrast, a patient with previous myocardial infarction, cerebral ischemia, existing coronary disease or lung disease may require a hemoglobin over 10 g/dl for a safe operation. A normal blood volume is more important than a normal hemoglobin concentration, and clinical judgement must balance the risk of transfusion against the risk of anemia.

Practical Considerations

Whole Blood

The only valid indication for whole blood is exsanguinating hemorrhage. While most authorities agree whole blood remains the treatment of choice here [4, 5], component therapy, that is, packed red cells with crystalloids and/or colloids can be used. Rapid flow of packed cells can be achieved by adding 100 ml of normal saline solution to the unit. Acute blood loss of less than 40% of blood volume can in fact be adequately treated with infusions of crystalloid alone, provided the infusion volume is 3–4 times the volume lost [5]. Certainly, in moderate to massive blood loss, as in elective aortic reconstruction surgery, component therapy is as efficacious as whole blood therapy [9]. In an emergency, un-cross-matched blood can be given; in one university hospital, 49 transfusions of un-cross-matched, group-specific (ABO and Rh) blood were given in 1 year without adverse effects. There is a potential danger, however, and when possible one should allow the extra 45 min for a cross-match [10].

The first goal in treating hemorrhagic shock is to restore blood volume. The crystalloid versus colloid controversy will be avoided here, except to say that giving albumin along with packed red cells is a poor idea. It is an expensive way to reconstitute whole blood, and one group was recently able to reduce albumin use 90% in their hospital by suggesting guidelines restricting its use for hemorrhage only in the first 2 h of bona fide shock, and then only after at least 1 liter of crystalloid solution had been given [11]. Albumin is probably preferable to plasma protein fraction for shock, because rapid infusion of some lots of plasma protein fraction has caused hypotension when Hageman-factor fragments generated bradykinin in the recipient. This problem may be corrected in current lots. This paradoxical hypotension could cause confusion in the treatment of hemorrhagic shock in the operating room or the intensive care unit [12]. The use of fresh frozen plasma plus packed red cells increases the risk of hepatitis compared to whole blood alone. Hydroxyethyl starch (a 6% solution in normal saline) is now commercially available and increasingly being used for colloidal therapy of hemorrhagic shock. Clinical results to date suggest it is hemodynamically comparable to albumin, does not adversely affect lung function, has few side effects, and is therefore a safe, inexpensive alternative to albumin as a plasma expander [13–15]. However, it may complicate cross-matching when large volumes are given.

Packed Red Blood Cells

A patient with chronic anemia should receive packed red cells, not whole blood, and should be transfused slowly. The patient's total blood volume is normal because of a compensatory increase in plasma volume, and a hemoglobin deficit that took months to occur need not be corrected in hours. As compared with whole blood, packed red cells reduce the hazard of circulatory overload, the severity of leukoagglutinin reactions and reactions to food or drug allergens, and the metabolic load of potassium, hydrogen, and ammonia. During the first 30 min of the transfusion, a slow drip (about 5 ml/min) should be used, and the transfusion should be stopped immediately at the first sign of an adverse reaction. Thereafter, unless there is a high risk of circulatory overload, the rate should be increased to 200–400 ml/h in adults. Elderly patients with severe anemia should be transfused very slowly throughout, possibly with diuretics, and watched very carefully for a rise in central venous pressure and clinical signs of incipient heart failure.

Frozen Blood

Frozen red cells have not found a large clinical role. Largely free of plasma, leukocytes, and platelets, they were considered theoretically hepatitis-free and nonsensitizing. Several early studies indeed suggested frozen cells were less likely to transmit hepatitis, but recently it has been shown they can transmit hepatitis B infection to chimpanzees [16]. A large clinical study has suggested they may *not* reduce the incidence of posttransfusion hepatitis in man [17]. Frozen cells still contain some viable lymphocytes that could cause graft-versus-host reaction in a susceptible recipient, and there are now few advantages for freezing of red cells [5]. They are still advocated when transfusion is required in a prospective recipient of a bone marrow transplant, but they are no longer given to patients awaiting renal transplants. Multiple random-donor transfusions aid engraftment of cadaveric renal transplants [18], and the best evidence to date suggests that this 'transplant benefit' is *not* achieved by transfusions of frozen red cells, but only by whole blood or packed red cells. Current policy now favors the pretransplant transfusion of 2–5 units given separately. The optimal interval between the transfusions and the transplantation is uncertain, and the mechanisms of the protection are unknown, but seem to involve both humoral and cell-mediated protection [19]. Given these drawbacks of frozen blood, the only remaining real advantage of freezing blood is to preserve selected units for provision of red cells to persons with rare blood types and for 'autotransfusion' to persons with multiple red cell alloantibodies.

Fresh Blood

There is no reason to insist on 'fresh whole blood' for massive hemorrhage, because blood is 'fresh' in the clinically important respects for at least 1 week. The red cells survive and circulate normally, and do not leak significant amounts of potassium. Only three clotting factors deteriorate in storage, and two of them, platelets and factor VIII, are more satisfactorily supplied as concentrates. The third, factor V, is only moderately labile on storage, and is still sufficient (over 50% of normal) in 1-week-old blood.

Physicians are concerned about the content of 2,3-diphosphoglycerate (DPG) in stored blood, because DPG modulates the release of oxygen from the red cell. DPG declines during storage, and the transfusion of massive amounts of blood depleted of DPG shifts the oxygen dissociation curve to the left and thereby inhibits delivery of oxygen to the tissues. Animal models, such as simulated carotid artery stenosis in the isolated canine brain, suggest that a left-shifted oxygen dissociation curve from massive amounts of DPG-depleted blood can cause rapid deterioration in cerebral oxygen consumption and in electroencephalogram patterns [20]. The clinical implications of these models, however, are not clear. There are many bodily adaptations that increase tissue oxygen delivery and largely offset any putative ill effects from low DPG. These include increased blood flow, increased oxygenation of arterial blood, a shift of the oxygen dissociation curve back to the right because of local acidosis, and microcirculatory and tissue adaptations to decrease the distance for oxygen diffusion and increase the extraction of oxygen from the blood.

Equally important, advances in storage have improved retention of DPG in bank blood. In modern anticoagulant-preservatives, DPG declines slowly, so blood 1 week or less in age is sufficient in DPG for all patients. Even if blood 2–3 weeks old is used (DPG 50% at 2 weeks and 30% or less at 3 weeks), there should be few clinical states in which the theoretical tissue hypoxia would not be immediately offset by the compensatory mechanisms discussed above. In addition, red cell DPG is rapidly regenerated in vivo; even when DPG is almost totally depleted, levels are 50% of normal in 4 h and 100% of normal in 24 h after transfusion. The physician may nonetheless be concerned about an occasional patient in whom even moderate reduction in DPG would bring theoretical risks; examples might include patients with fixed stenotic lesions of the carotid or coronary arteries; patients in shock with congestive heart failure and low, fixed cardiac output, and patients with low cardiac output and perfusion pressure that accompany cardiopulmonary resuscitation following arrest. For such patients, the physician needs to ascertain that all blood transfused is less than 1 week old.

Current State of Research on Blood Substitutes

Research on two proposed blood substitutes, hemoglobin solutions and perfluorochemicals, has reached the stage of pilot clinical trials in man. The term 'artificial blood' should not be used, since it gives potential blood donors the impression they are no longer needed, and since the substitutes are not interchangeable with real blood. The commercially available perfluorochemical Fluosol-DA, for example, which must be stored frozen and given with inspired oxygen, does only the work of hemoglobin, and its effects last only 3 days. Each substitute will probably find a different clinical role. Hemoglobin solutions, for example, could be used for field treatment of hemorrhagic shock in war or other catastrophes. Perfluorochemicals would seem suited for specific, hospital-based settings, such as treatment of hemorrhagic shock in patients who refuse blood or for whom no compatible blood can be found, for sickle cell crisis and carbon monoxide poisoning, and, with much more research, perhaps for early therapy of acute coronary or cerebral insufficiency [21, 22].

Hemoglobin Solutions

A recent clinical report of a patient with fulminant intravascular hemolysis from *Clostridium perfringens* septicemia, who maintained normal blood pressure, tissue oxygenation, and mentation, and survived longer than 4 h with a hematocrit value of 0% (and a plasma free hemoglobin of 5 g/dl) shows the potential of free hemoglobin for the maintenance of both intravascular volume and normal tissue oxygen delivery [23]. Purified hemoglobin solutions are not toxic to the kidneys, and have been given to volunteers with good results and with only mild and reversible diminutions in renal function [24], due in part to the dehydration caused by hemoglobin diuresis [25]. The two main drawbacks to hemoglobin solutions are the short half-life in circulation, about 3–4 h, because of rapid renal excretion and clearance by the reticuloendothelial system and the sharply compromised tissue offloading of oxygen, because of the high oxygen affinity of free hemoglobin, due to lack of DPG present in red cells [26, 27]. Current research is attemting to counter these problems by polymerization and stabilization of the hemoglobin tetramer. Another option would be to microencapsulate stroma-free hemoglobin in a cell-membrane substitute such as a 'neohemocyte' or in a capsule of cholesterol and lecithin [22]. Many different hemoglobin solutions are being researched, and the Army hopes to choose the two most promising for a field trial in 1989.

Perfluorochemicals

Oxygen is highly soluble in liquid perfluorochemicals – hydrocarbons or other organic chemicals in which all hydrogen atoms are replaced by fluorine atoms. Perfluorochemicals are water-insoluble and immiscible with blood, and must be emulsified with surfactants. Blood normally carries oxygen in two ways – bound to hemoglobin and dissolved in plasma. When perfluorochemicals are added to the blood, oxygen is also transported in a third way – dissolved in the perfluorochemical. Because perfluorochemicals carry oxygen only by direct solubility, a clinically significant rise in arterial oxygen content occurs only if the Pa_{O_2} is elevated by having the patient breathe 100% oxygen. At ambient oxygen tensions, then, Fluosol-DA, the commercially available perfluorochemical, acts only as a volume expander, whereas at tensions above 300 Torr it contributes substantially to the oxygen delivery system [28].

Fluosol-DA has been used extensively in Japan, but has been given to only 15 patients in the United States, including 1 patient who was reported twice [28, 29]. The most recent patients have been Jehovah's Witnesses with severe hemorrhagic anemia needing surgery. In these patients, Fluosol-DA has been generally well-tolerated, and has accounted for about 25% of their oxygen consumption [28]. Limitations include a short plasma half-life of 11 h, and the need to use a tight oxygen mask with 100% oxygen, to achieve a paO_2 over 300 Torr, which excludes its use in adult respiratory distress syndrome. Fluosol-DA may also activate complement and impair platelet function [30, 31]. Much more clinical research is needed before this product can be used widely. Implications that perfluorochemicals may reduce myocardial ischemic damage after coronary occlusion or acute cerebral ischemia during stroke have not gone beyond early animal models, and in the stroke model, Fluosol-DA was no more 'protective' than mannitol [32, 33].

The impression from the above clinical reports is that most of the Jehova's Witnesses receiving Fluosol-DA would have done equally well with conventional crystalloid therapy of hemorrhagic anemia, or perhaps, now that it is available, with hydroxyethyl starch therapy [34]. We have successfully treated major gastrointestinal hemorrhage with crystalloids alone in 3 such patients whose hemoglobin concentrations reached nadirs of 3–4 g/dl. *Ott and Cooley* [35] have reported a 20-year experience with major cardiovascular operations in a consecutive series of 542 Jehovah's Witnesses who received only crystalloids. Overall mortality (9.4%) was acceptably low, and, while postoperative anemia contributed to 12 deaths, only 3 deaths were related directly to loss of blood. Even major cardiac operations, then, can be performed safely without blood or colloid transfusion. Physicians face a special challenge in treating Jehovah's Witnesses and might gain a better understanding of this problem from a recent article pleading for treatment of the 'whole person' [36].

Complications

Massive Transfusion

The main complications of massive transfusion are abnormal hemostasis and the accumulation of microaggregates in the lungs. These will be discussed below. Citrate intoxication is rare in adults, but when transfusion is massive and rapid, the electrocardiogram should be monitored for signs of hypocalcemia, and 10 ml of 10% calcium gluconate should be given after the first 2,000 ml and after every 1,000 ml therafter. Rapid infusion of large amounts of cold blood, especially through a subclavian catheter, carries a risk of cardiac arrhythmia, and should be avoided by warming the blood during transfusion. Routine prophylactic bicarbonate therapy with massive transfusion is not necessary, and there is little danger of hyperkalemia from leakage of potassium from transfused red cells.

The major cause of abnormal bleeding after massive transfusion is thrombocytopenia. Platelets rapidly die in stored blood, and when a patient receives more than 15 units of blood (1.5 times blood volume) in less than 24 h, the platelet count falls in proportion to the amount of blood given (dilutional or washout thrombocytopenia). Factor V and VIII levels are usually normal in such patients, but individual patients may have low factor VIII levels, which may reflect low-grade disseminated intravascular coagulation rather than dilution by stored blood [37].

When a patient undergoes a massive transfusion, the platelet count should be followed and the physician should be alert for generalized oozing. If abnormal bleeding begins, or if the platelet count drops below 100,000/μl, the patient should receive platelet concentrates (if unavailable, fresh blood) as necessary to keep the platelet count above 100,000/μl. Giving platelets alone usually stops the diffuse microvascular bleeding. An occasional massively transfused patient will also need factor VIII, preferably as cryoprecipitate or a concentrate (if unavailable, fresh frozen plasma).

Controversy continues on the role of microaggregates of degenerating leukocytes and platelets in the genesis of 'shock lung', and on the proper use of microfilters (20 to 40-μm pores) compared to conventional blood filters (170-μm pores). Some studies suggest microfilters are clinically important; others suggest they are not. A recent study with homologous blood suggested subtle gas exchange alterations following blood transfusion are primarily reflected by increased dead-space ventilation secondary to vasoconstriction and occlusion of the pulmonary microvasculature with microaggregates larger than 90 μm in diameter [38]. Another study of patients with baseline pulmonary function abnormalities after elective coronary bypass showed no significant differences in posttransfusion tests of cardiopulmonary function in 25 patients who received blood through a 20-μm filter versus 25 who received blood through a 170-μm filter. It was concluded that microfilters were unnecessary for transfusions of 6–7 units [39]. A recent symposium [40] reviewed this controversy and offered practical guidelines: patients with severe lung disease should receive blood only through microfilters; patients without lung disease do not need microfilters until 2–5 units of blood (at the least) have been given; microfilters are contraindicated with fresh blood because they retain viable platelets, and in patients with massive bleeding, it is essential that microfilters do not hamper the adequate rate of transfusion.

Hemolytic and Other Transfusion Reactions

Hemolytic transfusion reactions are becoming increasingly rare (no more than 1 for every 6,000 units transfused). They have a female preponderance, are more likely to occur in patients with type O blood, and are more likely to be delayed than immediate [41]. Deaths from transfusion accidents, however, still occur, at the rate of 1 per million transfusions. All of 22 preventable primary fatalities in 1976–1978 were due to clerical errors resulting in a mismatch of ABO groups. 17 of these deaths were from a transfusion given to the wrong patient, usually in a surgical or intensive care facility, when established identification procedures were not followed because of human error [42].

There have been no recent changes in diagnosis or therapy of acute hemolytic transfusion reaction [43]. Signs and symptoms may include fever, chills, headaches, flushing, hot feeling in vein receiving blood, severe pain in chest, low back, and legs, dyspnea, wheezing, nausea, vomiting, hypotension, and oozing at surgery. If any adverse signs occur, the transfusion must be stopped, the line kept open with saline, and a sample of clotted blood from the patient, along with the blood bag, must be sent to the blood bank, where the serum is scanned for hemoglobin (pink, red, or brown) and a Coombs test is done. If hemoglobinemia is present and the direct Coombs test is positive, therapy consists of mannitol and fluids to maintain circulatory stability and urine output. One may also give furosemide to improve renal cortical blood flow and augment the diuresis. Nonimmune causes of intravascular hemolysis that could mimic a transfusion reaction are: thermal damage to the transfused cells; infusion of blood through a hypotonic solution such as dextrose and water; traumatic hemolysis from a heart valve; *Clostridium welchii* septicemia; brown recluse spider bite, and drug-induced or G-6-PD-deficient hemolysis [44]. The fever, chills, and brown serum seen in a reaction to intravenous iron dextran therapy can masquerade as an acute hemolytic transfusion reaction [45].

There is no way to predict or prevent delayed hemolytic transfusion reactions caused by anamnestic production of an alloantibody that destroys all the transfused cells 2–14 days after transfusion. Symptoms are low-grade and nonspecific, and misdiagnoses (assumed occult bleeding, sickle cell crisis, autoimmune hemolytic anemia) are common. Fortunately, major renal failure is uncommon and death rare (46–49].

Space does not permit consideration of many of the minor or rare transfusion reactions. Fever occurs with about 1% of transfusions, and 90% of the time does not signify hemolysis, but rather a leukoagglutinin reaction between transfused granulocytes and/or lymphocytes and an antibody in the recipient. Only about 15% of such patients will have a second febrile response; if so, they can thereafter be transfused with leukocyte-poor red cells, most easily obtained by inverted centrifugation technique [50]. The pulmonary leukoagglutinin reaction, the most severe form of the febrile complication, usually follows whole blood transfusion and can cause major respiratory distress. It can be mistaken for pulmonary edema from overtransfusion. The chest roentgenogram shows bilateral, multinodular, mainly perihilar infiltrates without cardiomegaly or pulmonary congestion (noncardiac pulmonary edema). This complication requires only nasal oxygen and supportive therapy; it abates within hours and the roentgenogram clears in 2–4 days [51–53].

Transmission of Infectious Disease

Infections transmitted by blood include: malaria, syphilis, brucellosis, babesiosis, toxoplasmosis, Rocky Mountain spotted fever, rubella, infectious mononucleosis, and cytomegalovirus disease. Hepatitis, however, remains the major threat. Non-A, non-B hepatitis now accounts for 90–95% of all cases of posttransfusion hepatitis. The most serious feature of the disease is its chronicity; posttransfusion hepatitis may progress to chronic active hepatitis and eventually to cirrhosis. About 50% of patients with non-A, non-B hepatitis following transfusion continue to have transaminase elevations 6 months after onset, and at least 20% have abnormalities beyond 1 year. Chronic liver disease may be more likely to develop in men than in women. In a 5-year, multicenter study that ended in 1979, 10% of 1,513 transfusion recipients developed non-A, non-B hepatitis, as defined by persistently elevated serum alanine aminotransferase levels. In contrast, only 1% developed hepatitis B and none developed hepatitis A [54]. The incidence of hepatitis was directly related to the alanine aminotransferase levels in blood donors in this and other studies [55, 56], and it has been estimated that the incidence of posttransfusion hepatitis could be reduced 30% if donor units with elevated levels of alanine aminotransferase were discarded. Such a decision would involve complex issues, but, in the absence of a specific test for the non-A, non-B agents, must be considered. Even with the exclusive use of volunteer blood, we can expect 150,000 cases of posttransfusion hepatitis every year in the United States.

Little is known about the ability of immune globulin to provide passive immunity against non-A, non-B hepatitis. In the late 1970s, three double-blind, randomized studies designed to evaluate this question were reported. In all three, no difference was seen between the incidence of anicteric non-A, non-B hepatitis cases among those who received immune globulin and those who did not. In two studies, however, there was a significant decrease in the incidence of icteric hepatitis cases among those who received immune globulin, suggesting the disease had been attenuated. One study also showed that less progression of acute hepatitis to chronic liver disease was seen in those patients who received preoperative immune globulin [57–59]. The timing, dose, and efficacy of immune globulin remain in doubt, however, and it is not routinely recommended at this time. The mortality rate of posttransfusion hepatitis is lower than formerly thought, but is not negligible.

Keeping blood as safe as possible requires eternal vigilance. For example, blood is not collected on Martha's Vineyard in the summer because healthy, asymptomatic donors can transmit babesiosis that can prove fatal [60]. Even more alarming, there is evidence suggesting that 1 infant and at least 1 adult may have acquired the 'new', frequently lethal, mysterious, acquired immunodeficiency syndrome from blood transfusion [61, 62]. There is also evidence suggesting hemophiliacs who receive factor VIII concentrates are in danger. Some communities have already asked homosexuals, a group at 'high risk' for acquired immunodeficiency syndrome, to refrain from donating blood. At this writing, a national advisory committee is meeting to weigh the public health menace and to consider what actions to take [2].

References

1 Sohmer, P.R.; Moore, G.L.; Beutler, E.; Peck, C.C.: In vivo viability of red blood cells stored in CPDA-2. Transfusion *22:* 479–484 (1982).

2 Check, W.A.: Preventing AIDS transmission: should blood donors be screened? J. Am. med. Ass. *249:* 567–570 (1983).

3 Diamond, L.K.: A history of blood transfusion; in Wintrobe, Blood, pure and eloquent, pp. 659–688 (McGraw-Hill, London 1980).

4 Katz, A.J.: Transfusion therapy: its role in the anemias. Hosp. Pract. *15:* 77–84 (1980).

5 Orlin, J.B.: Current trends in whole blood and red cell therapy. Postgrad. Med. *72:* 63–69 (1982).
6 Conley, C.L.; Lippman, S.M.; Ness, P.: Autoimmune hemolytic anemia with reticulocytopenia. J. Am. med. Ass. *244:* 1688–1690 (1980).
7 Schneider, A.J.; Stockman, J.A., III; Oski, R.A.: Transfusion nomogram: an application of physiology to clinical decisions regarding the use of blood. Crit. Care Med. *9:* 469–473 (1981).
8 Watson-Williams, E.J.: Hematologic and hemostatic considerations before surgery. Med. Clins N. Am. *63:* 1165–1189 (1979).
9 Shackford, S.R.; Virgilio, R.W.; Peters, R.M.: Whole blood versus packed cell transfusions. Ann. Surg. *193:* 337–340 (1981).
10 Blumberg, N.; Bove, J.R.: Un-cross-matched blood for emergency transfusion. J. Am. med. Ass. *240:* 2057–2059 (1978).
11 Alexander, M.R.; Alexander, B.; Mustion, A.L.; Spector, R.; Wright, C.B.: Therapeutic use of albumin: 2. J. Am. med. Ass. *247:* 831–833 (1982).
12 Alving, B.M.; Hojima, Y.; Pisano, J.J.; et al.: Hypotension associated with prekallikrein activator (Hageman-factor fragments) in plasma protein fraction. New Engl. J. Med. *299:* 66–70 (1978).
13 Lazrove, S.; Waxman, K.; Shippy, C.; Shoemaker, W.C.: Hemodynamic, blood volume, and oxygen transport responses to albumin and hydroxyethyl starch infusions in critically ill postoperative patients. Crit. Care Med. *8:* 302–306 (1980).
14 Puri, V.K.; Paidipathy, B.; White, L.: Hydroxyethyl starch for resuscitation of patients with hypovolemia and shock. Crit. Care Med. *9:* 833–837 (1981).
15 Haupt, M.T.; Rackow, E.C.: Colloid osmotic pressure and fluid resuscitation with hetastarch, albumin, and saline solutions. Crit. Care Med. *10:* 159–162 (1982).
16 Alter, H.J.; Tabor, E.; Meryman, H.T.; Hoofnagle, J.H.; Kahn, R.A.; Holland, P.V.; Gerety, R.J.; Barker, L.R.: Transmission of hepatitis B virus infection by transfusion of frozen-deglycerolized red blood cells. New Engl. J. Med. *298:* 637–642 (1978).
17 Haugen, R.K.: Hepatitis after the transfusion of frozen red cells and washed red cells. New Engl. J. Med. *301:* 393–395 (1979).
18 Strom, T.B.: Hepatitis B, transfusions, and renal transplantation – five years later. New Engl. J. Med. *307:* 1141–1142 (1982).
19 Moore, S.B.: The enigma of blood transfusions and kidney transplantation. Mayo Clin. Proc. *57:* 431–438 (1982).
20 Woodson, R.D.; Fitzpatrick, J.H., Jr.; Costello, D.J.; Gilboe, D.D.: Increased blood oxygen affinity decreases canine brain oxygen consumption. J. Lab. clin. Med. *100:* 411–424 (1982).
21 Which is the foreseeable clinical application of oxygen-carrying blood substitutes (fluorocarbons and hemoglobin solutions)? Which impact are they likely to have on the activity of blood services? Vox Sang. *42:* 97–109 (1982).
22 Cowart, V.S.: Blood substitutes: two ways to get there. J. Am. med. Ass. *249:* 159–164 (1983).
23 Terebelo, H.R.; McCue, R.L.; Lenneville, M.S.: Implication of plasma free hemoglobin in massive clostridial hemolysis. J. Am. med. Ass. *248:* 2028–2029 (1982).
24 Rosen, A.L.; Gould, S.A.; Sehgal, L.R.; Sehgal, H.L.; Rice, C.L.; Rushing, D.; Moss, G.S.: Hemoglobin solutions as red cell substitutes. Crit. Care Med. *10:* 275–278 (1982).

25 Friedman, H.E.; De Venuto, F.: Morphological effects of transfusions with hemoglobin solutions. Crit. Care med. *10:* 288–293 (1982).
26 Hauser, C.J.; Shoemaker, W.C.: Hemoglobin solution in the treatment of hemorrhagic shock. Crit. Care Med. *10:* 283–287 (1982).
27 De Venuto, F.: Hemoglobin solutions as oxygen-delivering resuscitation fluids. Crit. Care Med. *10:* 238–245 (1982).
28 Tremper, K.K.; Friedman, A.E.; Levine, E.M.; Lapin, R.; Camarillo, D.: The preoperative treatment of severely anemic patients with a perfluorochemical oxygen-transport fluid, fluosol-DA. New Engl. J. med. *307:* 277–283 (1982).
29 Tremper, K.K.; Lapin, R.; Levine, E.; Friedman, A.; Shoemaker, W.C.: Hemodynamic and oxygen transport effects of a perfluorochemical blood substitute, fluosol-DA. Crit. Care Med. *8:* 738–741 (1980).
30 Vercellotti, G.; Modelevsky, J.; Hammerschmidt, D.; et al.: Activation of plasma complement (C) by the synthetic erythrocyte substitute fluosol-DA: a mechanism of an adverse pulmonary reaction. Clin. Res. *28:* 731A (1980).
31 Colman, R.W.; Chang, L.K.; Mukherji, B.; et al.: Effects of a perfluoro erythrocyte substitute on platelets in vitro and in vivo. J. Lab. clin. Med. *95:* 553–557 (1980).
32 Glogar, D.H.; Kloner, R.A.; Muller, J.; De Boer, L.W.V.; Braunwald, E.: Fluorocarbons reduce myocardial ischemic damage after coronary occlusion. Science *211:* 1439–1441 (1981).
33 Peerless, S.J.; Ishikawa, R.; Hunter, I.G.; Peerless, M.J.: Protective effect of fluosol-DA in acute cerebral ischemia. Stroke *12:* 558–563 (1981).
34 Sassano, J.J.; Sladen, A.; Franklin, R.H.; Guntupalli, K.K.: Management of hemorrhagic shock with hydroxyethyl starch, total-dose imferon infusion, and mass spectrophotometry. Crit. Care Med. *10:* 484–485 (1982).
35 Ott, D.A.; Cooley, D.A.: Cardiovascular surgery in Jehovah's Witnesses. J. Am. med. Ass. *238:* 1256–1258 (1977).
36 Dixon, J.L.; Smalley, M.G.: Jehovah's Witnesses. The surgical/ethical challenge. J. Am. med. Ass. *246:* 2471–2472 (1981).
37 Counts, R.B.; Haisch, C.; Simon, T.L.; Maxwell, N.G.; Heimbach, D.M.; Carrico, C.J.: Hemostasis in massively transfused trauma patients. Ann. Surg. *190:* 91–99 (1979).
38 Robinson, N.B.; Heimbach, D.M.; Reynolds, L.O.; Pavlin, E.; Durtschi, M.B.; Reim, M.; Craig, K.: Ventilation and perfusion alterations following homologous blood transfusion. Surgery *92:* 183–191 (1982).
39 Snyder, E.L.; Hezzey, A.; Barash, P.G.; Palermo, G.: Microaggregate blood filtration in patients with compromised pulmonary function. Transfusion *22:* 21–25 (1982).
40 Lundsgaard-Hansen, P.: Symposium on microfiltration of blood and pulmonary function. Vox Sang. *39:* 46–59 (1980).
41 Pineda, A.A.; Brzica, S.M., Jr.; Taswell, H.F.: Hemolytic transfusion reaction. Recent experience in a large blood bank. Mayo Clin. Proc. *53:* 378–390 (1978).
42 Schmidt, P.J.: Transfusion mortality; with special reference to surgical and intensive care facilities. J. Fla med. Ass. *67:* 151–153 (1980).
43 Widmann, F.K.: Untoward effects of blood transfusion. Common problems and simple safeguards. Postgrad. Med. *69:* 40–53 (1981).
44 Sazama, K.; Klein, H.G.; Davey, R.J.; Corash, L.: Inoperative hemolysis. The initial manifestation of glucose-6-phosphate dehydrogenase deficiency. Archs intern. Med. *140:* 845–846 (1980).

45 Colburn, W.J.; Barnes, A.: Intravenous imferon masquerading as an acute hemolytic transfusion reaction. Transfusion *22:* 163–164 (1982).

46 Solanki, D.; McCurdy, P.R.: Delayed hemolytic transfusion reactions: an often missed entity. J. Am. med. Ass. *239:* 729–731 (1978).

47 Diamond, W.J.; Brown, F.L.; Bitterman, P.; et al.: Delayed hemolytic transfusion reaction presenting as sickle-cell crisis. Ann. intern. Med. *93:* 231–233 (1980).

48 Meltz, D.J.; Bertles, J.F.; David, D.S.; et al.: Delayed haemolytic transfusion reaction with renal failure. Lancet *ii:* 1348–1349 (1971).

49 Croucher, B.E.E.; Crookston, M.C.; Crookston, J.H.: Delayed hemolytic transfusion reactions simulating auto-immune hemolytic anemia. Vox Sang. *12:* 32 (1967).

50 Menitove, J.E.; McElligott, M.C.; Aster, R.H.: Febrile transfusion reaction: what blood component should be given next? Vox Sang. *42:* 318–321 (1981).

51 Ward, H.N.: Pulmonary infiltrates associated with leukoagglutinin transfusion reactions. Ann. intern. Med. *73:* 689–694 (1970).

52 Thompson, J.S.; Severson, C.D.; Parmely, M.J.; et al.: Pulmonary 'hypersensitivity' reactions induced by transfusion of non-HL-A leukoagglutinins. New Engl. J. Med. *284:* 1120–1125 (1971).

53 Wolf, C.F.W.; Canale, V.C.: Fatal pulmonary hypersensitivity reaction to HL-A incompatible blood transfusion: report of a case and review of the literature. Transfusion *16:* 135–140 (1976).

54 Aach, R.D.; Szmuness, W.; Mosley, J.W.; Hollinger, F.B.; Kahn, R.A.; Stevens, C.E.; Edwards, V.M.; Werch, J.: Serum alanine aminotransferase of donors in relation to the risk of non-A, non-B hepatitis in recipients. The transfusion-transmitted viruses study. New Engl. J. Med. *304:* 989–994 (1981).

55 Alter, H.J.; Purcell, R.H.; Holland, P.V.; Alling, D.W.; Koziol, D.E.: Donor transaminase and recipient hepatitis. J. Am. med. Ass. *246:* 630–634 (1981).

56 Hornbrook, M.C.; Dodd, R.Y.; Jacobs, P.; Friedman, L.I.; Sherman, K.E.: Reducing the incidence of non-A, non-B post-transfusion hepatitis by testing donor blood for alanine aminotransferase. New Engl. J. Med. *307:* 1315–1321 (1982).

57 Knodell, R.G.; Conrad, M.E.; Ishak, K.G.: Development of chronic liver disease after acute non-A, non-B post-transfusion hepatitis. Gastroenterology *72:* 902–909 (1977).

58 Gerety, R.J.; Aronson, D.L.: Plasma derivatives and viral hepatitis. Transfusion *22:* 347–351 (1982).

59 Czaja, A.J.; Davis, G.L.: Hepatitis non-A, non-B. Manifestations and implications of acute and chronic disease. Mayo Clin. Proc. *57:* 639–652 (1982).

60 Marcus, L.C.; Valigorsky, J.M.; Fanning, W.L.; Joseph, T.; Glick, B.: A case report of transfusion-induced babesiosis. J. Am. med. Ass. *248:* 465–467 (1982).

61 Possible transfusion-associated acquired immune deficiency syndrome (AIDS) – California. MMWR *31:* 652–654 (1982).

62 Jett, G.R.; Kuritsky, G.N.; Katzmann, G.A.; Homburger, H.A.: Acquired immunodeficiency syndrome associated with blood-product transfusion. Ann. intern. Med. *99:* 621–624 (1983).

E.R. Eichner, MD, University of Oklahoma Health Sciences Center,
Oklahoma City, OK 73106 (USA)

Renal System

Prog. crit. Care Med., vol. 2, pp. 133–150 (Karger, Basel 1985)

The Oliguric Patient

Leonard L. Vertuno

Loyola University Stritch School of Medicine, Maywood, Ill., USA

Oliguria, the failure to elaborate a urine flow of sufficient quantity to maintain homeostasis, is a frequent cause of admission to the intensive care unit. Oliguria is traditionally defined as a urine volume of less than 400 ml/day. This definition is derived from a consideration of the determinants of urine flow: (1) solute load; (2) osmolality of medullary interstitium, and (3) response to vasopressin.

The normal solute load requiring excretion ranges from 450 to 750 mosm/day, and the maximal urine osmolality is 1,200 mosm. Thus:

$$\frac{\text{(a minimal solute load)}}{\text{(maximal urinary concentration)}} \quad \frac{480\text{ mosm}}{1{,}200\text{ mosm}/1\text{ kg } H_2O} = 0.4\text{ kg } H_2O \text{ or } 400\text{ ml } H_2O.$$

Progressive azotemia often develops at urine flow rates higher than these minimal values because of high solute loads or inability to elaborate a maximally concentrated urine.

The development of oliguria does not imply renal failure and may occur in the presence of functionally intact kidneys, if the renal blood flow is sufficiently reduced (prerenal azotemia) or if an obstruction to urine flow is present (postrenal azotemia). Acute renal failure (ARF) is caused by renal parenchymal injury and is not reversible by manipulation of extrarenal factors.

An analysis of 2,500 cases of ARF from around the world indicates that 52% occurred in a surgical setting or following trauma, 26% in a medical setting, 13% in obstetrics, and 9% were due to nephrotoxins [1]. A more recent survey of hospital-acquired renal insufficiency revealed an incidence of 4.9% in 2,262 consecutive hospital admissions. In this series 42% were due to renal underperfusion, 18% followed major surgery, and 19% were due to contrast media or aminoglycoside administration. The incidence of oliguria in these patients with worsening renal function was 20%, yielding an incidence of approximately 1% in hospitalized patients [2].

Pathophysiology

An overview of the pathophysiology of oliguric syndromes is given in table I. Reduction of renal blood flow because of hypovolemia, reduced cardiac output, or renal vasoconstriction will decrease the glomerular filtration rate (GFR), increase filtration fraction and renal sodium absorption. In an attempt to conserve volume, the urine formed is low in sodium and concentrated with respect to plasma. Tubular urea reabsorption is enhanced by low urine flow, so urea clearance is decreased more than creatinine clearance. This is reflected by a greater rise in blood urea nitrogen (BUN) than serum creatinine. The urine sediment is normal or contains an increased number of hyaline casts. Restoration of circulatory factors to normal results in a prompt resolution of azotemia. Occasionally, patients with prerenal azotemia do not manifest oliguria. This is usually due to lack of appropriately concentrated medullary interstitium secondary to ageing [3], malnutrition, impaired delivery of sodium to Henle's loop, or preexisting renal disease [4]. Administration of diuretics may prevent equilibration of tubular fluid with medullary interstitium by increasing urine flow rate [5].

Obstruction to urine flow, if complete, results in anuria. Incomplete high-grade obstruction may result in oliguria, polyuria, or fluctuating urine flow rates. In early hydronephrosis, intratubular pressure rises, glomerular filtration falls, and the urine formed may be low in sodium, concentrated, and contain few sediment abnormalities. Thus, early obstruction may mimic prerenal azotemia. More prolonged obstruction results in an impaired capacity to absorb sodium and to respond to vasopressin, producing a sodium-rich, isosthenuric or hyposthenuric urine [6].

Renal functional impairment associated with obstruction is often reversible, so it must be excluded with confidence in any patient who presents with azotemia of uncertain etiology. Bladder outlet obstruction from prostatic disease is common in men. Bilateral ureteral obstruction occurs with retroperitoneal disease: idiopathic retroperitoneal fibrosis, lymphoma, and pelvic tumors. Ureteral injury may occur with pelvic surgery.

Table I. Oliguric syndromes

Prerenal	
Hypovolemia, congestive heart failure, liver disease	potentiation by prostaglandin synthetase inhibitors
Obstruction	
Intrarenal	uric acid nephropathy, myeloma
Extrarenal	bladder outlet, prostatism, retroperitoneal disease, surgery, calculi, clots, papillary necrosis
Intrinsic renal disease	
ARF syndrome	
Ischemic	all causes of prerenal azotemia
Nephrotoxic	radiological contrast media, aminoglycosides, chemotherapeutic agents, glycols, heavy metals, solvents
Pigment	
Hemoglobinuria	malaria, transfusion reactions, glucose-6-phosphate dehydrogenase deficiency, sepsis, valvular heart disease
Myoglobinuria	crush injuries, burns, alcohol, drugs, seizures, muscular activity, hypokalemia, viral
Acute glomerulonephritis	primary or systemic
Acute interstitial nephritis	penicillins, thiazide, rifampin, cimetidine, nonsteroidal anti-inflammatory agents
Arterial occlusions	
Microscopic	cortical necrosis, thrombotic thrombocytopenic purpura
Macroscopic	emboli, thrombosis, dissection
Venous occlusions	renal vein thrombosis

Renal calculi, papillary necrosis, or blood clots are occasional causes of bilateral obstruction. The presence of a solitary functioning kidney increases the potential for total urinary obstruction.

Intrinsic renal failure can occur as a consequence of prolonged ischemia, administration or exposure to nephrotoxins, or from the release of the heme pigments, hemoglobin or myoglobin. These forms of ARF, often misnamed acute tubular necrosis, may cause severe renal dysfunction in the absence of histopathologic manifestations of tubular necrosis. Several experimental models have elucidated the initiating and sustaining factors responsible for the prolonged reduction in GFR in these conditions [7]. Renal artery clamping, epinephrine infusion, and glycerol injection initiate ARF by ischemia. Early return of renal blood flow to or toward normal is not accompanied by an increase in GFR. Factors responsible for sustaining the reduced GFR in these models of ischemic ARF include tubular obstruction with cellular debris, backleak of filtrate through damaged tubules, and a decrease in the glomerular permeability coefficient, either a reduction in surface area or a decrease in hydraulic conductivity. The nephrotoxic models utilize uranyl nitrate or mercuric chloride to produce renal injury. Renal blood flow is more variable and it appears that renal ischemia is not necessary for the development of ARF. Direct cellular injury is the initiating factor. Again, tubular obstruction, backleak of filtrate, and decreased glomerular permeability coefficient are sustaining factors.

Ischemic ARF occurs in any setting that predisposes to prerenal azotemia: volume loss (hemorrhage, gastrointestinal losses, sequestration due to burns or pancreatitis) or reduced cardiac output (congestive heart failure, myocardial tamponade). Interruption of renal blood flow by aortic cross-clamping or rupture of an abdominal aortic aneurysm results in severe renal ischemia. The minimal stimulus required to produce ARF from ischemia varies widely among individuals. Renal injury may occur with a hypotensive episode so transient that it is unrecognized or a patient may endure several days of markedly reduced renal blood flow without developing parenchymal injury. The ageing kidney and concurrent administration of nephrotoxic medication may predispose to an earlier development of ARF. Inhibition of prostaglandin synthesis in the presence of reduced renal blood flow will predispose the kidneys to more severe ischemia [8]. The widespread use of nonsteroidal anti-inflammatory agents (ibuprofen, fenoprofen, naproxen, indomethacin, etc.) potentiates renal ischemia in patients with congestive heart failure, hepatic cirrhosis, and other clinical states of decreased renal blood flow [9–11].

The spectrum of nephrotoxic ARF has changed dramatically in recent years. Iatrogenic causes like radiological contrast media, aminoglycosides, and chemotherapeutic agents such as cisplatin have replaced industrial exposure and ingestion of toxic materials as the major causes of nephrotoxicity. Currently, radiocontrast administration and aminoglycosides may account for 20% of hospital-acquired renal insufficiency [2].

The high incidence of renal insufficiency following radiological contrast media administration has only been appreciated in recent years [12]. It occurs with all types of contrast study: intravenous urography, angiography, computerized tomography, and oral cholecystography. Prominent risk factors are advanced age, diabetes mellitus, prior renal insufficiency, multiple myeloma, and dehydration. Pathogenesis is uncertain, but renal vasoconstriction, direct nephrotoxicity, microcirculatory changes, immunologic reactions, and tubular obstruction with protein or uric acid crystals have all been implicated. Recent experiments demonstrate prolonged renal vasoconstriction with contrast media administration in the sodium-depleted subject [13]. Optimal hydration prior to the study is essential, but not necessarily protective. Mannitol and forced alkaline diuresis have been advocated as preventive measures, but their efficacy has not been proven. An occasional patient who develops oliguria will never have a return of function.

Aminoglycoside nephrotoxicity is also a common occurrence in the hospital setting [14]. These antibiotics are concentrated by renal tubular epithelium, and renal cortical concentrations may reach 20 times the serum level. This may account for cases of nephrotoxicity in which serum levels are not detected in the toxic range. Very early toxicity is manifested by tubular proteinuria and enzymuria. This is followed by cylindruria and other sediment abnormalities and then progressive azotemia. This type of renal failure is usually nonoliguric and may be associated with hypomagnesemia and hypocalcemia [15]. Factors contributing to the incidence of aminoglycoside renal injury include its administration in large doses to critically ill patients with uncertain renal function and the tendency of serum creatinine to overestimate the GFR in the elderly patient. Inappropriately high doses may be given which may result in toxic blood levels. Because individual pharmacokinetics are so variable, it is best to administer these drugs with careful monitoring of blood levels [16].

The chemotherapeutic agents represented by cisplatin are a third class of pharmaceuticals causing ARF. Toxicity of this heavy metal appears comparable to mercury [17]. Many cases are nonoliguric, although severe oliguria may occur. Renal magnesium wasting results in hypomagnesemia. Mannitol diuresis and perhaps chloride may reduce the severity of the nephrotoxicity [18]. Functional recovery is frequently incomplete.

More traditional causes of nephrotoxic ARF: heavy metals (lead, mercury, antimony, cadmium), organic solvents (tetrachloroethylene, carbon tetrachloride), and the glycols are seen less frequently today than iatrogenic causes.

Heme pigments, hemoglobin, and myoglobin may cause ARF. Neither substance appears nephrotoxic by itself; renal underperfusion is important in inducing nephrotoxicity. Hemoglobinuria occurs with intravascular hemolysis: transfusion reactions, clostridial sepsis, malaria, glucose-6-phosphate dehydrogenase deficiency, valvular heart disease, and hypotonic dialysate are examples. Myoglobinuria occurs massively with severe crush injuries and burns, but nontraumatic rhabdomyolysis associated with alcohol, drugs, seizures, intense muscular activity, hypokalemia, and viral syndromes is far more frequent. The clinical triad of elevated creatine phosphokinase, orthotolidine-positive urine, and the absence of red cells in urine is characteristic for myoglobinuria, but not very sensitive. The most severe elevations of creatinine, phosphorus, and uric acid are a feature of massive muscle destruction, but are not striking in the usual case [19].

Intrarenal tubular obstruction with uric acid crystals occurs after chemotherapy or radiation of leukemias or lymphoproliferative tumors [20]. Rapid cell lysis may result in severe hyperphosphatemia and hyperkalemia as well [21]. Pretreatment with the xanthine oxidase inhibitor allopurinol as well as a large volume alkaline diuresis may prevent this syndrome. Mannitol-induced solute diuresis is also helpful. Intrarenal tubular obstruction also occurs in multiple myeloma when Bence-Jones protein or light chains are precipitated by dehydration or contrast media.

Lastly, many primary renal diseases such as vascular, glomerular, or interstitial disease may present as oliguric ARF. Bilateral renal artery occlusion or occlusion of the glomerular microvasculature, as in thrombotic thrombocytopenia purpura or cortical necrosis, cause severe oligoanuria. Crescentic glomerulonephritis may be oliguric. Acute interstitial nephritis is characterized by ARF and occurs with administration of the penicillins, thiazides, furosemide, rifampin, and cimetidine [14]. The nonsteroidal anti-inflammatory agents also produce this renal injury.

Clinical Diagnostic Approach

Careful history and physical examination provide the cornerstones in evaluating the oliguric patient. Recent weight loss, fever, diarrhea, nasogastric suction, or 'third space' translocation of intravascular fluids occurring in burns or pancreatitis are clues to volume contraction. Renal blood flow may be compromised by hypotension, hypoxia, sepsis, congestive heart failure, or liver disease. Has there been an exposure to nephrotoxins or prostaglandin synthetase inhibitors? Fever, rash, and eosinophilia suggest an interstitial nephritis or systemic vasculitis. Smokey urine and hyper-

Table II. Urine sediment

Abnormality	Clinical correlation
Hyaline casts, finely granular casts	renal underperfusion without intrinsic renal injury
Tubular cell casts, tubular epithelial cells	intrinsic renal injury
Red blood cell casts	glomerulonephritis, cortical necrosis, thrombotic thrombocytopenic purpura, occasionally acute interstitial nephritis
White blood cell casts, sterile pyuria	interstitial nephritis, occasionally exudative glomerulonephritis
Pigmented acellular casts	hemoglobinuria, myoglobinuria
Crystalluria	
Uric acid	radiological contrast media, tumor dissolution
Calcium oxalate	glycol ingestion, methoxyfluorane
Cystine	cystinuria
Magnesium ammonium phosphate	infection

tension are clues to glomerulonephritis. Urinary flow patterns can suggest bladder outlet obstruction or a history of pelvic disease or surgery may provide a clue to bilateral ureteral obstruction. Congenital or surgical absence of a kidney makes obstructive uropathy a more likely possibility.

Postural hypotension and postural tachycardia, loss of skin turgor (best evaluated over the forehead or upper sternum), and the absence of axillary sweat – all point to volume contraction. Bladder outlet obstruction may be detected by percussion. It must be reliably excluded in every case, by catheterization if necessary.

Microscopic examination of the urine by the physician is an integral part of the physical examination (table II). The presence or absence of formed elements provide insight into the physical condition of the kidneys. Hyaline and finely granular casts suggest renal underperfusion without significant parenchymal injury. Many coarsely granular casts, renal tubular cell casts, and renal epithelial cells indicate intrinsic renal damage. Red

Table III. Urinary indices

	Renal underperfusion	Intrinsic renal injury
Concentrating ability		
Specific gravity	> 1.015	1.010
U/P, osm	> 1.5	0.90–1.10
Filtrate reabsorption		
U/P urea	> 10	< 3
U/P creatinine	> 40	< 10
Renal sodium handling		
U_{Na}, mEq/l	< 20	> 40
$FE_{Na}\left[\frac{U_{Na}}{P_{Na}} \times \frac{P_{cr}}{U_{cr}} \times 100\%\right]$, %	< 1	> 3
RFI $\left[\frac{U_{Na}}{U/P_{creatinine}}\right]$	< 1	> 3

Primary glomerular syndromes are characterized by proteinuria and frequently have indices characteristic of renal underperfusion. Early obstruction may mimic underperfusion; prolonged obstruction, intrinsic renal injury.

blood cell casts are especially suggestive of glomerular disease, but are occasionally seen with interstitial inflammation [22]. White blood cell casts occur with exudative glomerular lesions as well as interstitial inflammation. Urinary eosinophils (Wright's or Giemsa's stain) point to allergic interstitial nephritis. Orthotolidine-positive urine with pigmented casts, but without red blood cells, indicates hemoglobinuria or myoglobinuria. Crystalluria such as uric acid (tumor dissolution, contrast media), calcium oxalate (glycol ingestion, methoxyfluorane), cystine (cystinuria), and triple phosphate (infection) suggest distinctive etiologies as the cause of renal failure.

Renal integrity is then assessed by the use of urinary indices [23–25] (table III). The underperfused, but functionally intact kidney is able to reclaim glomerular filtrate, concentrate the urine, and conserve sodium. Simultaneous samples of urine and plasma analyzed for osmolality, sodium, creatinine, and urea will elucidate these features. Urinary concentrating ability (specific gravity, U/P osmolality), filtrate reabsorption (U/P creatinine, U/P urea), and renal handling of sodium (U_{Na}, FE_{Na}, renal failure index –RFI) are available from these simple tests. Because urinary concentrating ability and urine sodium concentration are insensitive discriminators between prerenal azotemia and ARF, the derived indices of sodium handling, such as fractional excretion of sodium (FE_{Na})

$$\frac{[U_{Na}\ P_{creatinine}]}{[P_{Na}\ U_{creatinine}]} \times 100\%$$

or the RFI

$$\frac{[U_{Na}]}{[U/P_{creatinine}]},$$

provide a more accurate guide to renal integrity. These indices usually provide excellent discrimination with an FE_{Na} less than 1% and RFI less than 1 in prerenal azotemia and over 3% or 3, respectively, in intrinsic renal failure.

Pitfalls occur in the interpretation of urine chemistries. Specific gravity is elevated by glucose, mannitol, and contrast media. Mannitol and loop diuretics interfere with sodium reabsorption and urinary concentration, so all studies should be obtained before their administration. Preexisting inability to concentrate the urine or conserve sodium occurs in malnutrition, in the ageing patient, or in chronic renal failure and will make the data less reliable. Clinical states with strong sodium avidity, such as cirrhosis of the liver and congestive heart failure, may have prerenal indices of sodium absorption despite intrinsic renal failure [26]. Urine sodium may be low in radiological contrast media injury, perhaps reflecting renal vasoconstriction [27]. Renal failure associated with burns is also associated with a very low fractional excretion of sodium [28]. Urine sediment in these cases reflects renal injury.

Patients with acute uric acid nephropathy consequent to tumor dissolution have very high urinary uric acid concentrations. This can be identified in a spot urine sample by a uric acid:creatinine ratio greater than unity [29]

$$\frac{U_{uric\ acid}}{U_{creatinine}} < 1.$$

Radiological techniques are necessary to assess kidney size, the presence or absence of hydronephrosis, and the presence of major arterial or venous occlusions. Plain abdominal films will identify radiopaque stones and often give a clue to kidney size. Intravenous pyelography yields a characteristic dense nephrogram in many cases of ARF, and delayed films – 12–24 h – will identify hydronephrosis with some precision. However, a substantial dose of contrast media is required [30]. The availability of B mode, gray-scale ultrasonography gives very accurate data regarding kidney size, the presence or absence of either kidney, and the presence of hydronephrosis [31]. Thus, intravenous pyelography and, especially, invasive retrograde pyelography are now rarely necessary in the investigation of oliguria.

Renal arteriography and venography identify bilateral arterial thrombosis and venous thrombosis, respectively. Sudden anuria with severe hypertension is the characteristic picture of bilateral arterial thrombosis. Its recognition is important because late revascularization may result in enough functional recovery to avoid end-stage renal failure [32]. Renal venography is indicated in situations where renal venous thrombosis is suspected, e.g., sudden deterioration of renal function in a nephrotic patient, ARF with dehydration in an infant, and acute oliguria associated with renal carcinoma. Radionuclide blood flow scans give an anephric tracing in cortical necrosis or arterial occlusions.

Renal biopsy is indicated in patients with (1) oligoanuria persisting longer than 3 weeks; (2) clinical signs and symptoms suggestive of glomerular, vascular, or systemic disease; (3) renal failure without an obvious cause, and (4) suspected drug-induced renal failure. Using these criteria, a significant proportion of biopsies will yield diagnostically useful information [32–34].

Management

During the initial phase of oliguria, identification and correction of remedial factors may prevent ARF. The combination of a plain abdominal film and ultrasonography will usually be adequate to diagnose obstructive uropathy. Cautious unilateral retrograde pyelography may be rarely necessary. Replacement of fluid losses and provision of maximal volume expansion may require invasive monitoring. In the critically ill patient with respiratory failure, sepsis, pulmonary edema, or coma, physical examination and chest film are often inadequate guides to the patient's hemodynamic status. Monitoring with a flow-directed balloon catheter may direct a change in therapy almost 50% of the time [35].

Only after adequate volume expansion is achieved should an attempt be made to re-establish urine flow with mannitol or a loop diuretic. Although there is no evidence that these substances increase GFR in the oliguric patient, re-establishment of urine flow may decrease tubular obstruction with cellular debris, and the clinical course of nonoliguric renal failure is shorter and has less morbidity and mortality than oliguric renal failure [36].

Mannitol, an inert osmotic nonelectrolyte confined to the extracellular space, increases intravascular volume, increases renal blood flow, and promotes an osmotic diuresis [37]. In situations where renal hemodynamics are altered, it may be effective when other diuretics are not. It is effective as prophylaxis against ARF in such high-risk situations as abdominal aortic surgery. Mannitol has a theoretical advantage in those situations where oliguria is maintained by intratubular obstruction. This would include all forms of ischemic ARF as well as uric acid and the pigment nephropathies. It has a lesser utility in nephrotoxic ARF. Its potential effectiveness in radiological contrast mediated ARF may be explained, because this is primarily a vasoconstrictive phenomenon. A test dose of 12.5 or 25 g of mannitol can be followed by an infusion of 10% mannitol in 0.45% NaCl to maintain a urine flow of 50–100 ml/h, if a diuresis is established. Hazards include the development of hyponatremia and intravascular volume expansion.

Alternatively, furosemide 240 mg, may be administered intravenously. If ineffective, 480 mg given 1 h later will constitute an adequate diuretic challenge. If diuresis ensues, adequate volume replacement is imperative, because further volume depletion will aggravate the original insult [38].

Further management of established oliguria requires correction of metabolic abnormalities, provision of adequate nutrition, and dialysis for uremia and its complications. Gastrointestinal hemorrhage, infection, and adverse drug reactions contribute to serious morbidity. Fluids should be restricted to 400 ml/day plus urine output in the absence of fever or external losses. A weight loss of 0.25–0.50 kg/day due to catabolism should be observed. The development of hyponatremia or weight gain indicate excessive fluid intake.

Hyperkalemia remains a major immediate life-threatening complication, although prompt recognition and treatment have rendered it no longer a major cause of mortality. The urine flow rate is a major determinant of potassium excretion, and hyperkalemia is a predictable consequence of oliguria. Because of similar effects on resting membrane potential, hyponatremia, hypocalcemia, and acidosis will potentiate the cardiotoxic effect of hyperkalemia. The progression of electrocardiographic changes – peaked T waves, prolongation of PR interval and QRS interval, and disappearance of P waves – correlates only roughly with serum potassium levels. Immediate administration of calcium chloride or calcium gluconate antagonizes the effect of hyperkalemia on resting membrane potential. Glucose and insulin (4 g/1 U) and sodium bicarbonate effect a transmembrane flux of potassium. These three maneuvers, while immediately effective, do not induce a negative potassium balance. Potassium removal requires binding with a cation exchange resin or dialysis.

Metabolic acidosis is a consequence of the kidneys' inability to excrete the nonvolatile hydrogen ion production. The average daily production of 1 mEq/kg/day results in an HCO_3 decrement of 1–2 mEq/l/day [39]. More rapidly progressive acidosis suggests hypercatabolism, superimposed lactic acidosis, or buffer loss. Reductions in serum bicarbonate to less than 15 mEq/l should be corrected to maintain an adequate buffer reserve.

Metabolic alkalosis or a combined metabolic and respiratory alkalosis occasionally leads to severe alkalemia in the oliguric patient. Metabolic alkalosis is generated by loss of HCl due to vomiting or nasogastric suction, administration of large amounts of base equivalent such as citrate in massive blood transfusions [40], or the administration of nonreabsorbable antacids with a cationic exchange resin or neutral phosphate [41]. The resultant bicarbonate excess will not be dissipated by nonfunctioning kidneys. Severe alkalemia predisposes to cardiac arrhythmias and seizures, and bicarbonate excess will interfere with weaning the ventilator-dependent patient. Cimetidine will reduce gastrointestinal loss of HCl in the patient requiring nasogastric suction [42]. Hydrochloric acid (0.1 *N*) can be administered via a central vein to titrate the bicarbonate excess [43]. Isolated ultrafiltration of bicarbonate-rich fluid with replacement with sodium chloride is very effective [44]. Commercially prepared dialytic solutions for either hemodialysis or peritoneal dialysis provide an excess of buffer to correct the more common acidosis, so specially prepared dialysate is required to correct this abnormality with dialysis alone [45].

Abnormalities of divalent cation metabolism include hyperphosphatemia, hypocalcemia, and hypermagnesemia. Hyperphosphatemia is controlled by phosphate binders (Dialume®, Amphogel®). Hypocalcemia is frequent, but is rarely symptomatic. Increased serum phosphate, decreased synthesis of 1,25-$(OH)_2$-cholecalciferol, and diminished end organ response to parathyroid hormone are etiologic factors [46]. Treatment is required only in the patient with tetany. Hypercalcemia may occur in the polyuric or recovery phase [47]. Hypermagnesemia of clinical importance is a consequence of magnesium administration as antacids, laxatives, or as an antihypertensive in severe toxemia. The best treatment is prevention.

Nutritional support of the critically ill patient unable to take adequate calories is provided by total parenteral nutrition. Early work in ARF suggested that a combination of essential amino acids and hypertonic glucose could shorten the course of ARF and improve survival [48]. A truly abbreviated course would imply that the reparative process is enhanced by total parenteral nutrition, and experimental support for this concept is provided by enhanced phospholipid synthesis in tubular cell membranes in uranyl nitrate induced ARF [49, 50].

Unfortunately, clinical studies have not borne out the impression of either a shortened course or improved survival [51]. Our current approach is to provide total parenteral nutrition to any patient who cannot receive an adequate supply of nutrients by other means. 30 kcal/kg provides the basal requirement for patients without excessive catabolism. This has to be revised upwards for severely catabolic patients with burns, sepsis, or crush injuries. 300–500 kcal/g nitrogen should be supplied. Nitrogen given as essential amino acids results in a lower urea appearance and less azotemia than a mixture of essential and nonessential amino acids, but the optimal solution is yet to be determined. Regardless of the type of amino acid preparation used, positive nitrogen balance is difficult to achieve in ARF. Electrolytes, trace elements, and vitamins are provided. Lipid is given weekly to avoid essential fatty acid deficiency. Complications include hyperglycemia, ketosis, profound hypophosphatemia, hypokalemia, and hypomagnesemia. Abrupt cessation of the infusion causes hypoglycemia. Liver dysfunction and steatosis may be consequences of intestinal overgrowth with colonic bacteria [52]. Infection due to long-term indwelling central venous catheters is avoided by skillful teams using meticulous aseptic technique.

Dialysis is required for volume overload, hyperkalemia, severe acidosis, uremic alterations in central nervous system function, pericarditis, or bleeding. Therapeutic decisions include considerations of early versus late dialysis, hemodialysis versus peritoneal dialysis, and the preferred circulatory access. Studies which critically evaluate the role of early versus late dialysis are surprisingly few, but do support the role of early dialysis [53]. We institute dialysis before the patient becomes severely azotemic (BUN $\cong$ 100 mg%) to allow adequate nutrition, prevent complications of severe azotemia, and to minimize the potential for uremic bleeding. The hypercatabolic patient, characterized by daily increase in BUN greater than 30 mg%, creatinine greater than 2 mg%, potassium greater than 1.0 mEq/l, and decrease in bicarbonate greater than 2.0 mEq/l will require daily dialysis. Frequent dialysis also allows provision of adequate nutrition. Dialysis access in the bleeding thrombocytopenic patient may be difficult to achieve safely. We have utilized the Cordis® Teflon introducer sheath system to introduce both dialysis catheters as well as flow-directed catheters for invasive monitoring [54]. This approach has been without complications and provides adequate dialysis. The need for systemic heparinization has been avoided by anticoagulation with prostacyclin [55] or citrate [56]. The dialytic technique of isolated ultrafiltration is useful in the oliguric, diuretic unresponsive patient with congestive heart failure. Fluid removal will lower elevated filling pressures and improve oxygenation and myocardial function [57]. As noted above, it is also effective in correcting metabolic alkalosis.

Peritoneal dialysis is especially useful in children, patients with unstable circulatory states, and in intraabdominal conditions that benefit from peritoneal lavage such as peritonitis or pancreatitis. Severely catabolic patients will not be adequately dialyzed by the peritoneal route.

Gastrointestinal hemorrhage, infection, and adverse drug reactions are serious complications. Gastrointestinal hemorrhage occurs in a very high percentage of patients who die in ARF [58]. Because abnormal platelet function is demonstrable at urea nitrogen levels as low as 60 mg%, early and frequent dialysis is advocated to prevent this complication [59]. Cimetidine is almost universally employed, although data to support its efficacy are sparse. Two new approaches to the control of uremic bleeding include infusion of cryoprecipitate [60] and 1-deamino-8-*D*-arginine vasopressin [61]. Their effectiveness suggests a role for factor VIII abnormalities in addition to platelet defects in uremia.

Nosocomial infection is frequent in the immunocompromised uremic patient in the intensive care setting. Two practical considerations are the avoidance of prophylactic antibiotics and long-term bladder catheterization. Bladder catheters do not contribute to management past the early period of volume expansion and attempts to induce a diuresis. Catheter-related infection is associated with a definite increase in mortality [62].

Adverse drug reactions occur in 24% of patients with a BUN over 40 mg% [63]. This toxicity can be reduced by eliminating all medications that are not absolutely necessary, basing dosage on timed creatinine clearances whenever possible, and using drugs the pharmacokinetics of which are well studied whenever possible. Drugs removed by dialysis need to be supplemented after dialysis in some instances [64].

References

1 Levinski, N.G.; Alexander, E.A.; Ventkachalam, M.A.: Acute renal failure; in Brenner, Rector, The kidney; 2nd ed., pp. 1181–1236 (Saunders, Philadelphia 1981).
2 Hou, S.H.; Bushinsky, D.A.; Wish, J.B.; Cohen, J.J.; Harrington, J.T.: Hospital-acquired renal insufficiency: a prospective study. Am. J. Med. *74:* 243–248 (1983).
3 Sporn, I.N.; Lanestremere, R.G.; Papper, S.: Differential diagnosis of oliguria in aged patients. New Engl. J. Med. *267:* 130–132 (1962).
4 Miller, P.D.; Krebs, R.A.; Neal, B.J.; McIntyre, D.O.: Polyuric prerenal failure. Archs intern. Med. *140:* 907–909 (1980).
5 Schrier, R.W.; Lehman, D.; Zacherle, B.; Earley, L.E.: Effect of furosemide on free water excretion in edematous patients with hyponatremia. Kidney int. *3:* 30–34 (1973).
6 Suki, W.; Eknoyan, G.; Rector, F.C.; Seldin, D.W.: Patterns of nephron perfusion in acute and chronic hydronephrosis. J. clin. Invest. *45:* 122–131 (1966).
7 Stein, J.H.; Lifschitz, M.D.; Barnes, L.D.: Current concepts on the pathophysiology of acute renal failure. Am. J. Physiol. F *234:* 171–181 (1978).
8 Henrich, W.L.; Anderson, R.J.; Berns, A.S.; McDonald, K.M.; Paulsen, P.J.; Berl, T.; Schrier, R.W.: The role of renal nerves and prostaglandins in control of renal hemodynamics and plasma renin activity during hypotensive hemorrhage in the dog. J. clin. Invest. *61:* 744–750 (1978).
9 Kimberly, R.P.; Bowden, R.E.; Keiser, H.R.; Plotz, P.H.: Reduction of renal function by newer nonsteroidal anti-inflammatory drugs. Am. J. Med. *64:* 804–813 (1978).
10 Walshe, J.J.; Venuto, R.C.: Acute oliguric renal failure induced by indomethacin: possible mechanism. Ann. intern. Med. *91:* 47–49 (1979).
11 Boyer, T.D.; Zia, P.; Reynolds, T.B.: Effect of indomethacin and prostaglandin A on renal function and plasma renin activity in alcoholic liver disease. Gastroenterology *77:* 215–222 (1979).
12 Byrd, L.; Sherman, R.L.: Radioconstrast-induced acute renal failure: a clinical and pathophysiologic review. Medicine *58:* 270–279 (1979).
13 Larson, T.S.; Hudson, K.; Mertz, J.I.; Romero, J.C.; Knox, F.G.: Renal vasoconstrictive response to contrast medium. The role of sodium balance and the renin-angiotensin system. J. Lab. clin. Med. *101:* 385–391 (1983).
14 Bennett, W.M.; Plam, C.; Porter, G.A.: Drug-related syndromes in clinical nephrology. Ann. intern. Med. *87:* 582–590 (1977).
15 Boi, R.S.; Wilson, H.E.; Mazzaferri, E.I.: Hypomagnesemic hypocalcemia secondary to renal magnesium wasting: a possible consequence of high dose gentamicin therapy. Ann. intern. Med. *82:* 646–649 (1975).
16 Zaske, D.E.; Irvine, P.; Strand, L.M.; Strate, R.G.; Cipolle, R.S.; Rotschafer, J.: Wide interpatient variations in gentamicin dose requirements for geriatric patients. J. Am. med. Ass. *248:* 3122–3126 (1982).
17 Madias, N.E.; Harrington, J.T.: Platinum nephrotoxicity. Am. J. Med. *65:* 307–314 (1978).
18 Blachley, J.D.; Hill, J.B.: Renal and electrolyte disturbances associated with cisplatin. Ann. intern. Med. *95:* 628–632 (1981).
19 Gabow, P.A.; Kaehny, W.D.; Kelleher, S.D.: The spectrum of rhabdomyolysis. Medicine *61:* 141–152 (1982).

20 Conger, J.D.; Falk, S.A.: Intrarenal dynamics in the pathogenesis and prevention of acute urate nephropathy. J. clin. Invest. *59:* 786–793 (1977).
21 Cohen, L.E.; Balow, J.E.; Magrath, J.T.; Poplack, D.G.; Ziegler, J.L.: Acute tumor lysis syndrome. Am. J. Med. *68:* 486–491 (1980).
22 Sigala, J.F.; Biava, C.G.; Hulter, H.N.: Red blood cell casts in acute interstitial nephritis. Archs intern. Med. *138:* 1419–1421 (1978).
23 Handa, S.P.; Marrin, P.A.F.: Diagnostic indices in acute renal failure. Can. med. Ass. J. *96:* 78–82 (1967).
24 Espinel, C.H.: The FE_{Na} test. J. Am. med. Ass. *236:* 579–581 (1976).
25 Miller, T.R.; Anderson, R.J.; Linas, S.L.; Henrich, W.L.; Berns, A.S.; Gabow, P.A.; Schrier, R.W.: Urinary diagnostic indices in acute renal failure. A prospective study. Ann. intern. Med. *89:* 47–50 (1978).
26 Diamond, J.R.; Yoburn, D.C.: Nonoliguric acute renal failure associated with a low fractional excretion of sodium. Ann. intern. Med. *96:* 597–600 (1982).
27 Fang, L.S.T.; Sirota, R.A.; Ebert, T.H.; Lichtenstein, N.S.: Low fractional excretion of sodium with contrast media-induced acute renal failure. Archs intern. Med. *140:* 531–533 (1980).
28 Planas, M.; Wachtel, T.; Frank, H.; Henderson, L.W.: Characterization of acute renal failure in the burned patient. Archs intern. Med. *142:* 2087–2091 (1982).
29 Kelton, J.; Kelley, W.N.; Holmes, E.W.: A rapid method for the diagnosis of acute uric acid nephropathy. Archs intern. Med. *138:* 612–615 (1978).
30 Cattell, W.R.; McIntosh, C.S.; Moseley, I.F.; Fry, I.K.: Excretion urography in acute renal failure. Br. med. J. *ii:* 575–578 (1973).
31 Ellenbogen, P.H.; Scheible, F.W.; Talner, L.B.; Leopold, G.R.: Sensitivity of gray scale ultrasound in detecting urinary tract obstruction. Am. J. Roentg. *130:* 731 (1978).
32 Wasser, W.G.; Krakoff, L.R.; Haimov, M.; Glabman, S.; Mitty, H.A.: Restoration of renal function after bilateral renal artery occlusion. Archs intern. Med. *141:* 1647–1651 (1981).
33 Sraer, J.D.; Kanfer, A.; Marjac, J.; Mignow, F.; Morel-Maroger, L.; Richet, G.; Whitworth, J.: Renal biopsy in acute renal failure. Kidney int. *8:* 60–61 (1975).
34 Wilson, D.M.; Turner, D.R.; Cameron, J.S.; Ogg, C.S.; Brown, C.B.; Chantler, C.: Value of renal biopsy in acute intrinsic renal failure. Br. med. J. *ii:* 459–461 (1976).
35 Conners, A.F., Jr.; McCaffree, D.R.; Gray, B.: Evaluation of right-heart catheterization in the critically ill patient without acute myocardial infarction. New Engl. J. Med. *308:* 263–267 (1983).
36 Anderson, R.J.; Linas, S.L.; Berns, A.S.; Henrich, W.L.; Miller, T.R.; Gabow, P.R.; Schrier, R.W.: Non-oliguric acute renal failure. New Engl. J. Med. *296:* 1134–1138 (1977).
37 Warren, S.E.; Blantz, R.C.: Mannitol. Archs intern. Med. *141:* 493–497 (1981).
38 Ufferman, R.C.; Jaenike, J.R.; Freeman, R.B.; Pabico, R.C.: Effects of furosemide on low-dose mercuric chloride acute renal failure in the rat. Kidney int. *8:* 362–367 (1975).
39 Van Ypersele de Strihou, C.; Frans, A.: The pattern of respiratory compensation in chronic uremic acidosis. Nephron *7:* 37–50 (1970).
40 Wilson, R.F.; Gibson, D.; Percinel, A.K.; Ali, M.A.; Baker, G.; Le Blanc, L.P.; Lucas,

C.: Severe alkalosis in critically ill surgical patients. Archs Surg. *105:* 197–203 (1972).
41 Madias, N.E.; Levey, A.J.: Metabolic alkalosis due to absorption of 'nonabsorbable' antacids. Am. J. Med. *74:* 155–160 (1983).
42 Barton, C.H.; Vaziri, N.D.; Ness, R.L.; Saike, J.K.; Mirahmadi, K.S.: Cimetidine in the management of metabolic alkalosis induced by nasogastric drainage. Archs Surg. *114:* 70 (1979).
43 Abouna, G.M.; Veazey, P.R.; Terry, D.B.: Intravenous infusion of hydrochloric acid for treatment of severe metabolic alkalosis. Surgery *75:* 194–202 (1975).
44 Kheirbeck, A.O.; Ing, T.S.; Viol, G.W.; Vilbar, R.M.; Bansal, V.K.; Gandhi, V.C.; Geis, W.P.; Hano, J.E.: Treatment of metabolic alkalosis with hemofiltration in patients with renal insufficiency. Nephron *24:* 91–92 (1979).
45 Ayus, J.C.; Olivero, J.J.; Adrogue, H.J.L.: Alkalemia associated with renal failure. Archs intern. Med. *140:* 513–515 (1980).
46 Llach, F.; Felsenfeld, A.J.; Haussler, M.R.: The pathophysiology of altered calcium metabolism in rhabdomyolysis-induced acute renal failure. New Engl. J. Med. *305:* 117–123 (1981).
47 Torrente, A. de; Berl, T.; Cohn, P.D.; Kawamoto, E.; Herts, P.; Schrier, R.W.: Hypercalcemia of acute renal failure. Clinical significance and pathogenesis. Am. J. Med. *61:* 119–123 (1976).
48 Abel, R.M.; Beck, C.H., Jr.; Abbott, W.M.; Ryan, J.A., Jr.; Barnett, G.O.; Fischer, J.E.: Improved survival from acute renal failure after treatment with intravenous l-amino acids and glucose. New Engl. J. Med. *288:* 695 (1973).
49 Toback, F.G.: Amino acid enhancement of renal regeneration after acute tubular necrosis. Kidney int. *12:* 193–198 (1977).
50 Toback, F.G.; Teegarden, D.E.; Havener, L.J.: Amino acid mediated stimulation of renal phospholipid biosynthesis after acute tubular necrosis. Kidney int. *15:* 542–547 (1979).
51 Feinstein, E.K.; Blumenkrantz, M.J.; Healy, M.; Koffler, A.; Silberman, H.; Massry, S.G.; Kopple, J.: Clinical and metabolic responses to parenteral nutrition in acute renal failure. Medicine *60:* 124–137 (1981).
52 Capron, J.P.; Gineston, J.L.; Herve, M.A.; Braillon, A.: Metronidazole in prevention of cholestasis associated with total parenteral nutrition. Lancet *i:* 446–447 (1983).
53 Conger, J.D.: A controlled evaluation of prophylactic dialysis in posttraumatic acute renal failure. J. Trauma *15:* 1056–1063 (1975).
54 Kozeny, G.; Vertuno, L.L.; Bansal, V.K.; Hano, J.E.: Rapid access for emergency dialysis. 11th Ann. Clin. Dialysis and Transplant Forum. Am. J. Kidney Dis. *1981:* 17.
55 Zusman, R.M.; Rubin, R.H.; Cato, H.E.; Cocchetto, D.M.; Crow, J.W.; Tolkoff-Rubin, N.: Hemodialysis using prostacyclin instead of heparin as the sole antithrombotic agent. New Engl. J. Med. *304:* 934–939 (1981).
56 Pinnick, R.V.; Wiegmann, T.B.; Diederich, D.A.: Regional citrate anticoagulation for hemodialysis in the patient at high risk for bleeding. New Engl. J. Med. *308:* 258–261 (1983).
57 Gerhardt, R.E.; Abdulla, A.M.; Mach, S.J.; Hudson, J.B.: Isolated ultrafiltration in the therapy of volume overload accompanying oliguric vascular shock states. Am. Heart J. *98:* 567–571 (1979).

58 Kleinknecht, D.; Jungers, P.; Chanard, J.; Barbanel, C.; Ganavel, D.: Uremic and non-uremic complications in acute renal failure: evaluation of early and frequent dialysis on prognosis. Kidney int. *1:* 190–196 (1972).
59 Eknoyan, G.; Wacksman, S.J.; Glueck, H.I.; Will, J.J.: Platelet function in renal failure. New Engl. J. Med. *280:* 677–681 (1969).
60 Janson, P.A.; Jubelirer, S.J.; Weinstein, M.J.; Deykin, D.: Treatment in uremia with cryoprecipitate. New Engl. J. Med. *303:* 1318–1322 (1980).
61 Mannucci, P.M.; Remuzzi, G.; Pusineri, F.; Lombardi, R.; Valsecchi, C.; Mecca, G.; Zimmerman, T.: Deamino-8-*D*-arginine vasopressin shortens the bleeding time in uremia. New Engl. J. Med. *308:* 8–11 (1983).
62 Platt, R.; Polk, B.F.; Murdock, B.; Rosner, B.: Mortality associated with nosocomial urinary tract infection. New Engl. J. Med. *307:* 637–642 (1982).
63 Smith, S.W.; Seidl, L.G.; Cluff, L.E.: Studies on the epidemiology of adverse drug reactions. V. Clinical factors influencing susceptibility. Ann. intern. Med. *65:* 629–640 (1966).
64 Anderson, R.J.; Bennett, W.M.; Gambertoglio, J.G.; Schrier, R.W.: Fate of drugs in renal failure; in Brenner, Rector, The kidney; 2nd ed., pp. 2659–2708 (Saunders, Philadelphia 1981).

L.L. Vertuno, MD, Renal Section, Loyola University Stritch School of Medicine, 2160 S. 1st Street, Maywood, IL 60153 (USA)

Prog. crit. Care Med., vol. 2, pp. 151–166 (Karger, Basel 1985)

Dialytic Therapy in the Intensive Care Unit

James A. Pederson

Department of Medicine, University of Oklahoma Health Sciences Center and Veterans Administration Medical Center, Oklahoma City, Okla., USA

Introduction

Hemodialysis or peritoneal dialysis is most frequently used to manage patients with renal failure. The basic technology employed may also be usefully applied in a diverse spectrum of disorders commonly managed in the intensive care unit (ICU).

Some of the common nonazotemic problems include acid-base, electrolyte, chemical, and volumetric imbalances. Less frequent situations are hypothermia, exogenous or endogenous intoxications, and necrotizing pancreatitis. If only rapid control of intravascular volume is required, hemofiltration may be employed [18]. This modified hemodialysis procedure sieves isotonic or slightly hypotonic water from the intravascular compartment producing little alteration in the concentration of most low molecular weight serum solutes. Another modified hemodialysis procedure, hemoperfusion, passes blood over adsorbent charcoals or resins and is the method of choice for detoxification in most severe drug overdoses or poisonings or for temporary reversal of hepatic coma. Suggested priority use of these techniques in the ICU is outlined in table I.

Hemodialysis and Peritoneal Dialysis

Hemodialysis and peritoneal dialysis effectively but temporarily correct intractable heart failure, electrolyte, chemical, and acid-base disorders.

Table I. Priority of dialysis technology in critical care

Hemodialysis	Peritoneal dialysis	Hemofiltration	Hemoperfusion
Hypercatabolic renal failure	Most cases of acute renal failure	Rapid correction of refractory overhydration	Most exogenous or endogenous intoxications
	Infants or aged		
Electrolyte/chemical imbalance	Bleeding		
	Brain injury		
	Shock		
Intoxications	Cardiovascular disease		
Salicylates			
Alcohols	Uremia with peritonitis		
Metals			
	Hemorrhagic pancreatitis		
	Hypothermia		
	Refractory overhydration		
	Electrolyte/chemical imbalance		

Peritoneal dialysis is usually the method of choice for management of these problems in an acute care setting [20, 22, 26, 32]. In many instances, the refractory nature of these conditions is the result of coexisting renal failure or a catabolic rate which exceeds the capacity of normal homeostatic mechanisms, i.e., lactic acidosis, ketoacidosis, rhabdomyolysis, etc. In such situations peritoneal dialysis using a specially prepared bicarbonate-based solution (30 mEq/l) may be the best means of sustaining a physiologic buffer capacity, until the inciting problem is controlled [35, 36]. Good results with peritoneal dialysis are reported even in surgical patients during the immediate postoperative period despite fresh incisions and abdominal drains [8, 31]. Even when hemodialysis is available, peritoneal dialysis is specifically indicated where rapid hemodynamic changes are hazardous, e.g., infants, the aged, and patients with an unstable cardiovascular system or where heparin is hazardous, e.g., bleeding disorders and recent head injuries. Peritoneal dialysis is also recommended for patients refusing transfusion. Because hemodialysis requires about 200 ml/min blood flow, peritoneal dialysis may be the only possible method when severe peripheral vascular disease is present.

Table II. Guidelines for initiation of dialysis

Parameter	Concentration	Rate increase/day
Blood urea nitrogen	> 150 mg%	20–30 mg%
Creatinine	> 10 mg%	1.0 mg%
Potassium	> 6.0 mEq/l	1.0 mEq/l
Calcium	> 14.0 mg%	1.0 mg%
Uric acid	> 18 mg%	3.0 mg%
pH	< 7.1	–

As one performs a paracentesis at the bedside, a rigid stylocath or Seldinger type of temporary peritoneal catheter (Cook Inc.) is entirely satisfactory for acute peritoneal dialysis. The flexible, cuffed Tenckhoff catheter is more cumbersome to implant and offers no clear advantage for short-term use unless automated, closed-system dialysate administration equipment is available [11].

Both clinical and laboratory criteria are used in uremic patients to gauge the need for dialysis. Clinical indications include uncontrollable heart failure, pericarditis, general clinical deterioration, preparation for procedures (intravenous pyelogram or biopsy) or surgery, and hemorrhagic or infectious problems complicating conservative care. Some evidence [17] suggests that prophylactic dialysis, i.e., before uremic symptoms begin or to preclude an excessive increase in the concentration of waste materials, improves survival in acute renal failure because of fewer problems from intestinal bleeding and sepsis. Table II offers guidelines for evaluating pertinent laboratory data with regard to initiating treatment in azotemic patients. With rapidly catabolic renal failure (ΔBUN > 30 mg%/day), hemodialysis is preferred [8, 22], but peritoneal dialysis can be initiated to good effect until the staff and equipment for hemodialysis are assembled.

A number of problems reported with both hemodialysis and peritoneal dialysis are summarized in table III. Fortunately, few of these complications are common, and most are easily remedied.

The advisability of initiating peritoneal dialysis is questioned in the situations listed in table IV, but there are no absolute contraindications to the procedure [30]. When catheter placement is considered hazardous, e.g., the scarred abdomen or a history of prior peritonitis, surgical exposure of the peritoneum with direct visual placement of the catheter is prudent.

Table III. Potential complications with acute dialysis

Hemodialysis	Peritoneal dialysis	Both methods
Mechanical	Mechanical	Metabolic problems
Blood leakage[1]	Failure to drain[1]	Glucose imbalance
Extracorporeal clotting	Dialysate leak	Electrolyte imbalance
Shunt failure	Visceral perforation	Osmolar imbalance
Air embolization	Dissection abdominal wall	Alkalosis[1]/acidosis
Thermal hemolysis	Scrotal edema	Hypermagnesemia
Osmolar hemolysis	Wound rupture	Neurologic
	Catheter loss	Convulsions
	Abdominal pain[1]	Disequilibrium
		Dementia
		Neuropathy
		Nausea/vomiting
		Muscle cramps
Inflammatory	Inflammatory	Inflammatory
Cannulation abscesses	Cannulation abscesses	Pyrogen reactions
Endovasculitis	Peritonitis	
Access pseudoaneurysms	Peritoneal fibrosis	
Cardiovascular	Cardiovascular	Cardiovascular
Steal syndrome	Congestive failure	Hypotension[1]
Hyperdynamic heart failure		Arrhythmia[1]
Endocarditis		Cardiac arrest
Pulmonary	Pulmonary	
Functional hypoxemia[1]	Atelectasis[1]	
	Pleural effusions	
	Pneumonia/bronchitis	
Metabolic		
Hypercalcemia		
Hypermagnesemia		
Hemorrhage		

[1] 5% acute procedures.

Table IV. Relative risk factors with peritoneal dialysis

Postoperative abdomen	Abdominal wall burns
Prior peritoneal dialysis	Abdominal wall ostomies
Abdominal wall abscesses	Generalized cachexia
Abdominal wall cellulitis	

Other common concerns about peritoneal dialysis include failure of the catheter to drain properly and the evaluation or treatment of peritonitis. Approaches to these problems are outlined in tables V and VI. Traditional treatment of dialysis-related peritonitis, consisting of rapid peritoneal lavage, requires large volumes of peritoneal dialysate containing antibiotic and is adapted from the surgical approach to postoperative peritonitis. Although usually satisfactory, the efficiency of this lavage technique has been challenged by experiences with peritonitis in continuous ambulatory peritoneal dialysis (CAPD) programs. The CAPD data indicate more rapid bacteriologic resolution of the peritonitis, if an antibiotic-containing peritoneal dialysis solution is permitted to dwell within the peritoneal cavity for 6 h

Table V. Peritoneal dialysate drainage failure

Problem	Causes	Diagnosis	Management
Malposition	Preperitoneal location	Subcutaneous swelling and slow inflow	Reposition
	Omental entrapment or uneven distribution of dialysate	Pain in mid or upper abdomen with aspiration Return increases with position change	
Catheter obstruction	Tissue, blood, fibrin obstructing lumen of catheter due to excessively large holes in the catheter	Dye injection under image intensifier or inspection after removal	Replace catheter, Obtain hemostasis in abdominal wall before puncture
	May have had asymptomatic infection with prior peritoneal dialysis	Pain with infusion, cloudy or bloody return, dye injection showing entrapment	Replace catheter under direct vision Culture Add antibiotic systemically and to dialysate
Constipation	Functional and reversible	Suspicion from flat plate abdomen or rectal examination	Bowel stimulant or purgative
Loss of siphon	Failure to obliterate air space, inadvertent installation of air into abdominal cavity	Abdomen soft, flow increases with manual compression of patient's abdomen or repositioning	Advance catheter or add more dialysate to abdominal volume to displace the air

Table VI. Diagnosis and treatment of peritonitis during peritoneal dialysis

Suspect if:
Peritoneal fluid becomes cloudy with or without:
  Fever or chills
  Abdominal pain and/or tenderness
  Diarrhea, nausea, or vomiting
  Peripheral polynuclear leukocytosis

Diagnosis if cloudy peritoneal fluid shows:
Organisms on gram stain with or without:
  100 polynuclear leukocytes/mm^3
  4.0 g% protein
Or culture reports identify bacterial agents

Treatment advised
Continue exchanges
  Rapid lavage exchanges times 3
  Heparin (1,000 U/l) added
  Reduce lavage volume for comfort if necessary
  Change to 4- to 6-hour dwell times with antibiotic containing dialysate solutions and continue until solution sterile for 4 days
Antibiotics per stain and culture
  Intraperitoneal, initially use broadspectrum drug or combinations
  Systemic, if severe or symptoms continue more than 24 h
  Change to specific antibiotics per culture results
Monitor antibiotic levels in blood and peritoneum
Culture peritoneal fluid daily
Reassess peritoneal integrity and fungal cultures, if signs or symptoms fail to indicate probable resolution within 3 days or if peritoneal cultures report mixed enteric organisms

[41]. The differences between lavage and long-dwell treatment of peritonitis are presently attributed to adverse effects on peritoneal phagocytic activity by repeated exposure to acidic and hyperosmolar peritoneal dialysis solutions [34]. Concentrations of selected antibiotics used to load the initial long-dwell exchange and each subsequent sustaining exchange for the intraperitoneal treatment of peritonitis are shown in table VII [40, 41].

Several reviews [1, 3, 5, 10] recommend adjustments in the dose of systemic medications in both acute and chronic dialysis. In general, either the frequency or dose size is adjusted in the dialysis patient receiving medications normally excreted in the urine. Table VIII offers guidelines for use of selected antibiotics in anephric patients, as well as those with less severe

Table VII. Intraperitoneal antibiotics for treatment of peritonitis [adapted from refs. 40 and 41]

	Loading dose per liter dialysate	Sustaining dose per liter dialysate
Initial drugs		
Cephalothin	500 mg	250 mg
Tobramycin	1.35 mg/kg	8 mg
Culture-specific alternatives		
Ampicillin	500 mg	50 mg
Cloxacillin	1,000 mg	100 mg
Ticarcillin	1,000 mg	100 mg
Septra (SMZ/TMP)	400/80 mg	25/5 mg
Clindamycin	300 mg	50 mg
Amikacin	250 mg	50 mg
Penicillin	1,000,000 U	50,000 U

renal insufficiency and those requiring treatment with either peritoneal dialysis or hemodialysis. Intraperitoneal antibiotics may be desired during treatment of systemic infections. Maintaining intraperitoneal antibiotic concentrations in the dialysate is intended to prevent dialytic depletion of systemic antibiotic levels. Drug augmentation is also required after hemodialysis to restore adequate systemic concentrations which are reduced by each treatment. The antibiotic schedule presented is based on a reduced dosage given at the frequency usually prescribed for normal patients after administering an appropriate systemic loading dose. The standard dose multiplied by the anephric dose fraction gives the adjusted dose for anephric patients. The dose fraction with lesser degrees of renal failure is approximated by the following equations [33]:

$$\text{males: dose fraction} = \frac{140 - \text{age}}{\text{serum creatinine (mg\%)}} \times 0.01.$$

females: dose fraction = 90% of above equation.

In all cases, serum concentration of the drug should be followed and appropriate adjustments in dosage made to obtain the desired level of antibacterial activity. Several other points must also be remembered: (1) some antibacterial agents are ineffective in renal failure, i.e., nitrofurantoin, nal-

Table VIII. Guidelines for antimicrobial use with renal insufficiency and dialysis [adapted from ref. 10]

Antimicrobials	Usual normal range per day	Fraction normal dose in anuria	Dose adjustment with renal insufficiency	Peritoneal dialysis mg/l dialysate	Hemodialysis adjustment per treatment mg/kg
Aminoglycosides					
Amikacin	1.5 g	0.03	give usual first dose	10	7–8
Gentamicin	180–350 mg	0.03	daily dose = normal	5–8	1–1.5
Kanamycin	1–1.5 g	0.03	daily dose times percent	10	7–8
Tobramycin	180–350 mg	0.04	normal renal function or dose fraction; repeat drug assays,	5–8	1–1.5
Vancomycin	1–2 g	0.03	monitor patient for	15	0–0.15
Cefazolin	1–4 g	0.07	toxicity and	15–25	15
Trimethoprim/			for response		
sulfamethoxazole	2–8 g			unknown	
Penicillin G	1–20 million U	0.01	give usual first dose, do not exceed high dose	10,000 to 50,000 U	1–5 million U
Ampicillin	1–8 g	0.09	adjusted for percent renal function or dose fraction, repeat drug	50	6–10
Carbenicillin	6–40 g	0.07	assay, adjust dose,	200	28
Cephalothin	2–8 g	0.20	monitor for toxicity and response	25–50	5–25
Erythromycin	1–4 g	0.40	no adjustment needed	none	none
Clindamycin	0.6–1.2 g	0.92	no adjustment needed	10	none
Chloramphenicol	1–6 g	0.60	no adjustment needed	none	8–15
Oxacillin	1–12 g	0.50	usual dose, assay and adjust	50	15
Methicillin	4–12 g	0.10	usually avoided in	100	15
Tetracycline	–	–	renal insufficiency	not recommended	
Amphotericin B	0.5–50 mg	0.60	begin with standard daily dose adjusted for	1.5	daily dose
Ethambutol	0.8–1.5 g	0.30	percent renal function or dose fractions;	none	15–25
INH (slow)	200–300 mg	0.25	patient must be followed closely for renal, hepatic, optic, acoustic, and hematologic toxicity;	none	1–2
INH (fast)	300–500 mg	0.75	assay if possible and follow response	none	2–4
Rifampin	600 mg	1.00	no adjustment needed	none	daily dose

idixic acid, and methenamine; (2) others inhibit anabolism and promote azotemia or diabetes insipidus, i.e., the tetracyclines except deoxycycline; (3) the penicillins and moxalactam antibiotics may potentiate a bleeding diathesis, especially in azotemic patients due to drug-induced platelet dysfunction [2, 37]; (4) the penicillins also contain sodium or potassium cations which may lead to electrolyte or fluid imbalances – sodium ranges from 3.1 mEq of oxacillin to 2.0 mEq/million units of penicillin G; (5) some drugs are best avoided entirely in renal failure due to toxicity, i.e., polymyxin B, colistin, and cephaloridine, and (6) drug combinations of aminoglycosides and penicillins, including carbenicillin, lead to subtherapeutic concentrations of the aminoglycoside due to amine formation with the combination.

Peritoneal Dialysis for Hemorrhagic Pancreatitis

Systemic absorption of pancreatic products, i.e., amylase, vasoactive peptides, lysosomes, methemalbumin, etc., is thought, in part, responsible for some of the symptoms and mortality noted in severe pancreatitis [13, 24]. Several experimental and clinical studies, comprehensively reviewed by *Glenn and Nolph* [14], note survival in 82 of 104 patients with acute pancreatitis treated by peritoneal dialysis. Specific indications for use of this technique in acute pancreatitis do not exist. Most reported cases are last resort attempts after other supportive modalities failed.

As described by *Ranson* et al. [27], the lavage mixture for acute pancreatitis is a typical isotonic peritoneal solution containing 1.5 g % dextrose, 4 mEq potassium, 500 U heparin, and 125 mg ampicillin per liter. Treatment begins within 48 h of admission, cycling 2-liter volumes of the solution per hour. Reported benefits include shorter intensive care time, earlier oral feeding, and shorter hospital stays. Addition of albumin to the lavage solution is reported to further improve survival in experimental studies [19].

Peritoneal Dialysis in Hypothermia

Hypothermia can follow extended water immersion in warm weather as well as general exposure in winter. Hypothermia depresses the sensorium, the medullary respiratory center, and the cardiovascular system [6].

Although systemic illness increases the mortality rate from hypothermia, the death rate is directly related to the degree of cooling which ranges from 17 to 34% at 32.2 °C compared to 4% above 32.2 °C [43]. Complications after rewarming including acidosis, coagulopathy, and renal or hepatic failure also contribute to the overall mortality. Death due to hypothermia per se, however, is uniformally attributed to refractory ventricular fibrillation at temperatures below 20 °C [6, 29].

The prognosis in hypothermia improves with rewarming and good supportive care [43]. At temperatures above 32.2 °C, surface rewarming, slowly at room temperatures for the elderly and more rapidly, using hot baths, in younger patients, is considered acceptable treatment [16, 23]. Core rewarming is strongly recommended at all ages with temperatures below 30 °C, or when the duration of hypothermia exceeds 12 h or when complications such as cardiac irritability, diabetes, uremia, acidosis, sepsis, embolization, myocardial infarction, bleeding, and trauma are present [16, 23, 28, 38, 39].

Either partial cardiac bypass [23, 38, 39] or peritoneal dialysis [16, 28] are the preferred methods of core rewarming in current use. Peritoneal dialysis has the advantages of the wider availability, easy initiation, and freedom from the bleeding problems reported with partial bypass.

Rewarming is conducted by routine peritoneal techniques using either a standard isotonic, potassium-free dialysate (1.5%) or lactated Ringer's solution alternated with 5% dextrose in water. The solutions are heated to 43 °C. Using 2-liter volumes cycled at 30-min intervals, rewarming is usually completed after 2 h (6–8 passes) [28]. Additional support is directed to correction of hypotension, respiratory insufficiency, hypoxia, drug intoxication, and coexisting primary medical problems.

Dialysis Techniques in Drug or Chemical Intoxication

Acute drug or chemical poisoning is a significant problem in many countries. Most patients admitted to hospitals are not severely poisoned, and their overall mortality rate is low: usually less than 1% [9]. Most deaths from overdoses and poisons occur prior to reaching the hospital or in those patients admitted with grade IV coma where death rates range from 5 to 26% [4, 44].

Aside from supportive care, treatment of the poisoned patient is directed at prevention of complications and, if possible, optimum elimination of the offending compound from the body. Renal clearance of only a few drugs, i.e., salicylate, phenobarbital, and amphetamines, is enhanced by diuresis and alteration of the urine pH. In the past, both peritoneal dialysis and hemodialysis were used to enhance elimination of some additional drugs and poisons. Today, except for intoxications with alcohols (methyl, ethyl, isopropyl, chloralhydrate, and ethylene glycol), salicylates, and several metals, where hemodialysis remains the method of choice for acute detoxification, hemoperfusion with either charcoal or a nonionic resin (Amberlite) offers far superior drug extraction for a greater number of compounds [7, 25, 42].

Table IX compares the various methods of enhancing clearance of selected drugs from the body. Charcoal binds both polar and nonpolar drugs and is the device most widely used in clinical overdoses. The resin columns are more specific binders of nonpolar lipophilic compounds and thus are less useful in situations where the agent causing the overdose is unknown or the possibility of multiple intoxicants exists. Another difference between the two types of devices is a more rapid saturation of adsorptive surfaces on the charcoal. Other clinical problems encountered with either type of hemoperfusion include hypoglycemia, hypocalcemia, thrombocytopenia, and a tendency to cause hypotension. The latter appears to result from adsorption of circulating sympathomimetic agents from the blood [15]. Similar phenomena explain the decreased glucose and calcium concentrations which are easily prevented or treated by intravenous infusion. Physical trapping of platelets is thought responsible for the thrombocytopenia. This usually reverses several hours after the procedure is complete and is seldom responsible for bleeding problems.

Neither dialysis nor hemoperfusion is intended to supplant good cardiovascular and pulmonary supportive care of the intoxicated patient. The vast majority of all overdose patients continue to be well managed without extracorporeal detoxification [21]. Criteria for considering the use of hemodialysis or hemoperfusion in a given patient are presented in table X [42]. If either hemoperfusion or dialysis are elected, initiation as soon after exposure as possible improves the possibility that a significant clinical response will be noted during treatment. Few drugs have been extensively studied clinically, but, based on the available literature, those compounds purported to be adsorbed by hemoperfusion are shown in table XI. It must be remembered that clinical responses may not coincide with serum or whole-blood drug concentrations, especially among drugs which are tightly protein bound or which are lipophilic.

Table IX. Dialysis techniques and comparative drug clearances [adapted from ref. 25]

Drugs	Ingested dose g	Serum level mg%	Induced diuresis ml/min	Peritoneal dialysis ml/min	Aqueous hemodialysis ml/min	Charcoal hemoperfusion ml/min	Resin hemoperfusion ml/min	Quantity drug removed g
Barbiturates								
Long-acting	5.0	8.0	17	10	15–30	44–300	280–300	1.5–6.6
Short-acting	5.0	8.0	17	10	50–80	44–300	280–300	1.5–6.6
Doriden	0.15/kg	3.0	18	5	20–80	66–200	140–300	0.3–1.8
Meprobamate	8–16	12.0	30	11	62–100	85–186	no data	1.5–4.5
Placidyl	10	7.0	23	18	64	114–140	184–287	1.5–2.5
Noludar	6	4.0	10	20	23	152–275	no data	2.0
Quaalude	120/kg	10.0	no data	7	20–80	150–275	195–200	10.0
Methanol	6,000	50–100	8	25	100–200	59–78	no data	80
Salicylate	0.3–0.5 kg	70.0	11	25	100	57–116	27–74	11–15
Acetominophen	15	200.0		3	120	125–190	no data	0.7–5.0
Digoxin	?	3.0 ng/ml	0	8	10–40	30–90	50–143	100–200 ng
Theophylline	2–24	2.0	21–60	no data	20–40	25–163	225	1.8–22

Table X. When to consider dialysis or hemoperfusion for drug intoxications [adapted from ref. 42]

1	Severe intoxication with abnormal vital signs, hypotension, apnea, hypothermia
2	Ingestion of a probable lethal dose
3	Potentially fatal blood level of drug
4	Impaired function of normal excretory routes for the drug (liver, kidney)
5	Presence of circulating toxins metabolizing to more noxious agents (methyl alcohol)
6	Clinical deterioration under good management
7	Drugs producing prolonged coma with increased attendant risks from pneumonia or sepsis
8	Underlying respiratory disease increasing the hazards of coma
9	Aspiration pneumonitis
10	Agents with delayed toxicity (paraquat, *Amanita phalloides,* acetominophen)

Table XI. Drugs reportedly adsorbed by hemoperfusion [adapted from ref. 42]

Barbiturates

Nonbarbiturate hypnotics

Sedatives, tranquilizers
- Placidyl
- Doriden
- Noludar
- Quaalude
- Phenothiazines
- Meprobamate

Antidepressants
- Amphetamines
- Tricyclic drugs (Tofranil, Elavil)
- Secondary amines (Pertofrane)

Analgesics
- Salicylates
- Acetominophen

Anticancer agents
- Methotrexate

Biologic toxins
- *Amanita phalloides*
- Paraquat
- Organophosphates

Cardiovascular agents
- Digoxin
- Procainamide
- Theophylline

Endogenous compounds
- Ammonia
- Bilirubin
- Thyroxin
- Triiodothyronine
- Insulin
- Growth hormone
- Epinephrine

Solvents
- Carbon tetrachloride

Hemoperfusion in Hepatic Coma

The similarities between renal failure and hepatic failure led to trials of dialytic treatment in hepatic coma. The cause of hepatic encephalopathy is uncertain. Temporary reversal of hepatic coma associated with reduced blood ammonia and plasma phenolic amino acid concentrations is reported with charcoal hemoperfusion [12]. The procedure, however, does not appear to alter the mortality from hepatic failure, and additional problems, including hypotension, thrombocytopenia, bleeding, and hypothermia, are common during hemoperfusion. At present, hemoperfusion seems to have a limited role in the treatment of hepatic coma.

References

1 Anderson, R.J., et al.: Clinical use of drugs in renal failure (Thomas, Springfield 1976).

2 Andrassy, K.; Llach, F.; Ritz, E.: Penicillin induced hemorrhage – a common complication of acute renal failure (Abstract). Kidney int. *23:* 200 (1983).

3 Appel, G.B.; Neu, H.C.: The use of drugs in renal failure. Disease-a-Month *25:* No. 11 (1979).

4 Arieff, A.I.; Friedman, E.A.: Coma following non-narcotic drug overdosage: management of 208 adult patients. Am. J. med. Sci. *266:* 405–426 (1973).

5 Bennett, W.M.; Singer, I.; Golper, T.; Feig, P.; Coggins, C.J.: Guidelines for drug therapy in renal failure. Ann. intern. Med. *86:* 754–783 (1977).

6 Black, P.R.; Van Devanter, S.; Cohn, L.H.: Effects of hypothermia on systemic and organ system metabolism and function. J. surg. Res. *20:* 49–63 (1976).

7 Burgess, E.D.; Blair, A.D.; Cutler, R.E.: Dialysis and hemoperfusion of drugs and poisons. Curr. Nephrol. *5:* 309–332 (1982).

8 Cameron, J.S., et al.: Peritoneal dialysis in hypercatabolic acute renal failure. Lancet *i:* 1188 (1969).

9 Clemmesen, C.; Nisson, E.: Therapeutic trends in the treatment of barbiturate poisoning: the Scandinavian method. Clin. Pharmacol. Ther. *2:* 220–229 (1961).

10 Cutler, R.E.; Krichman, K.H.; Blair, A.D.: Pharmacology of drugs in renal failure. Current Nephrol. *3:* 397–435 (1979).

11 Gastaldi, L.; Baratelli, L.; Cinquepalmi, M.; Naseinbene, E.; Piatti, L.: Peritoneal dialysis. Lancet *ii:* 845 (1978).

12 Gelfand, M.C.; Winchester, J.F.; Knepshield, J.H.; Cohan, S.L.; Schreiner, G.E.: Biochemical correlates of reversal of hepatic coma with charcoal hemoperfusion. Trans. Am. Soc. artif. internal Organs *24:* 239–242 (1978).

13 Geokas, M.C.; Olsen, H.; Carmack, C.; Rinkerknecht, H.: Studies on ascites and pleural effusion in acute pancreatitis (Abstract). Gastroenterology *58:* 950 (1970).

14 Glenn, L.D.; Nolph, K.D.: Treatment of acute pancreatitis with peritoneal dialysis. Peritoneal Dial. Bull. *2:* 63–68 (1982).

15 Horres, C.R.; Hill, J.B.; Ellis, F.W.: The adsorption of sympathomimetic agents by activated carbon hemoperfusion. Trans. Am. Soc. artif. internal Organs *22:* 425–430 (1976).
16 Johnson, L.A.: Accidental hypothermia: peritoneal dialysis. J. Am. Coll. Emerg. Physns *6:* 556 (1977).
17 Kleinknecht, D.; Jungers, P.; Chanard, J.; Barbanel, C.; Ganeval, D.; Rondon-Nuccte, M.: Factors influencing immediate prognosis in acute renal failure with special reference to prophylactic hemodialysis. Adv. Nephrol. *1:* 207–230 (1974).
18 Kramer, P.; Kaufhold, G.; Gronel, T.J.; Wigger, W.; Rieger, J.; Malthaei, D.; Stokke, T.; Burchard, H.; Scheler, F.: Management of anuric intensive care patients with arteriovenous hemofiltration. Int. J. artif. Organs *3:* 225–230 (1980).
19 Lankisch, P.G.; Hoop, H.; Winchkler, K.; Schmidt, H.: Continuous peritoneal dialysis as treatment of acute pancreatitis in the rat. I. Effect on length and rate of survival. Dig. Dis. Sci. *24:* 111–122 (1979).
20 Lindeman, R.D.; Papper, S.: Therapy of fluid and electrolyte disorders. Ann. intern. Med. *82:* 64–70 (1975).
21 Lorch, J.A.; Garella, S.: Hemoperfusion to treat intoxications. Ann. intern. Med. *91:* 301 (1979).
22 Merrill, J.P.: Dialysis in acute renal failure; in Drukker, Parsons, Maher, Replacement of renal function by dialysis, p. 328 (Nijhoff, The Hague 1968).
23 O'Keefe, K.M.: Accidental hypothermia: a review of 62 cases. J. Am. Coll. Emerg. Physns *6:* 491 (1977).
24 Pickford, I.R.; Blackett, R.L.; McMahon, M.J.: Early assessment of severity of acute pancreatitis using peritoneal lavage. Br. med. J. *ii:* 1377 (1977).
25 Pond, S.; Rosenberg, J.; Benowitz, N.L.; Takki, S.: Pharmacokinetics of haemoperfusion for drug overdose. Clin. Pharmacokinet. *4:* 329–354 (1979).
26 Raja, R.M.; Krasneff, S.O.; Moros, J.G.; Kramer, M.S.; Rosenbaum, R.L.: Repeated peritoneal dialysis in the treatment of heart failure. J. Am. med. Ass. *213:* 2268–2269 (1970).
27 Ranson, L.; Rifkind, K.M.; Turner, J.W.: Prognostic signs and non-operative peritoneal lavage in acute pancreatitis. Surgery Gynec. Obstet. *143:* 209–219 (1976).
28 Reuter, J.B.; Parker, R.A.: Peritoneal dialysis in the management of hypothermia. J. Am. med. Ass. *240:* 2289–2290 (1978).
29 Stine, R.J.: Accidental hypothermia. J. Am. Coll. Emerg. Physns *6:* 143 (1977).
30 Tenckhoff, H.: Peritoneal dialysis today: a new look. Nephron *12:* 420–436 (1974).
31 Tzamaloukas, A.H.; Garella, S.; Chazan, J.A.: Peritoneal dialysis for acute renal failure after major abdominal surgery. Archs Surg. *106:* 639–643 (1973).
32 Valk, T.W.: Peritoneal dialysis in acute renal failure: analysis of outcome and complications. Dialysis Transplant. *9:* 49 (1980).
33 Van Scoy, R.E.; Wilson, W.R.: Antimicrobial agents in patients with renal insufficiency. Mayo Clin. Proc. *52:* 704–710 (1977).
34 Vas, S.I.; Duwe, A.; Weatherhead, J.: Natural defense mechanisms of the peritoneum: studies on the effect of peritoneal fluid (dianeal) and polymorphonuclear cells; in Atkins, Thomson, Fanell, Peritoneal dialysis, pp. 41–51 (Churchill Livingstone, New York 1981).

35 Vaziri, N.D.; Ness, R.; Wellikson, L.; Barton, C.; Green, N.: Bicarbonate buffered peritoneal dialysis, an effective adjunct in the treatment of lactic acidosis. Am. J. Med. *67:* 392–396 (1979).
36 Warner, A.; Vaziri, N.D.: Treatment of lactic acidosis. Sth. med. J. *74:* 841–847 (1981).
37 Weitekamp, M.R.; Aber, R.C.: Prolonged bleeding times and bleeding diathesis associated with moxalactam administration. J. Am. med. Ass. *249:* 69–71 (1983).
38 Welton, D.E.; Mattox, K.L.; Miller, R.R.; Petmecku, F.F.: Treatment of profound hypothermia. J. Am. med. Ass. *240:* 2291–2292 (1978).
39 Wickstrom, P.; Ruiz, E.; Lilja, G.P.; Hinterkopf, J.P.; Haglin, J.J.: Accidental hypothermia: core rewarming with partial bypass. Am. J. Surg. *131:* 622–625 (1976).
40 William, P.: Loading doses of antibiotics for the treatment of peritonitis. Peritoneal Dial. Bull. *1:* 45 (1981).
41 Williams, P.; Khanna, R.; Vas, S.; Layne, S.; Pantalony, D.; Oreopoulous, D.G.: The treatment of peritonitis in patients on CAPD: to lavage or not. Peritoneal Dial. Bull. *1:* 14–17 (1980).
42 Winchester, J.F.: Dialysis and hemoperfusion for drug overdose. Clin. Pharmacokinet. *4:* 762 (1979).
43 Weyman, A.E.; Greenbaum, D.M.; Grace, W.J.: Accidental hypothermia in an alcoholic population. Am. J. Med. *56:* 13–21 (1974).
44 Young, R.K.B.; Campbell, D.; Reid, J.M.; Telfer, A.B.M.: Respiratory intensive care: a 10 year survey. Br. med. J. *i:* 307–310 (1974).

James A. Pederson, MD, Director Dialysis (111G1),
Veterans Administration Medical Center, 921 NE 13th Street,
Oklahoma City, OK 73104 (USA)

Prog. crit. Care Med., vol. 2, pp. 167–174 (Karger, Basel 1985)

Acute Upper Gastrointestinal Bleeding: Therapy and Prophylaxis

Robert A. Rankin

Department of Gastrointestinal Endoscopy, University of Oklahoma Health Sciences Center, Oklahoma City, Okla., USA

Introduction

Successful treatment of acute upper gastrointestinal bleeding must first be directed to a quick assessment of blood loss followed by stabilization of the patient's circulation. Once the patient is stabilized, localization of the bleeding site and definitive therapy should be initiated. Overall management of the patient seems best accomplished by a vigorous team approach. The team should be headed by the attending physician, and where available include a gastroenterologist, a radiologist and a surgeon.

Although bleeding stops spontaneously in approximately 80% of patients who present with a history of upper gastrointestinal bleeding, there are a number of patients who remain at high risk for continued or recurrent bleeding [2, 5]. These would include patients with peptic ulcer disease in whom a visible vessel is seen at the time of endoscopy, and the group of patients who are bleeding from esophageal or gastric varices. These patients will benefit the most from early diagnostic and therapeutic maneuvers. Remember, in patients with continued bleeding, the most common cause of dying is bleeding to death.

Early Patient Assessment

Initial evaluation is directed at estimating the severity of bleeding and the amount of blood loss. While shock indicates massive and usually ongoing blood loss, mild postural hypotension and tachycardia usually indicate a 20% decrease in circulating blood volume. Melenic stools can persist for 3 or 4 days after active bleeding has stopped, but, when accompanied with unstable vital signs, should indicate ongoing blood loss.

Interestingly, a complete blood count may be the least sensitive indicator of acute blood loss. Massive bleeding may have occurred in spite of a normal hemoglobin or hematocrit depending on the patient's original blood count and the extent of extravascular to intravascular fluid shifts. Hemodilution is only one-half complete at 8 h, so other parameters such as postural hypotension must always be taken into account.

Initial Therapy

General Measures

Although specific bleeding lesions may require different forms of therapy, many general measures are common to all causes of upper gatrointestinal bleeding. Blood should immediately be drawn for a complete blood count, white blood cell morphology, prothrombin time, platelet count, partial thromboplastin time, electrolytes, blood urea nitrogen, and creatinine. The patient's blood should be typed and cross-matched 4–6 units of whole blood or packed red blood cells. Fluid resuscitation and maintenance of adequate intravascular volume with crystalloid solutions, such as isotonic saline and Ringer's lactate or colloid solutions, such as albumin and plasma protein fraction, must be accomplished in all patients. A large-bore needle should be inserted for administration of isotonic fluids and blood. A separate central venous pressure line is recommended in the presence of shock.

A large-bore rubber or polyvinyl tube should be inserted into the stomach, preferably through the mouth. Aspiration through the tube is used as a means of detecting fresh or old blood, cleaning the stomach for diagnostic procedures, and for ice-water or ice-saline lavage. If no blood is aspirated through the tube, the gastric aspirate should be checked for bile. Since some duodenal ulcers bleed without blood refluxing into the stomach, the absence of blood and bile does not rule out an actively bleeding duodenal ulcer. This will occur in only a minority of actively bleeding duodenal ulcers. Large-bore tubes should not be left in place for prolonged periods of time, since they promote gastroesophageal reflux and pulmonary aspiration.

Transfusions

When blood becomes available for transfusion, it should be used in preference to or in addition to the isotonic solutions. Since many patients require replacement of several blood components (erythrocytes, clotting factors and platelets) as well as volume, fresh whole blood is convenient when it can be obtained. However, most blood banks at this time supply only blood components, such as packed cells and fresh frozen plasma. Packed red blood cells are more appropriate in stable patients, people who are bleeding at a slow rate and in those with congestive heart failure. One unit of packed red cell or whole blood should raise the hemoglobin approximately 1 g/dl or the hematocrit 3–4%. There is a tendency to undertransfuse patients based on the initial hemoglobin or hematocrit obtained during a time when hemodilution had not occurred. With moderate to severe hypotension, a unit of whole blood or packed cells should be given in a 15- to 30-min period and continued until the blood pressure and pulse return towards normal. If a central venous pressure line is in place, the pressure should be maintained around 12 cm of water. One should try to maintain a hemoglobin of 10 g/dl or a hematocrit of 30% in most patients, although in those with severe cardiovascular or chronic lung disease, it may be best to maintain their hemoglobin and hematocrit at higher values. Fresh frozen plasma can be given to patients in whom the prothrombin time or partial thromboplasin time are elevated and in whom whole blood is not available for transfusion.

Localization of the Bleeding Site

Hematemesis or bloody nasogastric aspirate indicates upper gastrointestinal bleeding. Even in patients who present with a history of melena, port wine colored stools, or bright red blood per rectum, a nasogastric or oral gastric tube should still be introduced to check for any evidence of upper gastrointestinal bleeding. In profound upper gastrointestinal bleeding with rapid intestinal transit, even bright red blood per rectum may indicate an upper gastrointestinal bleeding site. Also, an occasional duodenal ulcer may not reflux blood back through the pylorus. If bile is present in the gastric aspirate and no blood is detected, then either the bleeding is from a lower gastrointestinal site, active upper gastrointestinal bleeding has stopped or an ulcer near the ligament of Treitz is the site of active bleeding.

The history and physical examination may suggest a particular diagnosis but should not affect the diagnostic sequence of events. Even in patients with known esophageal varices from alcoholic liver disease, only about 40% are found to be bleeding from their varices. Bleeding from ulcers or gastritis will be found to be as frequent as bleeding from varices. On the other hand, patients with varices from nonalcoholic cirrhosis tend to bleed from their varices much more commonly than from peptic ulcer disease, and gastritis is rare. Although bleeding following prolonged and forceful vomiting suggests a mucosal tear (Mallory-Weiss), only about half of patients with this lesion present with a typical history.

Specific localization of a lesion should take place in the following order:

Esophagogastroduodenoscopy

Endoscopy is the primary method for localization of upper gastrointestinal hemorrhage with a diagnostic accuracy of 85–95% and a very low morbidity and mortality. If the patient stops bleeding and becomes hemodynamically stable, endoscopy should be performed within the initial 24 h of hospitalization. In patients with continued bleeding, adequate visualization may be impaired and thus the endoscopy should be performed preferably only after gastric lavage shows a pinkish return. A lesion will sometimes be missed at endoscopy because of the pool of blood and clots often found on the greater curve of the body and fundus. Although the patient can be repositioned during the procedure, sometimes it is necessary to repeat the endoscopy at a later date. Certain therapeutic maneuvers may be accomplished at the time of endoscopy and these will be discussed later in regard to individual lesions.

Abdominal Angiography

When bleeding is brisk or the stomach too full of blood for the endoscopist to localize the bleeding lesion, abdominal angiography can be performed. Success with this technique is most likely when the rate of bleeding is at least 0.5–1.0 ml/min at the time of procedure. Although this procedure will often define bleeding from gastritis, Mallory-Weiss tear or ulcers, it can only demonstrate that varices are present. Varices can be seen during the venous phase of arteriography, but a specific bleeding site from a varix is seldom documented.

Upper Gastrointestinal Barium Radiography

Barium studies have little if any usefulness in the early evaluation of the patient with upper gastrointestinal bleeding. Superficial mucosal lesions such as gastritis and Mallory-Weiss tear are not detected by routine barium studies. If blood is present in the stomach, it can hide lesions or sometimes be mistaken for carcinoma of the stomach. Even if a lesion is seen, the X-ray cannot confirm whether this is the bleeding lesion. Also, barium will interfere with both angiography and endoscopy.

Specific Therapy

Fortunately, bleeding ceases spontaneously in approximately 80% of patient with an upper gastrointestinal bleed. In these patients medical management should be started and continued until healing of the lesion occurs or surgery can be done. Since specific therapy is directed at different lesions, a correct diagnosis is mandatory. With the advent of therapeutic endoscopy and radiography, many things are possible today that were not available just a few years ago.

Recently, endoscopy has been used to cauterize bleeding lesions, direct a laser beam at a bleeding site and inject varices with sclerosing agents to stop active bleeding. Arteriography can be used to infuse vasopressin into the main artery feeding the bleeding lesion, infuse autologous clot or gel foam in an artery supplying a bleeding lesion or may be used through a percutaneous transhepatic approach to stop bleeding from esophageal varices. When bleeding continues, surgery plays an important role in patients with lesions amenable to surgery.

Esophagitis

Although esophagitis is not a common cause of a major upper gastrointestinal bleeding, bleeding may occur. The diagnosis should be made endoscopically and biopsies and brushings may be required if there is any suggestion that an infectious agent such as *Candida albicans* is the cause. Therapy should be medical and consist of a strict antireflux regimen. The head of the bed must be elevated 15–20 cm and cimetidine or ranitidine with or without antacids should be used to reduce the acid reflux into the esophagus.

Varices

The treatment of bleeding esophageal varices may include intraarterial superior mesenteric artery vasopressin infusion, intravenous vasopressin infusion, tamponade with a Sengstaken-Blakemore triple-lumen tube, endoscopic sclerosis of the varices or surgery. Surgery may attempt to decompress the varices or to transect the varices at the gastroesophageal junction with reanastomosis of the esophagus and stomach. The latter procedure is only performed on an emergency basis and portal decompressive surgery is often needed at a later date.

Peripheral venous vasopressin infusion is probably preferable as the first mode of therapy. Initially, 0.4 units/min (100 units in 250 ml of D_5W produces 0.4 units vasopressin/ml) is infused until bleeding is controlled and then the dosage slowly tapered down over the next 24–48 h. Higher levels of vasopressin (up to 1 unit/min) may be required for a short period of time. Since coronary artery vasoconstriction and decreased cardiac output can occur, cardiac parameters must be closely monitored. Infusion of vasopressin into the artery supplying the bleeding site can be tried if the peripheral venous route does not work, although it is doubtful that this route is any more effective.

In a patient who is exsanguinating, the Sengstaken-Blakemore tube should be used to help immediately control bleeding [7, 8]. The tube must first be checked for leaks and an 18 French nasogastric tube attached at the top end of the esophageal balloon. After the tube is passed and the gastric balloon is located in the stomach, it is inflated with 250 ml of air and the inlet clamped. Placement of the tube should be confirmed radiographically. Manual traction is applied to pull the gastric balloon against the gastroesophageal junction and is maintained by the use of a special helmet, a baseball catcher's mask, or foam blocks. The gastric tube is attached to continuous suction and the esophageal balloon inflated with sphygmomanometer monitoring to a pressure of 30–45 mm Hg. The nasogastric tube above the esophageal balloon is attached to low intermittent suction to remove swallowed secretions. If the inflated balloons should become displaced into the pharynx, there is danger of asphyxiation. Therefore, scissors must be kept at the bedside at all times so that the tube may be immediately transected to let the air out of the balloons. Tamponade should be maintained for 12–24 h. If bleeding has been controlled, the esophageal balloon can be deflated leaving the gastric ballon inflated for another 12–24 h. If no bleeding is noted, then the gastric balloon should be deflated and the tube removed.

Recently, scleroses of esophageal varices through either a flexible or a rigid esophagoscope has been used in patients acutely bleeding [1]. The technique employs an injector needle with a sclerosing agent such as sodium morrhuate or sodium tetradactyl, which is injected into the varices under direct vision. Some early studies show that approximately 85% of people acutely bleeding from esophageal varices can be controlled in this manner. Long-term efficacy is yet to be demonstrated.

Mallory-Weiss Tear

A Mallory-Weiss tear that continues to bleed can be treated either with left gastric artery infusion of vasopressin (if the bleeding is coming from this artery) or electrocautery through the endoscope. Laser therapy through the endoscope may also be used for this type of lesion. In a minority of patients who do not stop bleeding, surgery will be necessary.

Gastritis

Initially, medical therapy should be directed at neutralizing the acid in the stomach. Antacids seem to be the best choice and should be started immediately after the diagnosis is made. Because of its diffuse nature, endoscopic laser or electrocoagulation therapy is probably of little value. Arteriography with vasopressin infusion of the bleeding gastric artery can be used. Surgery should be performed as a last resort and opinion varies among surgeons as to the preferred procedure.

Gastric Ulcer

Medical management begins with either antacids or histamine-2 receptor blockers such as cimetidine. Should bleeding continue, endoscopic electrocoagulation or laser therapy can be used to help control or stop the bleeding [3, 4]. Occasionally arteriography may be useful, with vasopressin or autologous clot infusion through the artery supplying the bleeding ulcer. Should these fail and the patient is a surgical candidate, one should not hesitate to send the patient to surgery.

Duodenal Ulcer

Duodenal ulcers are treated in essentially the same manner as bleeding gastric ulcers. If the patient is a poor surgical risk or more time is needed to reduce surgical risks, endoscopic electrocoagulation can be attempted. Good surgical candidates who continue to bleed from a duodenal ulcer should go to surgery early in their course when it becomes obvious that medical therapy is failing. Because of the dual blood supply to duodenal ulcers, arterial perfusion with vasopressin, autologous clot, or gel foam is rarely useful.

Prophylaxis for Gastrointestinal Bleeding

Many patients who are extremely ill are at high risk for bleeding from stress gastritis. It has been documented that the patients with severe liver disease, burns, acute renal failure, sepsis, a need for prolonged respiratory support, jaundice and other acute illnesses, are at high risk for formation of stress gastritis and therefore bleeding. With three of these factors, the risk of bleeding is almost 40d% if no prophylactic treatment is given. In these patients, antacids are better than histamine-2 receptor blockers such as cimetidine for the prevention of bleeding [6]. These patients should have a nasogastric tube and be given hourly anacids at a dose sufficient to keep the gastric pH above 4. By doing this, the risk of bleeding and stress ulcer formation can be kept to a minimum and a potentially serious problem averted. If antacids are contraindicated, intravenous cimetidine can be used.

References

1 Fleig, W.E.; Stange, E.F.; Ruettenauer, K.; Ditschuneit, H.: Emergency endoscopic sclerotherapy for bleeding esophageal varices: a prospective study in patients not responding to balloon tamponade. Gatrointest. Endosc. *29:* 8–14 (1983).

2 Fleischer, D.: Etiology and prevalence of severe persistent upper gastrointestinal bleeding. Gastroenterology *84:* 538–548 (1983).

3 Gaisford, W.E.: Endoscopic electrohemostasis of active upper gastrointestinal bleeding. Am. J. Surg. *137:* 47–53 (1979).

4 Gilbert, D.A.; Protell, R.L.; Silverstein, F.E.; Auth, D.C.: Endoscopic treatment of nonvariceal upper gastrointestinal bleeding. J. clin. Gastroenterol. *2:* 139–143 (1980).

5 Griffiths, W.J.; Neumann, D.A.; Welsh, J.D.. The visible vessel as an indicator of uncontrolled or recurrent gastrointestinal bleeding. New Engl. J. Med. *300:* 1411–1413 (1979).

6 Hans, J.P.; Skillman, J.J.; Bushnell, L.S.; Long, P.C.; Silen, W.: Antacid versus cimetidine in preventing acute gastrointestinal bleeding. New Engl. J. Med. *302:* 426–430 (1980).

7 Hastings, P.R.; Skillman, J.J.; Bushnell, L.S.; Silen, W.: Antacid titration in the prevention of acute gastrointestinal bleeding. New Engl. J. Med. *298:* 1041–1045 (1978).

8 Pitcher, J.L.: Safety and effectiveness of the modified Sengstaken-Blakemore tube: prospective study. Gastroenterology *61:* 291–298 (1971).

Robert A. Rankin, MD, Assistant Professor of Medicine, Head,
Gastrointestinal Endoscopy, University of Oklahoma Health Sciences Center,
Oklahoma City, OK 73106 (USA)

Prog. crit. Care Med., vol. 2, pp. 175–185 (Karger, Basel 1985)

Nutrition in the Intensive Care Unit

Don P. Murray, Jack D. Welsh

Digestive Diseases and Nutrition Section, University of Oklahoma Health Sciences Center, Oklahoma City, Okla., USA

A resurgence of interest in nutrition has occurred over the past 10 years as a result of an increased awareness that the nutritional status of the patient bears heavily upon prognosis. As a result, we are becoming more adept at recognizing nutritional problems, and many improvements in the technology of nutritional therapy enable us to provide nutritional support for virtually every patient. These changes are perhaps most obvious in the intensive care unit (ICU).

Nutritional Status of ICU Patients

Approximately 25–50% of hospitalized patients have protein-calorie malnutrition (PCM) at the time of admission to the hospital or develop it during the course of hospitalization [1–3]. These patients may have a history of weight loss, a weight too low for height, loss of subcutaneous tissue, muscle wasting and/or decreased serum proteins reflecting nutritional depletion. Additionally, metabolic changes occurring during severe illness (trauma, sepsis) promote catabolism [4, 5]. There is a state of insulin resistance with increased levels of insulin, leading to inhibition of fat mobilization. Increased levels of catecholamines, glucocorticoids, glucagon and growth hormone promote skeletal muscle breakdown and utilization of these amino acids for gluconeogenesis, which in the absence of protein intake, leads to a negative nitrogen balance. This is compounded by the nature of the ICU patient's illness and his frequently limited oral intake. Because of the severity of derangements seen in these patients, the physician may be inclined to focus on one or two problems, with relative inattention to the patient's nutritional needs. *Driver and LeBrun* [6] found that 80–85% of patients requiring ventilatory support in one ICU had inadequate caloric or protein intake to meet their metabolic requirements.

Consequences of Protein-Calorie Malnutrition

The consequences of PCM are protean, but the most significant of these in the intensive care situation are impaired host resistance, delayed tissue repair and decreased respiratory muscle strength. There are defects in both humoral and delayed immunity, with anergy occurring in severe PCM [7, 8]. Wounds in malnourished patients heal poorly and there is decreased tensile strength of the tissue [9]. Patients with PCM have decreased respiratory muscle strength [10] and there is increasing evidence to support the concept that respiratory failure is frequently the result of respiratory muscle failure [11].

Although prospective studies examining the effects of nutritional support are not available as yet for many disease processes, it is known that such support can affect the outcome of patients in the ICU. Parenteral hyperalimentation has been shown to decrease postoperative morbidity and mortality [12], as well as mortality in patients with acute renal failure [13] and possibly in patients with chronic liver disease [14]. Nutritional support also increases the chances of successfully weaning patients from ventilators [15].

Nutritional Support

The requirements of any form of nutritional support include adequate nutrients (protein, fat, minerals, vitamins) to prevent deficiencies, and calorie sources (carbohydrate, fat) to meet energy demands. A rule of thumb for estimating protein requirements is that patients with normal serum proteins and no evidence of skeletal muscle wasting require 1–1.5 g/kg/day of protein, while those with depressed serum proteins and/or evidence of skeletal muscle wasting require 1.5–2.0 g/kg/day of protein. A more accurate method of determining protein requirements is to estimate nitrogen loss with a 24-hour urine collection for urea nitrogen and protein. Since nitrogen loss in the stool is 3–4 g/day, patients require 3–4 g of nitrogen

Table I. Correction factors for energy requirements

Long et al. [16]		*Blackburn and Bistrian*	
Activity factors[1]		Enteral therapy	1.5 × BEE
Confined to bed	1.2 × BEE	Parenteral therapy	1.75 × BEE
Out of bed	1.3 × BEE		
Injury factors[1]			
Minor operation	1.2 × BEE		
Skeletal trauma	1.35 × BEE		
Sepsis	1.6 × BEE		
Severe burns	2.1 × BEE		

BEE = Basal energy expenditure.
[1] Factors are cumulative, e.g. a patient in bed with sepsis: BEE × 1.2 × 1.6 = energy requirements.

more than that determined by the urine collection to remain in nitrogen balance, with amounts greater than this resulting in positive nitrogen balance.

Caloric requirements can be estimated by the Harris-Benedict equations for basal energy expenditure in healthy persons:

$$\text{women } 655 + (9.6 \times WT) + (1.8 \times HT) - (4.7 \times A),$$
$$\text{men } 66 + (13.7 \times WT) + (5.0 \times HT) - (6.8 \times A),$$

where WT = weight in kilograms, HT = height in centimeters and A = age in years. The basal energy expenditure is multiplied by the correction factors of *Long* et al. [16] or *Blackburn and Bistrian* [17] to determine the caloric requirements of the patient (table I).

Advances in enteral feeding formulas and parenteral feeding solutions have made several options of nutritional support available. One may supplement oral intake with an enteral formula, give an enteral formula via ube feeding (nasogastric, nasoduodenal, or needle jejunostomy) or support the patient parenterally.

Enteral Feeding

Oral supplements or tube feedings are indicated in patients who have an intact gastrointestinal (GI) tract but inadequate oral intake due to anorexia or problems swallowing. A variety of enteral formulas are available which fall into four categories: meal replacement or 'polymeric' formulas, elemental or 'monomeric' formulas, modular components and special formulas.

Meal replacement formulas are indicated for use in patients with normal proteolytic and lipolytic activity. They consist of proteins, fats and carbohydrates in high molecular weight form and have caloric densities of 1–2 cal/cm^3. The osmolality varies from 300 to 700 mosm and daily vitamin requirements are met at rates exceeding 1,500–2,000 cm^3/day.

Elemental formulas are indicated for use in patients with abnormalities of the gastrointestinal tract resulting in decreased lipolytic or proteolytic activity or mucosal surface area. These formulas consist of amino acids, oligosaccharides and medium-chain triglycerides, but little other fat. Therefore one should consider providing essential fatty acids in the form of safflower oil orally or lipid emulsions parenterally to prevent essential fatty acid deficiency when these mixtures are used for prolonged periods of time. The caloric density is usually 1 cal/cm^3 and the osmolality ranges from 450 to 800 mosm. Vitamin requirements are met at rates greater than 2,000–3,000 cm^3/day.

Modular components are concentrated sources of one nutrient (protein, carbohydrate, or fat) in high molecular weight form and may be useful in patients who require fluid restriction. Special formulas with specific amino acid profiles are available for use in patients with renal failure who are not being dialyzed or patients with hepatic encephalopathy.

Highly motivated patients may be able to take adequate amounts of a formula orally to meet their nutritional requirements or supplement their usual dietary intake. These formulas may also be given easily through weighted, small-bore (6–8 Fr.) nasoduodenal tubes, if oral intake is prohibited or inadequate. Many tubes are now self-lubricated and pass easily with the use of accompanying stylets. After the tube has been advanced into the stomach, placing the patient on his or her right side and giving one dose of metaclopramide 10 mg i.v. may facilitate passage of the tube into the duodenum. An abdominal X-ray should be taken to check the placement of the tube prior to feeding.

Tube feedings should start at a rate of 40–50 cm^3/h of an isotonic solution. Solutions having an osmolality of greater than 300 mosm can be diluted appropriately. The rate of feeding may be increased by 20–25 cm^3/h every 8–24 h as the patient's tolerance permits. When a rate is achieved which will deliver the desired volume per day, the formula may be changed to three-quarter strength for 24 h and then to full strength.

During enteral feeding one must monitor the patient for possible metabolic complications. This should include daily measurement of weight, records of intake and output and diabetic urinalyses. Electrolytes, blood urea nitrogen and glucose should be checked every 2–3 days until the patient has been shown to be stable and then on a weekly basis.

The most common complications of enteral feeding are the gastrointestinal symptoms of nausea, vomiting, bloating and diarrhea [18]. These symptoms are frequently the result of exceeding the absorptive capacity of the small bowel. This capacity is dependent upon the osmolality and rate of flow of the formula, and symptoms generally resolve with dilution of hyperosmolar formulas or decreasing the rate of flow for a period of time. Metabolic complications such as hyperglycemia or hypernatremia may occur, but are less common than gastrointestinal disturbances. The most serious of complications, aspiration, is fortunately rare. Elevation of the head of the bed and constant infusion of the formula into the small bowel rather than the stomach decrease the risk of aspiration.

Since enteral feeding mimics normal physiology more closely than parenteral feeding, it has several theoretical advantages. It is also economical. One may meet daily requirements for many individuals with meal replacement formulas for less than $ 5 per day, or with elemental diets for $ 10–15 per day. A parenteral feeding regimen will usually cost more than $ 100 per day [19].

Parenteral Feeding

If the integrity of the gastrointestinal tract is questionable or if it is anticipated that oral intake is precluded for 5 or more days, parenteral feeding is indicated. The physician must be careful, however, not to repeatedly postpone the initiation of parenteral feeding in anticipation of the return of gastrointestinal function. It is better to discontinue parenteral support earlier than was anticipated than to begin several days after it would have benefited the patient. However, when considering the use of parenteral hyperalimentation in a patient who has major metabolic abnormalities, a period of 12–24 h should be used to correct these abnormalities before beginning parenteral feeding.

In devising a parenteral regimen of feeding, the goal is, once again, to provide adequate nonprotein calories to meet energy needs and nutrients to prevent deficiencies. The calorie sources available are dextrose, which provides 3.4 cal/g (or 1.7 cal/cm^3 of a 50% solution) and lipid emulsions, which provide 1.1–2.0 cal/cm^3. There is some controversy concerning the

Table II. Usual electrolyte requirements during parenteral hyperalimentation

Sodium	60–150 mEq/day
Potassium	70–150 mEq/day (minimum of 5–6 mEq/g nitrogen)
Chloride	equal to sodium
Phosphate	10–15 mmol/1,000 calories
Calcium	0.25 mEq/kg/day (minimal requirement)
Magnesium	0.35 mEq/kg/day (minimal requirement)
Acetate	as needed (bicarbonate precursor)

use of lipid emulsions as a major source of calories in patients who are severely ill (e.g. sepsis) [20], and at this time, it is unclear what the optimal ratio of carbohydrate to lipid calories might be. When lipid is used as a calorie source, current recommendations are that dosage should not exceed 2.5 g/kg/day or 60% of calories per day. However, normal or moderately ill humans can clear up to 3.8 g/kg/day [21], and systems utilizing lipids for up to 83% of calories in moderately ill patients have resulted in positive nitrogen balance [22]. Lipid emulsions cannot be used in patients with hypertriglyceridemia and should be used with caution in patients with pancreatitis.

The protein sources for parenteral feeding are amino acid solutions which come in several concentrations, most frequently 5.0 or 5.5%, 8.5% or 10% solutions, and provide from 0.8 to 1.7 g of nitrogen per 100 cm^3. In most clinical situations, the optimal ratio of calories to nitrogen (in grams) that will ensure protein anabolism ranges from 130:1 to 250:1.

Daily sodium, potassium, chloride, magnesium, calcium and phosphate requirements for adults without renal impairment are highly variable [23–26], as shown in table II. Solutions of amino acids or dextrose with pre-mixed electrolytes are available and can be used with minor modifications in many instances. Current recommendations are that the trace elements zinc, copper, manganese and chromium be added to hyperalimentation solutions on a daily basis [27], in amounts for adults as listed in table III.

Vitamin requirements are met by adding 10 cm^3 of MVI-12 each day. Vitamin K is not included in this multivitamin preparation, and 10 mg should be given by the subcutaneous or intramuscular route each 1–2 weeks.

Other potential additives to the hyperalimentation solution itself are heparin and regular insulin. Heparin, 1,000 units/l, will prevent catheter

Table III. Trace element requirements during parenteral hyperalimentation

Zinc	2.5–4.0 mg/day
Copper	0.5–1.5 mg/day
Chromium	10–15 μg/day
Manganese	0.15–0.8 mg/day

occlusion in the event that flow is temporarily interrupted. This amount of heparin has no significant systemic effect on clotting mechanisms. When hyperlglycemia occurs, interval doses of subcutaneous regular insulin are given as required until the proper amount of regular insulin to be added to the solution is determined.

When lipid is not given daily as a calorie source, prevention of essential fatty acid deficiency is accomplished by giving 500 cm^3 of a 10% lipid emulsion twice weekly.

Traditionally, for total parenteral nutrition, 500 cm^3 of amino acid solution and 500 cm^3 of 50% dextrose solution are mixed together with the appropriate electrolytes and vitamins. This gives a final amino acid concentration of 2.5–5.0% and 25% dextrose. In situations where lipid is utilized as a calorie source, dextrose concentrations can be decreased by using $D_{40}W$ or $D_{30}W$ for the initial mixture.

Lipid emulsions are very useful as calorie sources for peripheral venous feeding. Amino acid solutions and dextrose are mixed to give solutions with 4.25–5.0% amino acid concentrations and 5–10% dextrose concentrations. The solution and 10% lipid emulsion are then infused at identical rates through a Y-connector at the site of the peripheral catheter. Infusion sites should be changed every 24 h to preserve the veins. Peripheral venous feeding may be a useful option in situations where central lines are contraindicated, but is not applicable in many intensive care situations because of problems with venous access.

The high osmolality of total parenteral nutrition solutions requires that they be given through central venous catheters. The catheter should be placed in a sterile manner, and an X-ray should be taken to confirm that the tip of the catheter is in the superior vena cava before beginning infusion of the hyperosmolar solution. Subclavian catheterization is the approach of choice because of the advantages it offers for catheter care. If a contraindication for transthoracic catheterization exists, silicon elastimer-coated central venous catheters are now available which can be placed via antecubital veins and remain in place for long periods of time. The hyperalimentation infusion line should have a micropore filter in place. Proper care of the catheter site requires placement of an occlusive dressing which is changed in a sterile manner every 72 h.

Complications of parenteral feeding include sepsis, hyperglycemia, hypophosphatemia, hypomagnesemia, acidosis, trace element deficiency, essential fatty acid deficiency, and increased pCO_2. The rate of complications is decreased with meticulous attention to aseptic placement and care of the hyperalimentation line, and careful monitoring of the patient. This should include daily weights, records of fluid intake and output, and diabetic urinalyses or Dextrostix every 6 h. Electrolytes, phosphate and glucose should be checked daily the first 3–5 days, since this is a period during which deficits are repleted. When these values have become stable, an SMA-18 may be drawn once a week, and electrolytes and glucose may be checked on alternate 3rd or 4th days.

Special Considerations

Severe Respiratory Disease

The respiratory quotient (CO_2 produced:O_2 utilized) varies for different fuels. Fat has a respiratory quotient of 0.7, while that of glucose is 1.0. When carbohydrate is given in excess of metabolic demands and fat synthesis occurs, the respiratory quotient exceeds 1.0 [28, 29]. Theoretically, patients with severe lung disease may not be able to increase ventilation adequately to excrete the increased CO_2 produced if large glucose loads are given. There are several largely anecdotal reports of precipitation of respiratory failure in such patients during hyperalimentation, and of difficulty in weaning patients from ventilators while receiving large glucose loads [30, 31]. When difficulty is encountered in weaning a patient from a respirator while on parenteral feeding, it may be useful to supply 50% of the calculated caloric requirement as lipid in hopes of decreasing CO_2 production.

Renal Failure

One of the derangements of metabolism in renal failure is the inability to excrete urea nitrogen and 'middle molecules' that are products of protein metabolism. Since the serum levels of these substances are directly proportional to protein intake, protein must be restricted if the patient is not being dialyzed. When these patients are given small amounts of high-quality protein (protein with large amounts of essential amino acids) and increased carbohydrate, studies have shown that urea nitrogen is utilized to produce nonessential amino acids [32, 33]. In this manner, serum urea nitrogen is stabilized or decreased while nitrogen balance is improved.

Utilizing such an approach for parenteral feeding in patients with acute or chronic end-stage renal failure who are not dialyzed, one may use 250 cm^3 of 5.5% amino acids with 500–750 cm^3 of $D_{70}W$. This will give 2 g of nitrogen and 1,190–1,785 cal for each 750 or 1,000 cm^3 delivered. Most patients will tolerate 2–4 g of nitrogen per day, with the volume of fluid delivered usually being the limiting factor. A 5.4% solution of essential amino acids plus histidine (Nephramine, McGaw Laboratories) is available for this purpose. Addition of electrolytes must of course be tailored for each patient, and one must monitor serum potassium and phosphate concentrations closely, since these will frequently drop as hyperalimentation proceeds.

Because of the obligatory loss of serum amino acids and proteins during dialysis, the protein requirements of patients undergoing dialysis are increased. Patients undergoing hemodialysis require 1 mg/kg/day of protein or more, while patients undergoing peritoneal dialysis often require 1.5–2.0 mg/kg/day.

Hepatic Disease

Patients with severe chronic liver disease frequently have an abnormality of the serum amino acid pattern characterized by decreased levels of branch-chain amino acids and increased levels of aromatic amino acids. It is felt that this abnormal amino acid pattern, either alone or in combination with elevations of ammonia or products of ammonia metabolism, contributes to development of hepatic encephalopathy [34]. It has been demonstrated that normalization of the serum amino acid pattern in patients with hepatic encephalopathy by feeding or infusion of appropriate amino acids can reverse encephalopathy. A formula for enteral use (Hepatic-Aid, McGaw Laboratories) and a solution for parenteral use (Hepatamine, McGaw Laboratories) that are high in branched-chain amino acids and low in aromatic amino acids are available for use in patients with hepatic encephalopathy or a history of protein intolerance. It is unclear at this time whether manipulation of serum amino acids is useful in patients with hepatic encephalopathy due to acute fulminant hepatic necrosis.

References

1 Bistrian, B.; Blackburn, G.; Hollowel, E.; Heddle, R.: Protein status of general surgical patients. J. Am. med. Ass. *230:* 858–860 (1974).

2 Bistrian, B.; Blackburn, B.; Vitale, J. ; Cochran, D.; Naylor, J.: Prevalence of malnutrition in general medical patients. J. Am. med. Ass. *235:* 1567–1570 (1976).

3 Weinsier, R.; Hunker, E.; Krundieck, G.; Butterworth, C., Jr.: A prospective evaluation of general medical patients during the course of evaluation. Am. J. clin. Nutr. *32:* 418–426 (1979).

4 Siegel, J.; Cerra, F.; Coleman, B.; Giovannini, I.; Shetye, M.; Border, J.; McMenamy, R.: Physiologic and metabolic correlations in human sepsis. Surgery *86:* 163–193 (1979).

5 Wilmore, D.; Kinney, J.: Panel report on nutritional support of patients with trauma or infection. Am. J. clin. Nutr. *34:* 1213–1222 (1981).

6 Driver, A.; LeBrun, M.: Iatrogenic malnutrition in patients receiving ventilatory support. J. Am. med. Ass. *244:* 2195–2196 (1980).

7 Law, D.; Dudrick, S.; Adbou, N.: Immunocompetence of patients with protein-calorie malnutrition. The effects of nutritional repletion. Ann. intern. Med. *79:* 545–550 (1973).

8 Spanier, A.; Meakins, J.; MacLean, L.; Shizgal, H.: The relationship between immune competence and nutrition. Surg. Forum *27:* 332–336 (1976).

9 Vasantha, L.; Srikantia, S.; Gopalan, C.: Biochemical changes in the skin in kwashiorkor. Am. J. clin. Nutr. *23:* 78–82 (1970).

10 Arora, N.; Rochester, D.: Respiratory muscle strength and maximal voluntary ventilation in undernourished patients. Am. Rev. resp. Dis. *126:* 5–8 (1982).

11 Roussos, C.; Macklem, P.: The respiratory muscles. New Engl. J. Med. *307:* 786–797 (1982).

12 Mullen, J.; Buzby, G.; Matthews, D.; Smale, B.; Rosato, E.: Reduction of operative morbidity and mortality by combined preoperative and postoperative nutritional support. Ann. Surg. *192:* 604–613 (1980).

13 Able, R.; Beck, C.; Abbott, W.; Ryan, R.; Barnett, G.; Tisher, J.: Improved survival from acute renal failure after treatment with essential l-amino acids and glucose. New Engl. J. Med. *288:* 695–699 (1973).

14 Freund, H.; Dienstag, J.; Lehrich, J.; Yoshimura, N.; Bradford, R.; Rosen, H,; Atamian, S.; Slimmer, E.; Holroyde, J.; Fisher, J.: Infusion of branched chain amino acid solution in patients with hepatic encephalopathy. Ann. Surg. *196:* 209–220 (1982).

15 Bassili, H.; Deitel, M.: Effect of nutritional support on weaning patients off mechanical ventilators. J. parenter. enter. Nutr. *5:* 161–163 (1981).

16 Long, C.; Schaffel, N.; Geiger, J.; Schiller, W.; Blakemore, W.: Metabolic response to injury and illness; estimation of energy and protein needs from indirect calorimetry and nitrogen balance. J. parenter. enter Nutr. *3:* 452–456 (1979).

17 Blackburn, G.; Bistrian, B.: Nutritional support resources in hospital practice; in Schneider, Anderson, Coursin, Nutritional support of medical practice, pp. 139–151 (Harper & Row, New York 1977).

18 Heymsfield, S.; Bethel, R.; Ansley, J.; Nixon, D.; Rudman, D.: Enteral hyperalimentation: an alternative to central venous hyperalimentation. Ann. intern. Med. *90:* 63–71 (1979).

19 Michel, L.; Serrano, A.; Malt, R.: Nutritional support of hospitalized patients. New Engl. J. Med. *304:* 1147–1152 (1981).
20 Woolfson, A.; Heatley, R.; Allison, S.: Insulin to inhibit protein catabolism after injury. New Engl. J. Med. *300:* 14–17 (1979).
21 Wretlind, A.: Complete intravenous nutrition. Nutr. Metab. *14:* suppl. 1, pp. 1–57 (1972).
22 Jeejeebhoy, K.; Anderson, G.; Nakhooda, A.; Greenberg, G.; Sanderson, I.; Marlis, E.: Metabolic studies in total parenteral nutrition in man. J. clin. Invest. *57:* 125–136 (1976).
23 Grant, J.: Administration of parenteral nutrition solutions; in Grant, Handbook of total parenteral nutrition, pp. 92–117 (Saunders, Philadelphia 1980).
24 Sheldon, G.; Grzyb, S.: Phosphate depletion and repletion relation to parenteral nutrition and oxygen transport. Ann. Surg. *182:* 683–689 (1975).
25 Jones, J.; Manalo, R.; Flink, E.: Magnesium requirements in adults. Am. J. clin. Nutr. *20:* 632–635 (1967).
26 Wittine, M.; Freeman, J.: Calcium requirements during total parenteral nutrition in well-nourished individuals. J. parenter. enter. Nutr. *1:* 152–155 (1977).
27 AMA Department of Foods and Nutrition: Guidelines for essential trace element preparations for parenteral use. A statement by an expert panel. J. Am. med. Ass. *241:* 2051–2054 (1979).
28 Askanazi, J.; Rosenbaum, S.; Hyman, A.; Silverberg, P.; Milic-Emili, J.; Kinney, J.: Respiratory changes induced by the large glucose loads of total parenteral nutrition. J. Am. med. Ass. *243:* 1444–1447 (1980).
29 Askanazi, J.; Carpentier, Y.; Elwyn, D.; Nordenstrom, J.; Jeevanandam, M.; Rosenbaum, S.; Gump, F.; Kinney, J.: Influence of total parenteral nutrition of fuel utilization in injury and sepsis. Ann. Surg. *191:* 40–46 (1979).
30 Askanazi, J.; Elwyn, D.; Silverberg, P.; Rosenbaum, S.; Kinney, J.: Respiratory distress secondary to a high carbohydrate load: a case report. Surgery *87:* 596–598 (1980).
31 Covelli, H.; Black, J.; Olsen, M.; Beekman, J.: Respiratory failure precipitated by high carbohydrate loads. Ann. intern. Med. *95:* 579–581 (1981).
32 Giordano, C.: Use of exogenous and endogenous urea for protein synthesis in normal and uremic subjects. J. Lab. clin. Med. *62:* 231–246 (1963).
33 Giovannetti, S.; Maggiore, Q.: A low nitrogen diet with proteins of high biological value for severe chronic uremia. Lancet *i:* 1000–1003 (1964).
34 James, J.; Jeppsson, B.; Ziparo, V.; Fischer, J.: Hyperammonemia, plasma amino acid imbalance, and blood-brain amino acid transport: a unified theory of portal-systemic encephalopathy. Lancet *ii:* 772–775 (1979).

Don P. Murray, MD, Digestive Diseases and Nutrition Section,
University of Oklahoma Health Sciences Center, Post Office Box 26901,
Oklahoma City, OK 73190 (USA)

Prog. crit. Care Med., vol. 2, pp. 186–205 (Karger, Basel 1985)

Disorders of Potassium, Calcium, Magnesium, and Phosphorus

Christian E. Kaufman, Jr.

The University of Oklahoma Health Sciences Center, Oklahoma City, Okla., USA

Overview

Considering the important role of potassium and divalent ion equilibrium, it comes as no surprise that dysfunction of almost every organ can result from severe perturbations of intracellular or extracellular ion concentrations. Until recently, serum calcium and phosphorus levels were not routinely monitored in the critically ill and even today, magnesium levels are rarely determined in these patients. Consequently, abnormalities of these ions often go unrecognized or are ignored because their clinical significance is not readily apparent. Clearly this is a mistake. Hemodynamic and respiratory derangements may demand first priority but they are often caused or aggravated by disordered potassium, calcium, phosphorus, or magnesium metabolism. Therefore, prompt attention should be given to the consequences and correction of disordered potassium and divalent ion metabolism, especially in the critically ill patient.

Potassium

Hyperkalemia

Pathogenesis

Hyperkalemia results from either excessive intake, impaired excretion, or a net shift of potassium out of cells (table I).

Table I. Mechanisms of hyperkalemia

Exogenous load	*Transcellular shift*
Oral potassium supplements	Acidosis
'Salt substitutes'	Hypoaldosteronism
Intravenous potassium therapy	Insulin deficiency
Potassium-containing drugs	Alpha-adrenergic activity
Blood transfusions	Beta-adrenergic insufficiency
Geophagia	Hyperosmolality (hyperglycemia)
	Diffuse cellular injury
Impaired excretion	Drugs (succinylcholine, arginine HCl)
Renal failure	Digitalis poisoning
Hypoaldosteronism	Familial periodic paralysis
Potassium-sparing diuretics	
Primary defect in potassium secretion	

Exogenous Potassium Load

An excessive intake is rarely the only cause of hyperkalemia. However, even ordinary intake may contribute to life-threatening hyperkalemia in patients with impairment of renal excretory function. The hazards of oral potassium supplements and salt substitutes are often overlooked. These agents may cause dangerous potassium elevations especially when used with potassium-sparing diuretics [1]. When potassium additives pool in the dependent portions of parenteral fluid containers, the consequent infusion of a concentrated potassium solution may result in fatal hyperkalemia [2]. The rapid intravenous infusion of high-dose penicillin is an additional source of potentially fatal hyperkalemia [3]. The potassium load from blood transfusions is also important to consider and is significantly greater if aged blood is used. A 21-day-old unit of packed red blood cells provides about 5 mEq of potassium. Within 24 h after transfusion, an additional 3 mEq is released into the extracellular space from in vivo hemolysis. With fresh blood, a load of only about 1 mEq of potassium results [4].

Impaired Excretion

Patients with oliguric renal failure are prone to hyperkalemia primarily because a low urine flow rate markedly limits potassium excretion. Additionally, acidosis and increased catabolism provide an important endogenous potassium load. In nonoliguric acute renal failure, hyperkalemia is also common but is usually less severe and more easily managed [5].

In chronic renal failure, significant hyperkalemia is much less common, probably because of the higher urine flow rate. In addition, hyperaldosteronism [6] and other adaptations permit each remaining nephron to excrete a greater quantity of potassium [7]. Hence, hyperkalemia in a patient with chronic renal failure should prompt a thorough search for additional causes. Hyporeninemic hypoaldosteronism is relatively common in patients with mild renal disease, in particular diabetics [8]. In these patients hyperkalemia may result from the combined effects of hypoaldosteronism, reduced renal mass, and in some cases, insulin deficiency. Adrenal insufficiency without renal disease can also cause hyperkalemia but this is unusual if cortisone replacement is adequate. Potassium-sparing diuretics including spironolactone, triamterene, and amelioride may cause severe hyperkalemia. These agents block renal tubular secretion of potassium and therefore limit urinary potassium loss. They are hazardous in patients with renal disease or in combination with potassium supplements.

Transcellular Shifts

The most important mechanisms of acute hyperkalemia do not involve excessive potassium intake or impaired excretion but a net shift of small quantities of potassium into the extracellular fluid [9]. Metabolic acidosis is the most common cause of such shifts. However, not all types of acidosis are associated with changes in serum potassium, suggesting that factors other than pH may be involved [10, 11]. Aldosterone favors skeletal muscle uptake of potassium and the hyperkalemia seen in states of mineralocorticoid deficiency may be partially related to lack of this effect. Insulin deficiency likewise results in loss of intracellular potassium and may be an important factor contributing to hyperkalemia [12]. Alpha-adrenergic stimulation or beta-adrenergic blockage favor a loss of potassium into the extracellular fluid [13, 14]. Although the clinical importance of these adrenergic mechanisms is unsettled at present, beta-adrenergic blocking agents should be used cautiously in patients prone to hyperkalemia and avoided if possible in the presence of frank elevations in the serum potassium concentration. Hyperosmolality, including the hyperglycemic variety, may also shift potassium out of cells [15]. Numerous types of diffuse tissue injury may contribute to hyperkalemia. In rhabdomyolysis, renal failure is common but the release of potassium from cells contributes to the severe hyperkalemia which is often observed [16]. The effect of drugs [17, 18] including digitalis poisoning [19] and the syndrome of familial hyperkalemic periodic paralysis [20] represent unusual examples of hyperkalemia due to maldistribution across cell membranes.

Clinical Consequences of Hyperkalemia

Severe hyperkalemia may produce weakness, paresthesia, agitation, and a sense of 'impending doom'. On a rare occasion, flaccid paralysis may occur. However, the cardiac toxicity of hyperkalemia which may occur without any other symptoms is of greatest concern. Cardiac toxicity is related to the serum potassium level but the correlation is a crude one. Other factors which influence the effect of hyperkalemia on the heart include underlying heart disease, the rate of rise of serum potassium, and the concentration of sodium and calcium in the extracellular fluid. Usually the T waves show the earliest electrocardiographic changes. Classically, they become tall, narrow, and pointed but this occurs in a minority of cases. More commonly the T waves merely increase in amplitude and resemble those seen in a variety of other conditions and some normal individuals [21]. Another early electrocardiographic change of hyperkalemia is shortening of the Q-T interval. Changes in atrioventricular (A-V) conduction also occur when the plasma potassium is modestly elevated. At levels of 6.0–6.5 mEq/l, A-V conduction is often accelerated while at higher levels of potassium, it is progressively impaired [22]. When the plasma potassium exceeds 6.5 mEq/l, progressive widening of the QRS complex may be noted. The amplitude of the P wave begins to diminish when the potassium exceeds 7 mEq/l and as the plasma concentration increases further, P waves progressively flatten and broaden and the P-R interval increases. At plasma levels of about 9 mEq/l, P waves may disappear entirely, ST segment deviations occur and may suggest ischemic injury or pericarditis. At this point, death is imminent and may occur from either asystole or ventricular fibrillation [23].

Management of Hyperkalemia

Prophylactic measures can often be instituted before a significant rise in plasma potassium occurs. Patients with oliguric renal failure, for example, should receive a low potassium diet (40–60 mEq/day) and additional sources of exogenous potassium should be avoided. The plasma potassium usually increases by less than 0.5 mEq/l/day in acute renal failure and control is not difficult if begun early [24]. As a rule, therapy should begin when the plasma potassium is about 5.5 mEq/l or earlier if a rapidly rising level is

Table II. Treatment of hyperkalemia

Reverse cardiac toxicity (< 5 min)	↓ *Intake*
↑ Plasma calcium concentration	
↑ Plasma sodium concentration	↑ *Elimination* (2–12 h)
Transvenous pacemaker	↑ Urinary excretion
	Kayexalate and sorbitol
Shift potassium into cells (30–60 min)	Dialysis
Hypertonic $NaHCO_3$	
Glucose and insulin	

anticipated. However, the plasma potassium may increase by 1–2 mEq/l in a few hours in patients with tissue trauma, large hematomas, or sepsis [25, 26]. In these circumstances, aggressive therapy should be started as early as possible.

The four primary strategies for treatment of hyperkalemia are listed in table II. Which modalities to employ depends on the mechanisms of the hyperkalemia, the plasma potassium level, and the presence or absence of cardiac toxicity. Symptoms or electrocardiographic changes associated with a serum potassium greater than 6.5 mEq/l represent a medical emergency. When QRS or P wave changes occur or A-V block is noted, immediate action is indicated. The first priority is to reverse cardiac toxicity and calcium is the most effective agent. It should be given as calcium gluconate, 10 ml of a 10% solution intravenously over 3–5 min. This dose may be repeated once or twice if necessary. Raising the sodium concentration in the extracellular fluid also antagonizes hyperkalemic cardiac toxicity. Therefore, intravenous hypertonic sodium bicarbonate should be given (50–100 cm^3 of a 7.5% solution) if hyponatremia is also present. A transvenous pacemaker should be placed if A-V block or other causes of bradycardia are not reversed within minutes by these measures.

The second line of defense against severe hyperkalemia is to shift potassium into the intracellular space. Sodium bicarbonate and/or insulin and glucose should be used if cardiac toxicity is noted or the plasma potassium exceeds 7.0–7.5 mEq/l. 2 ampules of sodium bicarbonate (100 mEq) will expand the extracellular volume by about 500 ml, hence, caution should prevail when using large doses of this agent. Hypertonic glucose and insulin therapy does not significantly expand the extracellular compartment. Therefore, 100 cm^3 of 50% glucose and 15–20 U of regular insulin is the preferred therapy when volume overload is present. Potassium intake should also be restricted whenever hyperkalemia is noted.

Efforts to enhance potassium elimination should be initiated only after attention has been directed to measures described above. When hyperkalemia is mild, the kaliuretic effect of thiazide or loop diuretics may be used beneficially. Patients with congestive heart failure, for example, may be suited to this approach. Sodium polysulfonate resin (Kayexalate®) can effectively remove potassium over a period of hours to days. Kayexalate is given in doses of 50–60 g in 200 cm^3 of tap water as a retention enema. Careful placement of a Foley catheter well into the sigmoid colon allows the solution to be more easily retained and enhances its effectiveness. Although usually given at 4- to 6-hour intervals, the dose may be repeated every 1–2 h if necessary.

Dialysis is the most effective means of removing excess potassium. While peritoneal dialysis will not remove potassium rapidly, it is effective in hyperkalemia because it simultaneously corrects acidosis and supplies a glucose load (stimulating endogenous insulin). To provide an optimal diffusion gradient a potassium-free dialysis solution should be used. Hemodialysis is the most rapid means of removing potassium and is indicated when peritoneal dialysis cannot be done or when renal failure and hyperkalemia are associated with greatly accelerated catabolism [24]. A more detailed discussion of the technical aspects of dialysis is given in the chapter on 'Dialytic Therapy in the Intensive Care Unit'.

Hypokalemia

Hypokalemia may reflect a total body deficit or simply a shift of potassium into cells, but when chronic or moderately severe (serum potassium less than 3.0 mEq/l), a significant deficit is generally present. In the critical care setting, the differential diagnosis of hypokalemia (table III) is of less concern than the consequences and management of the hypokalemic state. Therefore, these issues will be discussed in some detail; readers interested in the pathogenesis of hypokalemia should consult other sources [27, 28].

Clinical Consequences of Hypokalemia

Potassium depletion and hypokalemia may result in a variety of sequelae (table IV) of which the neuromuscular and cardiovascular are most prominent.

Table III. Mechanisms of hypokalemia

Inadequate intake	*Excessive urinary loss*	*Transcellular shifts*
	Diuretics	Alkalosis
Gastrointestinal loss	Metabolic alkalosis	Insulin therapy
Vomiting and gastric drainage	Mineralocorticoid effect	Treatment of megaloblastic anemia
	Tubulointerstitial renal disease	
Diarrhea	Renal tubular acidosis	Periodic paralysis
Laxative abuse	Diabetic ketoacidosis	Barium poisoning
Ureterosigmoidostomy	Antibiotics	
	Magnesium depletion	
	Acute leukemia	
	Bartter's syndrome	
	Liddle's syndrome	

Table IV. Effects of potassium depletion

Neuromuscular	*Cardiac*	*Renal*
Adynamic ileus	Electrocardiographic changes	Concentrating defect
Weakness		Chronic renal failure
Rhabdomyolysis	Arrhythmias	
Encephalopathy	Myocardial necrosis (fibrosis)	*Metabolic*
		Carbohydrate intolerance
		Alkalosis

Neuromuscular

Impairment of gastrointestinal motility is a well-known feature of hypokalemia but potassium depletion can also profoundly affect skeletal muscle. Weakness is common and may on occasion progress to frank paralysis. Overt rhabdomyolysis may occur in severely potassium-depleted individuals [29]. Confusion and depression have been described but such nonspecific symptoms should not be attributed to hypokalemia without a thorough search for other explanations.

Cardiac

The electrocardiogram typically shows ST segment depression, T wave flattening, and prominence of the U wave. A variety of ectopic rhythms including atrial tachycardia, ventricular tachycardia, and ventricular fibrillation may occur [22]. These arrhythmias are more likely in patients with underlying heart disease or those taking digitalis but can occur in the absence of these conditions. The electrocardiographic changes and arrhythmias usually resolve when the potassium deficit is corrected, but with severe depletion, myocardial necrosis and fibrosis may result.

Treatment of Hypokalemia

The degree of potassium depletion should be estimated by considering the factors listed in tables I and II and the serum potassium concentration. As a general rule, a fall in serum potassium from 4 to 3 mEq/l represents a loss of about 150 mEq and for each further drop of 1 mEq in serum level, an additional deficit of about 300 mEq exists. Therefore, plasma levels of about 2 mEq/l would signify a deficit of approximately 400–500 mEq of potassium.

Whether or not potassium depletion represents an urgent problem needs careful consideration. Whereas patients with life-threatening arrhythmias or muscular paralysis deserve aggressive potassium repletion, a more gradual approach is usually warranted. Whenever possible, the potassium deficit should be replaced slowly and by the oral route. When intravenous replacement is indicated because of intestinal dysfunction or the presence of a life-threatening condition such as cardiac arrhythmias, several guidelines should be followed. First, the potassium concentration should be relatively low; 60–80 mEq/l is the maximum concentration recommended but usually less than 40 mEq/l is employed. High concentrations of potassium will cause pain and sclerosis of peripheral veins and increase the chances that a 'bolus' of potassium will be inadvertently given. The infusion rate should be carefully controlled by an infusion pump when concentrated solutions are used. When more than 10 mEq/h is given, electrocardiograph monitoring is warranted. With high rates of potassium infusion (10–20 mEq/h), the response is difficult to predict and serum levels should be monitored every few hours if not more frequently.

Calcium

Of the normal total serum calcium concentration of approximately 10 mg/dl, only half, the ionized fraction, is biologically active. 40–45% is protein bound; the remaining 5% is complexed to citrate and other anions and hence is also physiologically inert. The concentration of ionized calcium is normally kept within narrow limits by the action of parathyroid

Table V. Signs and symptoms of hypercalcemia

Neuromuscular	*Cardiovascular*	*Gastrointestinal*	*Genitourinary*
Lethargy	Hypertension	Polydipsia	Polyuria
Confusion	Digitalis toxicity	Vomiting	Stones
Obtundation		Constipation	Renal failure
Muscle weakness		Peptic ulcers	
		Pancreatitis	

hormone on bone and kidney. Parathyroid hormone also enhances the conversion of 25-hydroxycholecalciferol to 1,25-dihydroxycholecalciferol, the major regulator of intestinal calcium absorption. Despite these potent homeostatic mechanisms, wide fluctuation in the serum calcium concentration may be seen in numerous disease states with important clinical consequences.

Hypercalcemia

Hypercalcemia is usually due to malignancy or hyperparathyroidism, although vitamin D intoxication and a variety of unusual causes should also be considered in the differential diagnosis [30]. Patients with hypercalcemia are unusual in the critical care setting but on occasion the sequela of a high serum calcium may dominate the clinical picture.

Clinical Manifestations of Hypercalcemia

Hypercalcemia is often mild and the symptoms are subtle. However, moderate to severe elevations of serum calcium (12.5–20 mEq/l) may have major consequences (table V). Acidosis and hypoalbuminemia by increasing the ionized fraction enhance the toxicity of any level of total serum calcium. Likewise, the rate of rise of serum calcium and the effect of associated electrolyte abnormalities may contribute to the severe toxicity which is sometimes seen at relatively modest (12–13 mg%) serum levels.

Treatment of Hypercalcemia

The cause of hypercalcemia is usually readily apparent if a careful history, some skeletal radiographs, and routine blood studies are done. In symptomatic patients, early aggressive therapy should take precedence over any additional diagnostic considerations. Most hypercalcemic patients are volume depleted because of the combined effects of inadequate intake, vomiting, and impaired renal conservation of salt and water. These deficits should be replaced by intravenous saline infusions beginning with isotonic saline and progressing to more hypotonic solutions as needed to restore the extracellular fluid volume and the serum sodium concentration to normal. If acute renal failure has not supervened, potassium replacement may also be needed. Once these fluid and electrolyte deficits have been corrected, repeated doses of intravenous furosemide should be given to induce a brisk diuresis which will markedly enhance urinary calcium losses. The ongoing sodium, potassium, and water losses will need to be replaced as judged by the urine output and spot urine electrolyte determinations. Furosemide-saline therapy, although a popular and effective means of lowering the plasma calcium, is not without hazard in elderly patients and those with underlying cardiac or renal impairment. In these patients, central venous or pulmonary capillary wedge pressure should be monitored in order to prevent fluid overload and pulmonary edema. On occasion hypercalcemia is refractory to the furosemide-saline regimen. In this situation or in patients with advanced renal failure, mithramycin and/or hemodialysis should be employed. A small dose of mithramycin (25 μg/kg body weight) will usually lower the serum calcium for several days. However, its effect is usually not apparent for 24–48 h after the intravenous administration. Hemodialysis with a calcium-free bath is an effective means of rapidly lowering the serum calcium although the benefits may be quite transient. Other measures including calcitonin, intravenous phosphorus, and ethylenediaminetetraacetic acid (EDTA) are less effective or more difficult to use but might be considered under special circumstances. In addition, efforts to treat the underlying cause are of great importance. Patients thought to have sarcoidosis or vitamin D intoxication should receive corticosteroids and those with malignancies, radiation or chemotherapy as indicated. The rare patient with severe hypercalcemia due to hyperparathyroidism should undergo neck exploration as soon as the metabolic status permits.

Hypocalcemia

Protein binding of calcium and the formation of calcium complexes in the extracellular fluid need to be considered when interpreting a low serum calcium concentration. For example, hypocalcemia can be associated with a normal ionized calcium if serum protein concentrations are sufficiently reduced. (As a rule of thumb, a decrease in the concentration of serum albumin of 1 g/100 ml will lower the total calcium by about 0.8 mg/dl without significantly influencing the concentration of ionized calcium.) Most hypocalcemia which is not explained by low serum proteins is due to hypoparathyroidism, magnesium depletion, malabsorption syndrome, or acute pancreatitis [31]. Extreme alkalosis or a high concentration of citrate will reduce the ionized calcium concentration without changing the total serum calcium. The latter circumstance may be important when massive transfusions of citrated blood are employed, especially when hepatic clearance of citrate is reduced by liver disease or hypoperfusion. Without measuring the ionized calcium, however, there is no easy way to estimate the role of these factors in lowering its concentration. Nonetheless, calcium complexing and changes in pH and protein concentration of the blood as well as the rate of fall in serum calcium may help to explain the variability in clinical manifestations resulting from a given serum concentration.

Clinical Consequences of Hypocalcemia

The most dramatic manifestation of hypocalcemia is tetany. While muscle cramps and carpopedal spasms are relatively benign consequences of hypocalcemia, generalized seizures and spasms can have dire consequences. The usual cardiac manifestation of hypocalcemia is prolongation of the Q-T interval. This finding may provide a helpful indication that the ionized calcium is reduced in those situations where hypoproteinemia or other factors make such an assessment difficult. With acute hypocalcemia, hypotension may occur and it may be refractory to vasoactive drugs. The mechanisms probably involve a decrease in vascular tone and a negative inotropic effect. Impairment in myocardial contractility may be sufficient to precipitate congestive heart failure [32].

Treatment of Hypocalcemia

Asymptomatic hypocalcemia does not require treatment unless the serum level is falling rapidly, in which case symptoms can be anticipated. In acute symptomatic hypocalcemia, which is usually the result of surgical hypoparathyroidism, an intravenous infusion of calcium is recommended. In adults, 10–20 ml of 10% calcium gluconate can be given intravenously over 5–10 min. The benefits will be transient and if symptoms recur, a continuous infusion of calcium is advisable. The proper rate of calcium infusion must be determined empirically, but as a starting point, 10–20 ml of 10% calcium gluconate (4.5–9.0 mEq of calcium) can be added to 500 cm^3 of intravenous fluids every 6 h. Patients with surgical hypoparathyroidism may require larger calcium doses because of rapid skeletal uptake by the 'hungry bones' in response to lower levels of parathyroid hormone. The serum calcium level and clinical response should be monitored closely and special caution must be given patients with renal failure or those receiving digitalis glycosides. Likewise, any associated hypomagnesemia should be corrected simultaneously because magnesium depletion will make correction of hypocalcemia more difficult. Vitamin D and oral calcium supplements are indicated when the hypocalcemia state is likely to persist beyond 24–48 h.

Magnesium

Hypermagnesemia

Clinical significant hypermagnesemia is rarely seen in patients with normal renal function, except during treatment of preeclampsia or eclampsia when aggressive magnesium sulfate administration often elevates plasma levels to 6–8 mEq/l. With impairment of renal function, however, the ability to excrete a magnesium load is markedly diminished [33]. Even so, symptomatic hypermagnesemia is rarely seen unless the patient is receiving an exogenous magnesium load. However, magnesium-containing antacids, cathartics, and enemas are in widespread use and magnesium intoxication is not a rare event when patients with renal failure are exposed to these preparations [33].

Clinical Consequences of Hypermagnesemia

Clinical manifestations first become evident at serum levels of about 4 mEq/l at which point deep tendon reflexes are usually depressed. At 5–6 mEq/l a drop in blood pressure and depression of central nervous system function may be noted. With progressively higher serum levels, nausea, vomiting, respiratory depression, dilated pupils, refractory hypotension, neuromuscular paralysis, and cardiac dysrhythmias, including complete heart block and cardiac arrest, may occur. As a rule, healthy individuals with experimental hypermagnesemia and preeclamptic women receiving magnesium therapy tolerate hypermagnesemia better than patients with renal disease and multiple electrolyte abnormalities. In this latter group, serious

Table VI. Common causes of hypomagnesemia

Gastrointestinal disorders	*Renal disease*
Malabsorption	Renal tubular acidosis
Prolonged diarrhea	Tubulointerstitial disease
Vomiting or nasogastric drainage	Recovery phase of acute renal failure
Pancreatitis	
Fistulae	*Diuretics*
Hyperalimentation	Thiazides
	Loop diuretics
Endocrine	Osmotic diuretics
Hyperparathyroidism	Alcoholism
Hypoparathyroidism	
Diabetic ketoacidosis	

arrhythmias, refractory hypotension, respiratory depression, and coma have occurred with serum concentrations in the range of 5–7 mEq/l [34].

Treatment of Hypermagnesemia

In many cases no treatment other than elimination of exogenous sources of magnesium will be needed. However, respiratory depression, hypotension, profound muscle weakness, cardiac arrhythmias, or conduction disturbances indicate the need for aggressive intervention. Intravenous calcium (5–10 ml of 10% calcium gluconate over 3–5 min) should be given to directly counteract the toxic effect of hypermagnesemia [33]. Infusion of glucose and insulin may also be used to drive magnesium into cells, although the value of this method is unproven. Hypotension should be counteracted by volume expansion and vasopressor agents but it may be refractory to these measures [35]. Hemodialysis with a magnesium-free solution is the most effective therapy and should be employed on an emergency basis in patients with renal failure and symptomatic hypermagnesemia. For patients with good renal function, a saline-furosemide diuresis may provide an effective alternative means of lowering the serum magnesium level.

Hypomagnesemia

Clinically significant hypomagnesemia is common in critically ill patients particularly in groups with a high incidence of alcoholism. In normal individuals, the plasma or extracellular concentration of magnesium is closely regulated between 1.6–2.1 mEq/l. As is the case in other largely intracellular cations, the plasma concentration can only provide a crude estimate of total body stores [36]. In symptomatic hypomagnesemia, the serum level is usually less than 1.0 mEq/l. While many circumstances have been associated with magnesium depletion (table VI) most symptomatic hypomagnesemia, like symptomatic hypophosphatemia, is related to alcoholism, diabetic ketoacidosis, or refeeding after nutritional deprivation. However, almost any condition which leads to potassium depletion can also produce magnesium depletion. Often multiple mechanisms are involved [36].

Consequences of Hypomagnesemia

The major clinical sequelae of hypomagnesemia are related to cardiac arrhythmias and neurologic dysfunction. Magnesium depletion like potassium depletion enhances cardiac toxicity of digitalis glycosides [37], but even in the absence of digitalis, ventricular ectopy including ventricular tachycardia may result [38]. The central nervous system manifestations of hypomagnesemia resemble the alcohol withdrawal syndrome with which it is often associated. Tremor, disorientation, hyperactive deep tendon reflexes, ataxia, and generalized seizures may occur. Because magnesium depletion impairs the release of parathyroid hormone and may block its action in the periphery, hypocalcemia is also often present [39]. Although hypocalcemia may potentiate the effects of low magnesium, all of these neurologic features (except perhaps for tetany) can occur with magnesium depletion alone [36].

Treatment of Magnesium Depletion

Symptomatic hypomagnesemia usually will require parenteral magnesium replacement. In patients with normal renal function, *Flink* [40] recommends giving 6 g of magnesium sulfate (49 mEq) in 1 liter of intravenous fluids over 3 h as an initial measure. Following this, 49 mEq of magnesium can be distributed throughout each day's intravenous fluids until the deficit is corrected. Alternatively, 1–2 ml of 50% magnesium sulfate (8.1–16.3 mEq of Mg) can be given every 4 h intramuscularly. In either case, these large doses of magnesium are justified only for symptomatic or severe hypomagnesemia (serum level less than 1.0 mEq/l) and require frequent monitoring of the serum concentration. Patients with renal failure and hypomagnesemia should receive significantly smaller doses and more frequent monitoring of the serum concentration should be carried out.

Table VII. Mechanisms of hypophosphatemia

Decreased intake/absorption	*Transcellular shift*
Phosphate-binding antacids[1]	Hyperalimentation[1]
Vomiting	Carbohydrate or insulin administration
Starvation	Alkalosis (especially respiratory)[1]
Malabsorption	Liver disease
	Pregnancy
Urinary loss	Sepsis
Hyperparathyroidism	Estrogens/androgens
Diuretics (especially thiazides)	Epinephrine
Volume expansion	
Hypomagnesemia	*Mixed mechanisms*
Hypokalemia	Alcoholism[1]
Acidemia	Diabetic ketoacidosis[1]
Renal tubular defects	
X-linked hypophosphatemic rickets	
Tumor phosphaturia	

[1] May reduce serum phosphorus to less than 1.0 mg.

Phosphorus

In the critically ill patient, hyperphosphatemia is rarely of clinical importance except as an indication of renal failure which is usually the cause. Severe hypophosphatemia (serum level less than 1.0 mg/dl) in contrast may result in serious morbidity.

Mechanisms of Severe Hypophosphatemia

Hypophosphatemia can result from inadequate intake, excessive loss or a redistribution into cells. While a great variety of factors have the potential to lower the serum phosphorus, relatively few clinical circumstances (table VII) are associated with severe hypophosphatemia [41]. In most patients with severe hypophosphatemia inadequate intake and/or excessive loss is coupled with factors which drive phosphate into cells, i.e. alkalosis or the administration of carbohydrate or insulin. The hypophosphatemia develops after a delay period which is somewhat characteristic (fig. 1) for each of the major causes.

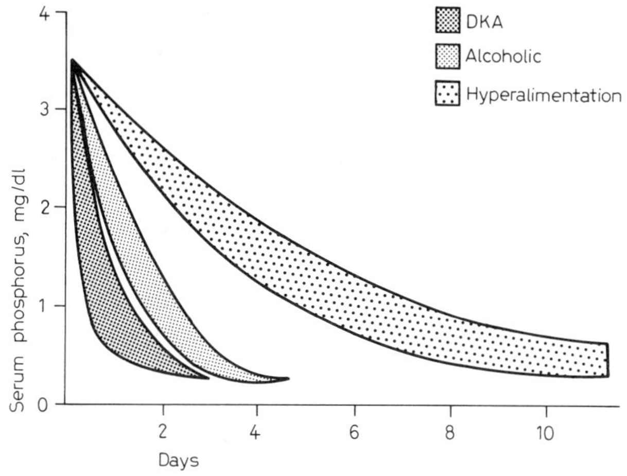

Fig. 1. Approximate time when severe hypophosphatemia appears during treatment for diabetic ketoacidosis (DKA), alcoholic withdrawal, and hyperalimentation [from ref. 42, with permission].

Consequences of Severe Hypophosphatemia

The importance of high energy compounds (ADP, ATP) in the metabolism of all cells suggests that profound hypophosphatemia can functionally impair every organ system. However, the tissues which are most profoundly affected seem to be skeletal and cardiac muscle, the hematopoietic system, and the brain. The neurologic effects are the most common, often leading to tremor, paresthesias, lethargy, and on occasion, convulsions and coma [42]. The effects on skeletal muscle may be equally striking, muscle weakness and frank rhabdomyolysis being well described [41]. Weakness of respiratory muscles may be so profound that acute respiratory failure can result [43]. The myocardium may be affected in a similar way, and a reversible impairment of cardiac performance is known to occur [44]. Congestive heart failure has also been attributed to hypophosphatemia [45]. The hematologic consequences of hypophosphatemia are more subtle although overt hemolysis has been reported [46]. Whereas intracellular ATP rarely falls low enough to cause hemolysis, the concomitant reduction in levels of 2,3-diphosphoglycerate (2,3-DPG) impairs the release of oxygen in peripheral tissues [47]. The function of leukocytes [48] and platelets [49] is also impaired by severe hypophosphatemia although the clinical relevance of these observations remains unclear.

Treatment of Severe Hypophosphatemia

Since phosphorus may rapidly shift between the extracellular and intracellular or bone compartments, the magnitude of body deficits cannot be estimated from the serum phosphorus levels. Therefore, correction of hypophosphatemia must be based on a close follow-up of the serum levels. Oral phosphate may be appropriate for asymptomatic patients, but critically ill patients with severe hypophosphatemia require intravenous phosphorus therapy. The hazards of intravenous phosphorus administration include hypocalcemia, hypotension, and metastatic calcifications as well as hyperkalemia from the potassium salts [50]. However, with controlled infusions of small doses of phosphorus and careful monitoring of the serum concentration these complications can be avoided. An initial dose of 0.08–0.16 m*M*/kg body weight given over 6 h has been recommended [51]. A similar dose (0.10–0.17 m*M*/kg given every 12 h) has proved safe and effective in a small series of patients. However, with this regimen it took up to 36 h to raise the serum phosphorus about 1.0 mg/dl in some patients [52].

References

1 Lawson, D.H.: Adverse reactions to potassium chloride. Q. Jl Med. *171:* 433–440 (1974).

2 Lankton, J.W.; Siler, J.N.; Neigh, J.L.: Hyperkalemia after administration of potassium from nonrigid parenteral-fluid containers. Anesthesiology *39:* 660–661 (1973).

3 Mercer, C.W.; Logic, J.R.: Cardiac arrest due to hyperkalemia following intravenous penicillin administration. Chest *64:* 358–359 (1973).

4 Simon, G.E.; Bove, J.R.: The potassium load from blood transfusion. Postgrad. Med. *49:* 61–64 (1971).

5 Anderson, R.J.; Linas, S.L.; Berns, A.S.; Henrich, W.L.; Miller, T.R.; Gabow, P.A.; Schrier, R.W.: Nonoliguric acute renal failure. New Engl. J. Med. *296:* 1134–1138 (1977).

6 Weidmann, P.; Maxwell, M.H.; Lupu, A.N.: Plasma aldosterone in terminal renal failure. Ann. intern. Med. *78:* 13–18 (1973).

7 Schultze, R.G.; Taggart, D.D.; Shapiro, H.; Pennell, J.P.; Caglar, S.; Bricker, N.S.: On the adaptation in potassium excretion associated with nephron reduction in the dog. J. clin. Invest. *50:* 1061–1068 (1971).

8 Knochel, J.P.: The syndrome of hyporeninemic hypoaldosteronism. Annu. Rev. Med. *30:* 145–153 (1979).

9 Sterns, R.H.; Cox, M.; Feig, P.U.; Singer, I.: Internal potassium balance and the control of the plasma potassium concentration. Medicine *60:* 339–354 (1981).

10 Adrogue, H.J.; Madias, N.E.: Changes in plasma potassium concentration during acute acid-base disturbances. Am. J. Med. *71:* 456–467 (1981).

11 Fulop, M.: Serum potassium in lactic acidosis and ketoacidosis. New Engl. J. Med. *300:* 1087–1089 (1979).

12 Cox, M.; Sterns, R.H.; Singer, I.: The defense against hyperkalemia: the roles of insulin and aldosterone. New Engl. J. Med. *299:* 525–532 (1978).

13 Bia, M.J.; DeFronzo, R.A.: Extrarenal potassium homeostasis. Am. J. Physiol. *240:* F257–F268 (1981).

14 Rosa, R.M.; Silva, P.; Young, J.B.; Landsberg, L.; Brown, R.S.; Rowe, J.W.; Epstein, F.H.: Adrenergic modulation of extrarenal potassium disposal. New Engl. J. Med. *302:* 431–434 (1980).

15 Moreno, M.; Murphy, C.; Goldsmith, C.: Increase in serum potassium resulting from the administration of hypertonic mannitol and other solutions. J. Lab. clin. Med. *73:* 291–298 (1969).

16 Koffler, A.; Freidler, R.M.; Massry, S.G.: Acute renal failure due to nontraumatic rhabdomyolysis. Ann. intern. Med. *85:* 23–28 (1975).

17 Bushinsky, D.A.; Gennari, F.J.: Life-threatening hyperkalemia induced by arginine. Ann. intern. Med. *89:* 632–634 (1978).

18 Cooperman, L.H.; Strobel, G.E.; Kennell, E.M.: Massive hyperkalemia after administration of succinylcholine. Anesthesiology *32:* 161–164 (1970).

19 Reza, M.J.; Kovick, R.B.; Shine, K.I.; Pearch, M.L.: Massive intravenous digoxin overdosage. New Engl. J. Med. *291:* 777 (1974).

20 Pearson, C.M.; Kalyanaraman, K.: The periodic paralyses; in Stanbury, Wyngaarden, Fredrickson, Metabolic basis of inherited disease (McGraw-Hill, Maidenhead 1972).

21 Braun, H.A.; Surawicz, B.; Bellet, S.: T waves in hyperpotassemia. Am. J. med. Sci. *230:* 147 (1955).

22 Fisch, C.: Relation of electrolyte disturbances to cardiac arrhythmias. Circulation *47:* 408–419 (1973).

23 Ettinger, P.O.; Regan, T.J.; Oldewurtel, H.A.: Hyperkalemia, cardiac conduction, and the electrocardiogram: a review. Am. Heart J. *88:* 360–371 (1974).

24 Lordon, R.E.; Burton, J.R.: Post-traumatic renal failure in military personnel in southeast Asia. Am. J. Med. *53:* 137–147 (1972).

25 Teschan, P.E.; Post, R.S.; Smith, L.H.; Abernathy, R.S.; Davis, J.H.; Gray, D.M.; Howard, J.M.; Johnson, K.E.; Klopp, E.; Mundy, R.L.; O'Meara, M.P.; Rush, B.F.: Post-traumatic renal insufficiency in military casualties. Am. J. Med. *18:* 172–186 (1955).

26 Maher, J.F.; Schreiner, G.E.: Cause of death in acute renal failure. Archs intern. Med. *110:* 493–504 (1962).

27 Kunau, R.T.; Stein, J.H.: Disorders of hypo- and hyperkalemia. Clin. Nephrol. *7:* 173–190 (1977).

28 Nardone, D.A.; McDonald, W.J.; Girard, D.E.: Mechanisms in hypokalemia: clinical correlation. Medicine *57:* 435–446 (1978).
29 Campion, D.S.; Arias, J.M.; Carter, N.W.: Rhabdomyolysis and myoglobinuria associated with hypokalemia of renal tubular acidosis. J. Am. med. Ass. *220:* 967–969 (1972).
30 Parfitt, A.M.; Kleerekoper, M.: Clinical disorders of calcium, phosphorus, and magnesium metabolism; in Maxwell, Kleeman, Clinical disorders of fluid and electrolyte metabolism (McGraw-Hill, Maidenhead 1980).
31 Schneider, A.B.; Sherwood, L.M.: Progress in endocrinology and metabolism: pathogenesis and management of hypoparathyroidism and other hypocalcemic disorders. Metabolism *24:* 871–898 (1975).
32 Troughton, O.; Singh, S.P.: Heart failure and neonatal hypocalcaemia. Br. med. J. *iv:* 76–79 (1972).
33 Mordes, J.P.; Wacker, W.E.C.: Excess magnesium. Pharmac. Rev. *29:* 273–300 (1978).
34 Randall, R.E.; Cohen, M.D.; Spray, C.C.; Rossmeisl, E.C.: Hypermagnesemia in renal failure. Ann. intern. Med. *61:* 73–88 (1964).
35 Ferdinandus, J.; Pederson, J.A.; Whang, R.: Hypermagnesemia as a cause of refractory hypotension, respiratory depression and coma. Archs intern. Med. *141:* 669 (1981).
36 Wacker, W.E.C.; Parisi, A.F.: Magnesium metabolism. New Engl. J. Med. *278:* 658–663 (1968).
37 Seller, R.H.; Cangiano, J.; Kim, K.E.; Mendelssohn, S.; Brest, A.N.; Swartz, C.: Digitalis toxicity and hypomagnesemia. Am. Heart J. *79:* 57–68 (1970).
38 Iseri, L.T.; Freed, J.; Bures, A.R.: Magnesium deficiency and cardiac disorders. Am. J. Med. *58:* 837–846 (1975).
39 Massry, S.G.: The clinical pathophysiology of magnesium. Contr. Nephrol., vol. 14, pp. 64–73 (Karger, Basel 1978).
40 Flink, E.B.: Therapy of magnesium deficiency. Ann. N.Y. Acad. Sci. *162:* 901–917 (1969).
41 Fitzgerald, F.T.: Hypophosphatemia. Adv. internal Med. 137–157 (1978).
42 Knochel, J.P.: The pathophysiology and clinical characteristics of severe hypophosphatemia. Archs intern. Med. *137:* 203–220 (1977).
43 Newman, J.H.; Neff, T.A.; Ziporin, P.: Acute respiratory failure associated with hypophosphatemia. New Engl. J. Med. *296:* 1101–1103 (1977).
44 O'Connor, L.R.; Wheeler, W.S.; Bethune, J.E.: Effect of hypophosphatemia on myocardial performance in man. New Engl. J. Med. *297:* 901–903 (1977).
45 Darsee, J.R.; Nutter, D.O.: Reversible severe congestive cardiomyopathy in three cases of hypophosphatemia. Ann. intern. Med. *89:* 867–870 (1978).
46 Jacob, H.S.; Amsden, T.: Acute hemolytic anemia with rigid red cells in hypophosphatemia. New Engl. J. Med. *285:* 1446–1450 (1971).
47 Lichtman, M.A.; Miller, D.R.; Cohen, J.; Waterhouse, C.: Reduced red cell glycolysis, 2,3-diphosphoglycerate and adenosine triphosphate concentration, and increased hemoglobin-oxygen affinity caused by hypophosphatemia. Ann. intern. Med. *74:* 562–568 (1971).
48 Craddock, P.R.; Yawata, Y.; VanSanten, L.; Gilberstadt, S.; Silvis, S.; Jacob, H.S.: Acquired phagocyte dysfunction: a complication of the hypophosphatemia of parenteral hyperalimentation. New Engl. J. Med. *290:* 1403–1407 (1974).

49 Yawata, Y.; Hebbel, R.P.; Silvis, S.; Howe, R.; Jacob, H.: Blood cell abnormalities complicating the hypophosphatemia of hyperalimentation: erythrocyte and platelet ATP deficiency associated with hemolytic anemia and bleeding in hyperalimented dogs. J. Lab. clin. Med. *84:* 643–653 (1974).

50 Shackney, S.; Hasson, J.: Precipitous fall in serum calcium, hypotension, and acute renal failure after intravenous phosphate therapy for hypercalcemia. Ann. intern. Med. *66:* 906–916 (1967).

51 Lentz, R.D.; Brown, D.M.; Kjellstrand, C.M.: Treatment of severe hypophosphatemia. Ann. intern. Med. *89:* 941–944 (1978).

52 Vannatta, J.B.; Whang, R.; Papper, S.: Efficacy of intravenous phosphorus therapy in the severely hypophosphatemic patient. Archs intern. Med. *141:* 885–887 (1981).

C.E. Kaufman, Jr., MD, The University of Oklahoma Health Sciences Center, Oklahoma City, OK 73106 (USA)

Prog. crit. Care Med., vol. 2, pp. 206–217 (Karger, Basel 1985)

Hyponatremia

Christian E. Kaufman, Jr.
University of Oklahoma Health Sciences Center, Oklahoma City, Okla., USA

Relationship to Hypoosmolality

Hyponatremia, or a serum sodium concentration below 135 mEq/l, is one of the most common disturbances observed in critically ill patients. Since sodium is the most abundant cation in the extracellular fluid, hyponatremia usually indicates a reduced osmolality of this fluid compartment. Virtually all somatic cells are freely permeable to water, hence, hypoosmolality of the extracellular fluid is accompanied by a similar dilution of intracellular solute. This hypoosmolar state must be distinguished from two other situations where the serum sodium concentration is also reduced. The more important of these situations can occur when a high concentration of glucose or other small molecular weight compound such as mannitol is present in the extracellular fluid. As a result of osmotic forces, water moves out from the intracellular space diluting the extracellular sodium and lowering its concentration. This effect of hyperglycemia will reduce the serum sodium concentration by 1.6 mEq/l for each 100 mg/dl elevation of the blood glucose. A less common reason for hyponatremia not associated with hypoosmolality is 'pseudohyponatremia', which may be noted with severe hyperlipidemia or hyperproteinemia. Plasma water is displaced by excess lipids or protein thereby reducing the amount of sodium (which is dissolved only in the water) in a given quantity of serum or plasma. To exclude these spurious or nonhypoosmolar circumstances, measurement of plasma osmolality should be a routine part of the evaluation of hyponatremia. The remainder of this discussion will focus on the more typical situation when hyponatremia is associated with a comparable degree of hypoosmolality of the body fluids.

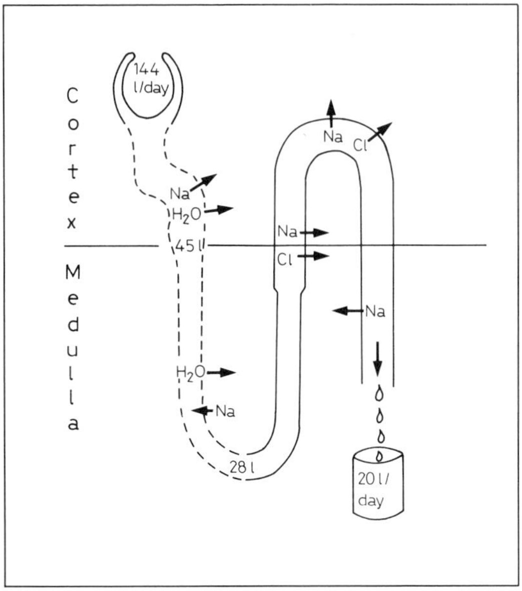

Fig. 1. Renal diluting mechanisms. The sites of sodium chloride and water reabsorption in the absence of ADH are indicated in this composite nephron. With a glomerular filtration of 144 liters/day, approximately 45 liters of filtrate would remain at the end of the proximal tubule and 28 liters would remain at the tip of Henle's loop. In the absence of ADH very little water is reabsorbed beyond this point, and up to 20 liters of solute-free water can be excreted in the urine. --- = Water-permeable; —— = water-impermeable [from ref. 16, with permission].

Physiologic Control of the Serum Sodium Concentration

An understanding of the pathogenesis of hyponatremia requires a clear perception of the physiologic pathways which regulate the osmolality of body fluids and maintain the serum sodium concentration between 137 and 143 mEq/l. This control depends on the two factors which influence water balance: water intake and water losses. Since most people do not curtail fluid intake in response to hyponatremia, the major system for preventing dilution of body fluids involves adjustments in water loss. This is achieved by renal excretion of the excess water which in turn depends upon a variety of factors, including suppression of antidiuretic hormone (ADH) secretion, intact intrarenal hemodynamics and sodium handling and excretion of an adequate urinary solute load. The sensitivity of the normal hypothalamic-pituitary axis is such that a 1–2% depression of serum osmolality (serum sodium about 135 mEq/l) will suppress ADH to undetectable levels. Under these circumstances, normally functioning kidneys can excrete up to 20 liters a day of solute-free water (fig. 1). Hence, hyponatremia will not occur unless water intake exceeds this rate or the renal excretion of water is impaired.

Pathogenesis of Hyponatremia

With these considerations in mind, the pathogenesis of hyponatremia can be understood in terms of the mechanisms listed in table I. Of these, excessive water intake (as the sole explanation for the development of hyponatremia) is probably the least common. However, a fresh water drowning victim can ingest and aspirate a large volume of water which enters the extracellular fluid and temporarily overwhelms the renal capacity to excrete it. A similar situation occasionally is seen in psychotic patients, who can ingest huge quantities of water and rapidly become hyponatremic [1, 2]. More commonly, a relatively generous intake of water contributes to the development of hyponatremia in patients whose modest impairment of water excretion would not otherwise be a sufficient cause for their dilutional state.

The normal diluting mechanisms are quite sensitive to disorders of circulatory and endocrine physiology. Hence, a great variety of conditions can impair the urinary diluting ability and predispose to the development of hyponatremia [3]. For example, any factor which reduces glomerular filtration rate may reduce the rate of fluid delivery to the distal nephron and limit the maximum rate of urine flow and water excretion. Similarly, conditions which reduce the effective arterial blood volume will enhance the reabsorption of filtrate in the proximal tubule and limit distal delivery of filtrate and maximum urine flow rate. Examples include volume depletion, congestive heart failure and decompensated cirrhosis. Despite a normal rate of delivery of filtrate to the distal nephron, impairment of sodium and chloride transport in the ascending limb and distal convoluted tubule may also impair dilution of the urine. Both loop diuretics and thiazide diuretics share this mechanism for impairing free water clearance. Another important but often subtle factor impairing urinary dilution is the presence of ADH. The distal convoluted tubule and collecting duct are exquisitely sen-

Table I. Mechanisms of hypoosmolality (hyponatremia)

1. Excessive water intake (> 20 liters)
2. Impaired water excretion
a. ↓ Glomerular filtration rate
b. ↑ Proximal reabsorption
c. Impaired sodium transport in distal nephron
d. Antidiuretic hormone effect
e. ↓ Solute load
3. Potassium depletion

sitive to the hydroosmotic effects of ADH. Hence, ADH concentrations below the detection level of a sensitive radioimmunoassay can enhance the back diffusion of water in the distal tubule and collecting duct. As a result, normal minimal urine osmolality of about 50 mosm will not be achieved and free water clearance impaired. A variety of hemodynamic, pharmacologic and emotional stimuli may also trigger ADH secretion [3, 4]. Hence, an important role for ADH in the pathogenesis of hyponatremia is common, particularly in the critical care setting.

Finally, since many normal individuals cannot dilute the urine much below 50 mosm/kg, the rate of solute excretion provides another factor which limits free water clearance. Normally, about 600 mosm/kg of solute are excreted in the urine each day. A urine osmolality of 30 mosm/kg (which can be achieved by some perfectly healthy people) would therefore be required to excrete 20 liters of water. Under these conditions, a minimum urine osmolality of 60 mosm/kg would only permit 10 liters of water excretion (60 mosm/kg × 10 liters = 600 mosm/24 h). However, the rate of urinary solute excretion may be markedly diminished in patients on a low protein and low sodium intake. In such patients, maximum rates of free water clearance will be diminished in proportion to the decrease in solute load even if a normal minimum urine osmolality can be achieved. For example, with a reduction in solute excretion to 300 mosm/24 h and a urine osmolality of 50 mosm/kg, a maximum urine volume of only 6 liters/24 h could be expected. Water intoxication due to beer potomania can be explained by this mechanism. Since beer is low in sodium and essentially free of protein, the intake of large quantities to the exclusion of other foods has led to severe hyponatremia due to the combined effects of high fluid intake and impaired free water clearance [5].

Potassium depletion may also play a role in the pathogenesis of hyponatremia. In patients with thiazide-induced hyponatremia, the depression in serum sodium concentration cannot be entirely accounted for by sodium loss or water retention. These patients show evidence of major potassium deficits, which might allow entry of sodium into cells to restore osmotic equilibrium between the extracellular and intracellular fluid compartments [6]. The potential importance of potassium depletion in the pathogenesis of hyponatremia is supported by studies [7] demonstrating a linear relationship between serum sodium concentration or osmolality and total body sodium potassium and water according to this equation:

$$[Na^+] \sim \frac{Na_e + K_e}{\text{Total body water}},$$

where $[Na^+]$ = sodium concentration or osmolality of body fluids, Na_e = exchangeable sodium and K_e = exchangeable potassium.

In many patients, particularly in the critical care setting, the combination of several of these mechanisms may be operative. Since these physiologic derangements occur in a great variety of illnesses, it is not surprising that hyponatremia is so common in the critically ill patient.

Clinical Approach to Hyponatremia

Understanding the pathogenesis of hypoosmolar states is particularly helpful when the origin of hyponatremia is obscure or multifactorial. However, most clinicians have adopted a straightforward approach to the differential diagnosis of hyponatremia based on a clinical estimate of the extracellular fluid volume (table II). There are two practical reasons for this approach. First, like any classification, this one is helpful in simplifying the differential diagnosis. For example, having determined that a hyponatremic patient demonstrates an expanded extracellular volume, one can initially consider the conditions in that category instead of the total array of possibilities. Secondly, since the decision to administer sodium to a hyponatremic patient is dependent primarily on the state of extracellular fluid volume, therapeutic strategies are based on this approach. Thus, even if one cannot determine the exact mechanism(s) of hyponatremia when a patient demonstrates evidence of volume depletion, isotonic saline administration would be indicated. In contrast, patients with an expanded extracellular

Table II. A classification of hyponatremia (hypoosmolality)

1. Associated with an expanded extracellular fluid volume		
	Congestive heart failure	
	Cirrhosis	
	Renal failure	
	Nephrotic syndrome	
2. Associated with a contracted extracellular fluid volume		
	Gastrointestinal losses	
		Vomiting or nasogastric drainage
		Diarrhea
		Sequestration of fluid in retroperitoneal or peritoneal space
		Drainage of pancreatic, biliary or small bowel fluid
	Urinary sodium losses	
		Renal disease
		Diuretic therapy
		Osmotic diuresis
		Adrenal insufficiency
3. Associated with an 'apparently' normal extracellular fluid volume		
	'Occult volume depletion'	
	Drugs (including thiazides)	
	Mechanical ventilation	
	Myxedema	
	Syndrome of inappropriate ADH	

volume have an excess total body sodium and would not be candidates, as a general rule, for sodium administration. Therefore, the first step in differential diagnosis and management of hypoosmolar states is to assess the extracellular fluid space, classifying the patient as having an expanded, contracted or 'apparently normal' extracellular fluid volume.

Hyponatremia with an Expanded Extracellular Fluid Volume

Dependent or generalized edema is the hallmark of an expanded extracellular compartment and indicates an excess of total body sodium even in the hyponatremic patient. Neck vein distention or an S3 sound may also indicate an expanded extracellular space, but edema is usually present as well. However, in patients with advanced renal failure with minimal or no edema, hypertension may on occasion be the major clue to an expanded extracellular fluid volume. Only rarely must one rely on measurements of the central venous, right atrial or pulmonary capillary wedge pressure to accurately identify an expanded extracellular fluid compartment. Since total body sodium is increased, water restriction is the cornerstone of management for these patients. The appropriate degree of restriction depends upon the severity of the impairment of water excretion. The anuric patient for example, might be able to tolerate no more than 500 cm^3 of free water without developing hyponatremia. Under these conditions, a restriction to 500 cm^3/day would maintain the status quo, but correction of hyponatremia would usually require dialysis therapy. Typically, however, water losses are sufficient so that a restriction of 500–1,000 cm^3/day will be associated with a negative water balance and correction of the hyponatremic state.

Hyponatremia Associated with a Contracted Extracellular Fluid Volume

A 10% reduction in blood volume provides a stimulus of ADH secretion so that ADH levels will persist despite the feedback inhibition that hypoosmolality should provide. 'The body preserves volume at the expense of osmolality.' Volume depletion is also often associated with a reduction in glomerular filtration rate and enhanced proximal reabsorption of filtrate, both limiting further free water clearance. For these reasons, the volume-depleted patient is obligated to excrete small quantities of relatively concentrated urine. Ordinary intake of water which continues on the basis of habit or due to therapeutic measures can easily lead to hyponatremia in this circumstance.

Volume depletion is recognized primarily by a careful history looking for clues to the cause of salt loss (table II). (A minimal decrease in extracellular volume is sufficient to limit urinary sodium excretion to less than 10 mEq/24 h. Since nonrenal losses of sodium amount to very little in otherwise healthy people, inadequate intake of sodium is not a sufficient explanation for the development of a contracted extracellular fluid volume or hyponatremia.) Volume depletion is usually apparent on physical examination where orthostatic hypotension and tachycardia are the most reliable signs. Laboratory findings of prerenal azotemia and hemoconcentration may likewise be helpful in suggesting a state of volume depletion. Management of these patients is relatively straightforward. Correction of the volume deficit with isotonic saline will restore free water clearance and correct the hyponatremia. (Failure to correct hyponatremia in response to volume repletion indicates that other mechanisms may be involved.) It is important to realize that the development of hyponatremia in the volume-depleted patient is dependent upon continued water intake and that correction of the hypoosmolar state will be delayed if this water intake is not controlled. Therefore, in addition to providing isotonic saline to correct the volume deficit, dextrose solutions and dietary fluids should be temporarily limited.

Hyponatremia with an Apparently Normal Extracellular Fluid Volume

In these patients, subclinical volume depletion must also be considered. A random urine specimen for determination of sodium concentration may be helpful since a value greater than 20 mEq/l in the absence of renal disease or recent use of diuretics indicates an adequate extracellular fluid volume. A brief trial of isotonic saline administration may also be of diagnostic help. (In the absence of volume depletion, the salt load will be rapidly excreted and the hyponatremia will persist.)

Multiple pathways may impair water excretion in these disorders. ADH secretion is often incompletely suppressed in response to pain, emotional distress or the effects of drugs [4]. The patient with respiratory failure requiring ventilatory support is particularly prone to hyponatremia [8, 9]. Renal perfusion may be impaired and ADH secretion stimulated by the detrimental effects of positive pressure ventilation on cardiac output. Additionally, hypoxemia and hypercapnia stimulate ADH release and may perturb intrarenal hemodynamics further impairing free water clearance [10]. Not only is respiratory water loss eliminated, but the patient may gain 300 cm^3 of water per day from the ventilation nebulization system, further accentuating positive water balance [11]. Finally, the clinician's zeal to liquefy bronchial secretion with infusions of dextrose and water may contribute to the dilution of body fluids and precipitate severe water intoxication. Since these patients have a normal or slightly expanded extracellular volume, water restriction and not sodium administration should be the main therapeutic tool.

Consequences and Management of Symptomatic Hyponatremia

On occasion, a low serum sodium concentration may be the first clue to an unsuspected disorder such as adrenal insufficiency. However, the importance of hyponatremia is usually related to the neurologic sequelae (table III) which may result from the associated overhydration of brain cells. Although there is considerable overlap of serum sodium values between

Table III. Consequences of hypoosmolality

Headache	Coma
Nausea and vomiting	Seizures
Lethargy	Permanent central nervous system damage
Stupor	Death

symptomatic and asymptomatic patients, a sodium level of less than 125 mEq/l is generally required for symptoms to develop (fig. 2). However, some patients remain asymptomatic with sodium levels chronically less than 115 mEq/l. In contrast, when severe hyponatremia develops acutely (less than 24 h) mortality is approximately 50% (fig. 3). An explanation for these observations is provided by experiments in rabbits which indicate that brain water increases very little with chronic hyponatremia, but with comparable degrees of acute (2 h) hyponatremia, seizures and death ensue [12].

Most hyponatremic patients have no signs or symptoms which can be directly attributed to the hypoosmolar state. In these individuals, the appropriate use of water restriction and isotonic saline infusions as outlined earlier will prove to be safe and effective management. Patients symptomatic from hyponatremia justify a more aggressive approach. However, the clinical manifestations of the hypoosmolar state are nonspecific and it may be particularly difficult to determine the role of hypoosmolality in critically ill patients with multiple organ failure. Nonetheless, encephalopathy or seizures in a patient with a serum sodium level less than 120 mEq/l should be managed as outlined below unless another explanation for the clinical manifestations is readily apparent. A serum sodium of less than 110 mEq associated with central nervous system dysfunction is a clear indication for rapid and aggressive therapy even in patients with other explanations for the brain dysfunction because it is impossible to exclude an additive role of the hyponatremia. The therapeutic strategy in these symptomatic patients is to correct the hyponatremia rapidly, since this will not only reverse the clinical manifestations but will provide the best opportunity for recovery without permanent neurologic sequelae [13]. A guideline should be the restoration of the sodium concentration to above 125 mEq/l within 12–18 h. This can be achieved in most patients by the proper use of hypertonic saline and furosemide combined with careful water restriction [14]. As a rule for adults, the infusion of 500–800 mEq of sodium chloride as a 3 or 5% solu-

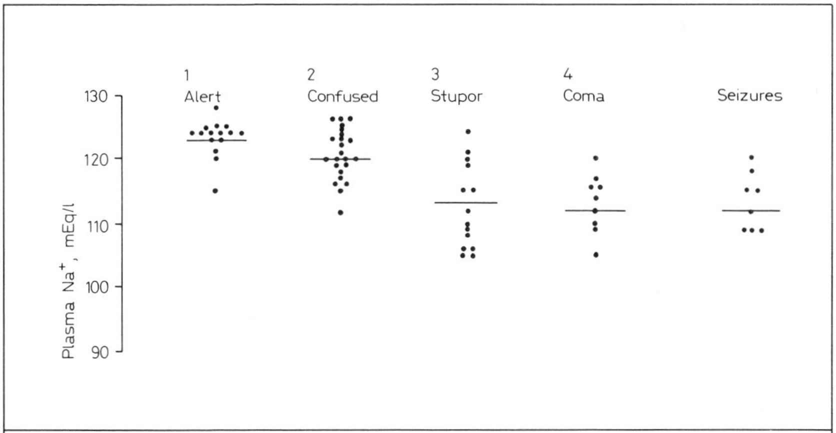

2

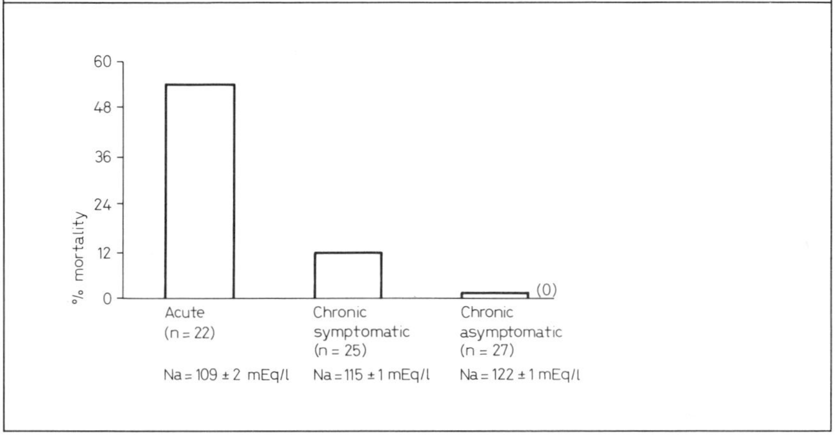

3

Fig. 2. Mental status of 65 consecutive patients with serum Na^+ of 128 mEq/l or less. $r = 0.64$, $n = 65$, $p < 0.01$ [from ref. 12, with permission].

Fig. 3. Mortality in 74 adult patients with hyponatremia. A mortality rate of 55% in adults with acute hyponatremia is contrasted with a 12% mortality rate in symptomatic adults with chronic hyponatremia. No deaths were seen in adults with chronic asymptomatic hyponatremia [from ref. 17, with permission].

tion given over 12–15 h is appropriate. If a concomitant furosemide diuresis is induced, the serum sodium concentration should rise by about 2 mEq/l per hour [15].

Pulmonary edema owing to expansion of the extracellular fluid compartment is an obvious potential hazard of this therapy. Therefore, careful assessment of the extracellular fluid volume by the clinical parameters outlined earlier is essential. This assessment forms the basis for a 'target' urine flow rate which can be achieved by frequent doses of intravenous furosemide. In this way, patients with volume depletion are initially treated with the hypertonic saline infusion until extracellular volume is restored, then furosemide diuresis is initiated while the saline infusion is continued. Patients with volume expansion require a more brisk diuresis at the outset of therapy to assure that sodium excretion exceeds the rate of intravenous sodium infusion. In those with an approximately normal extracellular volume, the goal is to achieve a urinary sodium excretion rate which is approximately equal to the rate of sodium administration. As a first approximation, the urine can be considered to have about 50–80 mEq/l and spot specimens are sampled at occasional intervals during the diuresis to improve the precision of these estimates.

It is apparent that patients with oliguric renal failure or end-stage chronic renal disease are not candidates for this type of therapy. In these individuals hypertonic saline can still be administered, but when the extracellular volume is expanded, dialysis (hemo- or peritoneal) is needed to remove the excess sodium. In the hyponatremic patient, either method of dialysis will also remove water in excess of sodium and rapidly speed recovery. Although peritoneal dialysis is effective in this situation, acute hemodialysis provides the most rapid means of correcting severe life-threatening hyponatremia.

References

1 Langgard, H.; Smith, W.O.: Self-induced water intoxication without predisposing illness. Report of two cases. New Engl. J. Med. *266:* 378–381 (1962).
2 Hariprasad, M.K.; Eisinger, R.P., Nadler, I.M.; Padmanabhan, C.S.; Nidus, B.D.: Hyponatremia in psychogenic polydipsia. Archs intern. Med. *140:* 1639–1642 (1980).
3 Schrier, R.W.; Berl, T.: Nonosmolar factors affecting renal water excretion. New Engl. J. Med. *292:* 81–88 (1975).
4 Miller, M.; Moses, A.M.: Drug-induced states of impaired water excretion. Kidney int. *10:* 96–103 (1976).
5 Demanet, J.C.; Bonnyns, M.; Bleiberg, H.; Stevens-Rocmans, C.: Coma due to water intoxication in beer drinkers. Lancet *ii:* 1115–1117 (1971).
6 Fichman, M.P.; Vorherr, H.; Kleeman, C.R.; Telfer, N.: Diuretic-induced hyponatremia. Ann. intern. Med. *75:* 853–863 (1971).
7 Edelman, I.S.; Leibman, J.; O'Meara, M.P.; Birkenfeld, L.W.: Interrelations between serum sodium concentration, serum osmolarity and total exchangeable sodium, total exchangeable potassium and total body water. J. clin. Invest. *37:* 1236–1256 (1958).

8 Murdaugh, H.V.; Sieker, H.O.; Manfredi, F.: Effect of altered intrathoracic pressure on renal hemodynamics, electrolyte excretion and water clearance. J. clin. Invest. *38:* 834–842 (1959).
9 Farber, M.O.; Bright, T.P.; Strawbridge, R.A.; Robertson, G.L.; Manfredi, F.: Impaired water handling in chronic obstructive lung disease. J. Lab. clin. Med. *85:* 41–49 (1975).
10 Anderson, R.J.; Pluss, R.G.; Berns, A.S.; Jackson, J.T.; Arnold, P.E.; Schrier, R.W.; McDonald, K.M.: Mechanism of effect of hypoxia on renal water excretion. J. clin. Invest. *62:* 769–777 (1978).
11 Sladen, A.; Laver, M.B.; Pontoppidan, H.: Pulmonary complications and water retention in prolonged mechanical ventilation. New Engl. J. Med. *279:* 448–453 (1968).
12 Arieff, A.I.; Llach, F.; Massry, S.G.: Neurological manifestations and morbidity of hyponatremia: correlation with brain water and electrolytes. Medicine *55:* 121–129 (1976).
13 Ashraf, N.; Locksley, R.; Arieff, A.I.: Thiazide-induced hyponatremia associated with death or neurologic damage in outpatients. Am. J. Med. *70:* 1163–1168 (1981).
14 Hantman, D.; Rossier, B.; Zohlman, R.; Schrier, R.: Rapid correction of hyponatremia in the syndrome of inappropriate secretion of antidiuretic hormone. Ann. intern. Med. *78:* 870–875 (1973).
15 Ayus, J.C.; Olivero, J.J.; Frommer, J.P.: Rapid correction of severe hyponatremia with intravenous hypertonic saline solution. Am. J. Med. *72:* 43–48 (1982).
16 Kaufman, C.E.: Disorders of sodium and water metabolism; in Kaufman, Papper, Review of pathophysiology (Little, Brown, Boston 1983).
17 Covey, C.M.; Arieff, A.I.: Disorders of sodium and water metabolism and their effects on the nervous system; in Brenner, Stein, Sodium and water homeostasis (Churchill Livingstone, Edinburgh 1978).

C.E. Kaufman, Jr., MD, University of Oklahoma Health Sciences Center,
Oklahoma City, OK 73106 (USA)

Prog. crit. Care Med., vol. 2, pp. 218–228 (Karger, Basel 1985)

Hyperosmolar States

Charles R. Rost, David C. Kem

Endocrinology, Metabolism and Hypertension Section,
University of Oklahoma Health Sciences Center, Oklahoma City, Okla., USA

Introduction

Several clinical situations are associated with the development of increased serum osmolality. These hyperosmolar states are characterized by the increased plasma accumulation of endogenous solutes, such as glucose or sodium, or the administration of exogenous solutes, such as mannitol or hyperalimentation solutions. As serum osmolality increases, resultant intracellular dehydration and compensatory changes in cellular constituents produce functional alterations. Cells of the central nervous system (CNS) are particularly sensitive to changes in extracellular osmolality and their dysfunction produces a spectrum of neurological findings.

Hyperglycemic hyperosmolality, with or without ketoacidosis, is frequently encountered in clinical practice. Nonketotic hyperglycemic hyperosmolar coma (NKHHC) accounts for 5–15% of cases of diabetic coma requiring critical care and many more patients without coma suffer from uncontrolled hyperglycemia and hyperosmolality. Hypernatremia is often a contributing factor to NKHHC. In addition, euglycemic hypernatremic hyperosmolality is not uncommonly seen in young children and the elderly. The effects of disordered sodium metabolism on CNS function have recently been reviewed by *Covey and Arieff* [4]. This chapter will focus on NKHHC. The pathophysiology, clinical manifestations, and therapy will be reviewed and contrasted to those of diabetic ketoacidosis (DKA). NKHHC will be used as a model to describe the effects of hyperosmolality on CNS function. Where differences exist, proposed mechanisms of CNS dysfunction in NKHHC will be compared to postulated mechanisms in other hyperosmolar states.

Pathophysiology

Metabolic Abnormalities

In NKHHC, the primary hormonal abnormality appears to be a relative deficiency of insulin. Plasma insulin concentrations in patients with untreated NKHHC are as low as those observed in patients with untreated DKA [7]. Plasma glucagon concentrations have been reported to be elevated in both conditions [14]. As described elsewhere in this volume, the combination of increased glucagon and decreased insulin concentrations leads to increased hepatic gluconeogenesis and decreased peripheral glucose utilization with subsequent hyperglycemia. Glycosuria develops when the blood glucose concentration exceeds the renal threshold for glucose. The subsequent osmotic diuresis results in substantial water and electrolyte losses. Water losses are in excess of electrolyte losses resulting in volume depletion and hyperosmolality. Most patients who develop NKHHC are unable or fail to maintain adequate fluid and electrolyte intake. In addition, many of these patients have underlying renal insufficiency. The combination of volume depletion and renal insufficiency results in a decrease in the glomerular filtration rate and an increase in the renal threshold for glucose. As a consequence, blood glucose concentrations rise. In the fully developed case of NKHHC, the plasma glucose concentration is usually greater than 600–800 mg/dl and the serum osmolality is over 350 mosm/kg [16]. However, osmolality greater than 400 mosm/kg and plasma glucose concentrations as high as 4,800 mg/100 ml have been reported [13].

It continues to be an unresolved question why some patients with uncontrolled diabetes develop NKHHC while others develop DKA. The biochemical and physiological basis of ketogenesis has been outlined elsewhere in this volume. Two major hypotheses are offered to explain why patients with NKHHC do not develop ketosis. Ketogenesis is dependent upon the delivery of free fatty acids (FFA) to the liver. In DKA, the plasma concentrations of lipolytic hormones, particularly cortisol and growth hormone, are elevated [7, 18]. However, plasma cortisol and growth hormone levels in patients with NKHHC are significantly lower than in DKA and this is associated with significantly lower concentrations of FFA [7]. Also, the combined effects of hyperosmolality and dehydration have been demonstrated to decrease the release of FFA from adipose tissue [8, 19]. The reduced delivery of ketogenic substrate to the liver is postulated as one reason for the lack of ketogenesis in NKHHC.

Although the plasma FFA concentrations are lower in NKHHC than in DKA, these levels are significantly higher than those observed in fasting normal people [7]. Thus decreased delivery of FFA to the liver does not fully account for the lack of ketosis in NKHHC. An intrahepatic inhibition of ketogenesis may also be present [9, 10]. Portal vein plasma insulin concentrations are significantly higher in NKHHC than in DKA. In both conditions, the peripheral plasma insulin concentrations are low. It is postulated that the high ratio of portal vein to peripheral plasma insulin levels in NKHHC is indicative of increased hepatic insulin uptake. The hepatic insulin levels are sufficient to inhibit ketogenesis, perhaps by preventing elevation of carnitine concentrations and, thereby, inhibiting the activity of carnitine acyltransferase I, the control point for entry of FFA into the beta-oxidation pathway. However, the hepatic insulin levels are believed to be insufficient to inhibit counterregulatory hormone-stimulated gluconeogenesis. Thus, the decreased delivery of FFA coupled with the inhibition of hepatic ketogenesis results in the nonketotic state while hepatic gluconeogenesis and decreased peripheral glucose disposal result in marked hyperglycemia and hyperosmolality.

CNS Alterations

The various neurological manifestations of NKHHC and the altered sensorium seen in both DKA and NKHHC correlate strongly with serum hyperosmolality [1, 6, 15]. This is emphasized by the observation that despite plasma glucose concentrations in excess of 600 mg/dl, coma seldom occurs in NKHHC when plasma osmolality is less than 350 mosm/kg [1]. The reason for the association of CNS signs with hyperosmolality is not known. However, studies in animals with experimentally induced hyperosmolality suggest that cerebral dehydration is not the cause. When hyperosmolality is induced by sodium or glucose administration, there is an initial loss of brain water content followed by a return to control values by 4–6 h of continued hyperosmolality [1]. Measurements of osmotically active constituents of the brain reveal an initial increase in Na^+ and K^+ accounting for an increase in CNS osmolality preserving brain water content. However, after 4 h of continued hyperosmolality the Na^+ and K^+ concentrations decrease to control levels. The increased CNS osmolality is maintained by unmeasured 'idiogenic' osmoles [1]. Under conditions of hyperosmolality due to hypernatremia the idiogenic osmoles appear to be newly synthesized amino acids. When the hyperosmolality is caused by hyperglycemia, brain amino acid content is not increased over control. The exact nature of the idiogenic osmoles in the latter situation is not known [1]. In either case, the development of idiogenic osmoles seems to be a response to the hypernatremia or hyperglycemia and not a response to the hyperosmolality. If hyperosmolality is induced by infusion of mannitol, the brain does not accumulate idiogenic osmoles and is unable to defend against loss of water [1].

Clinical Manifestations

Neurological Signs and Symptoms

The patient with NKHHC may present with a variety of neurological signs and symptoms. Most of these are reversible with appropriate therapy of the hyperosmolar state. Up to 15% of patients with NKHHC have grand mal or focal seizures or transient hemiparesis believed to be caused by the hyperosmolality [1, 15, 16]. In contrast, patients with DKA rarely present with neurological signs other than altered mental status, even when serum osmolality is elevated to levels found in NKHHC. The difference in frequency of neurological signs between NKHHC and DKA may reflect the underlying status of the CNS. Patients who develop NKHHC are generally older, and subclinical CNS pathology may become evident during the hyperosmolar period. However, it has not been proven that this hypothesis is true for all, or even most, of the neurological findings usually observed.

The reversible neurological signs most frequently observed in NKHHC are listed in table I. Alterations of consciousness, grand mal seizures, alterations of respiratory rate, and hyperthermia are the most serious. Fatal respiratory failure is usually preceded by hyperpnea. Hyperthermia is a poor prognostic sign. The presence of meningeal signs, especially in the hyperthermic patient, may confound appropriate diagnosis. A lumbar puncture will reveal increased pressure with elevated cerebrospinal fluid osmolality and glucose and chloride concentrations. Pleocytosis and bacteriologic evidence of infection will be absent. Pupillary abnormalities and signs of peripheral neuropathy are occasionally observed. These findings are generally not reversible and are not likely related to the hyperosmolality [15].

Nonneurological Clinical Findings

NKHHC typically occurs in older individuals with underlying chronic disease. Cardiovascular pathology and renal insufficiency are commonly found. Patients usually have non insulin-dependent diabetes

Table I. Neurological signs associated with nonketotic hyperglycemic hyperosmolar coma [adapted from ref. 15]

Alteration of consciousness
Gradual onset from lethargy to deep coma
More frequent when plasma glucose over 600 mg/dl and serum osmolality over 350 mosm/kg

Hallucinations
Precede development of stupor
Usually visual, including false impression of objects or shadows in the periphery of visual fields

Focal neurological signs
Aphasia, homonymous hemianopia, hemisensory deficits, hemiparesis, unilateral hyperreflexia, and Babinski's sign

Seizures
Grand mal or focal
Preceded or followed by focal neurological signs
Resistant to usual anticonvulsant therapy but respond to adequate insulin and fluid administration

Myoclonic twitches

Abnormal muscle tone

Vestibular dysfunction
Tonic eye deviation and nystagmus

Hyperpnea or accelerated respiratory rate

Hyperthermia

Meningeal signs
Nuchal rigidity, Kernig's sign, photophobia
CSF usually normal except for increased glucose, chloride, and osmolality

Psychopathological states
Depression, apathy, irritability

EEG abnormalities
Nonparoxysmal: slowing of background, disappearance of alpha rhythm, medium to high voltage continuous theta-delta activity
Paroxysmal: focal spike and wave discharges, focal medium to high voltage theta-delta transients, and synchronous generalized slow bursts
Correct with correction of metabolic status, but correction of nonparoxysmal changes lags behind clinical improvement

mellitus which has been adequately controlled with diet alone or diet and oral hypoglycemic agents. It is not uncommon for NKHHC to be the initial presentation of noninsulin-dependent diabetes mellitus in elderly individuals. Most patients are chronically debilitated and are unable to respond to normal thirst mechanisms to maintain fluid intake. Therapy with either diphenylhydantoin, thiazide diuretics, diazoxide, propranolol, cimetidine, or furosemide has been associated with the development of NKHHC [16].

Nonneurological clinical findings represent a combination of signs and symptoms produced by associated illnesses and the hyperglycemic hyperosmolar state. All patients with NKHHC are severely volume-depleted and dehydrated. The skin and mucous membranes reflect the dehydration. Hypotension and tachycardia with major orthostatic components are indicators of the severe hypovolemia. Body temperature is usually low. The eyes are usually sunken and soft with funduscopy revealing normal retina or varying stages of diabetic retinopathy. Lipemia retinalis may be present if there is marked hyperlipemia. Even in the presence of pneumonitis, the lungs are usually clear on auscultation. Rales may become evident as therapy progresses. Rarely, pleural or pericardial friction rubs may be detected [16]. Abdominal discomfort and tenderness are seen frequently and may represent intraabdominal pathology requiring close observation and occasionally surgical intervention. Gastric stasis and ileus occur in over 50% of patients with NKHHC and gastrointestinal bleeding is common in this group [16].

Laboratory

Plasma glucose concentrations greater than 600–800 mg/dl are observed at diagnosis. In pure NKHHC, the serum sodium is usually normal or slightly elevated. Occasionally, the plasma glucose will not be markedly elevated and hypernatremia coexists contributing to the hyperosmolality. In this situation, serum sodium concentrations exceed 150 mEq/l and may even exceed 210 mEq/l [16]. The serum osmolality may be measured or calculated by the formula

$$\text{Osmolality} = 2\,[\text{Na} + \text{K}] + \frac{[\text{glucose}]}{18} + \frac{[\text{BUN}]}{2.8}$$

and is in excess of 350 mosm/kg. Values exceeding 400 mosm/kg are not uncommon. Symptoms associated with hyperosmolality may be present in some individuals when the calculated serum osmolality is less than 350 mosm/kg. Appropriate therapy should be initiated despite the absence of this diagnostic criterion. Serum creatinine and BUN levels are uniformly elevated.

The lack of hepatic ketogenesis is associated with absence of significant ketonemia and an arterial pH greater than 7.3 pH units. The nonketogenic liver continues to synthesize fatty acids and triglycerides resulting in the accumulation of fat in the liver. In addition, as the liver secretes very low density lipoproteins there is a marked elevation of serum triglycerides and cholesterol. Chylomicronemia is a frequent finding.

The differential diagnosis of coma in the diabetic patient is outlined elsewhere in this volume. It is important to reemphasize that any pathological condition which can produce coma in the nondiabetic can also produce coma in the diabetic. Most patients with NKHHC have other medical conditions, many of which can produce nondiabetes-related coma. A meticulous search for concurrent illness as well as for conditions which could have precipitated acute metabolic decompensation is a critical component of the initial evaluation.

Therapy

The management of NKHHC in the intensive care unit is very similar to the management of DKA. The major emphasis is on appropriate supportive care and the prompt, rational administration of fluids, insulin, and potassium. Treatment of precipitating conditions, concurrent illnesses, gastric distension, and hypothermia should be initiated simultaneously with NKHHC-specific therapy. Mental status, vital signs, physical findings, and laboratory parameters, including central venous or pulmonary artery pressures in patients with cardiovascular disease, must be monitored frequently. During the first 12–24 h of therapy, blood glucose, serum electrolytes, BUN, urine output, and calculated serum osmolality should be monitored every 1–2 h. Close observation by the physician with meticulous attention to the clinical course is the single most important factor determining successful treatment.

Fluid administration is the most important aspect of NKHHC-specific therapy. Repletion and maintenance of adequate intravascular volume is essential to prevent vascular thrombotic complications [3]. As hypovolemia is corrected, renal perfusion improves. With increased renal perfusion the effective glomerular filtration rate also improves and there is increased delivery of glucose to the proximal tubule. This results in increased glycosuria and net glucose disposal through the kidneys. Adequate fluid therapy alone will produce a reduction in serum glucose concentration and serum osmolality [20]. The reduction of serum glucose concentration associated with fluid therapy can be accounted for totally by the increase in urinary glucose excretion [17].

The fluid deficit in NKHHC is approximately 100 ml water/kg body weight. This is associated with marked intracellular and extracellular dehydration. It is often necessary to administer 4–7 liters of fluid in the first 6–8 h of therapy. Whether initial fluid replacement should be isotonic or hypotonic is a matter of some controversy. It is argued that use of hypotonic solutions will allow a more rapid replacement of intracellular water and correction of the total body water deficit. On the other hand, isotonic solutions, which are hypotonic to existing body fluids, may provide better repletion of intravascular volume. In addition, dextrose-free hypotonic solutions may not be readily available when initial fluid therapy is instituted. We recommend the use of 0.9% NaCl as the initial fluid replacement and volume expander.

Fluid should be administered as rapidly as possible, consistent with the status of the patient. An initial rate of 1,000 cm^3/h is recommended for most patients. After the first 1,000–1,500 cm^3 of fluid is infused, the infusion rate should be decreased to 500 cm^3/h. At this time, we recommend changing to hypotonic solutions. The use of 0.45% NaCl provides the excess of free water needed to correct intracellular and extracellular hypertonicity. Alternatively, 2.5% dextrose in 0.45% NaCl provides a near-isotonic infusate with generation of free water as the glucose is utilized. This solution may be preferred when the hyperosmolality is caused by the combination of mild hyperglycemia and moderate or severe hypernatremia. When the serum glucose concentration decreases to 250–300 mg/dl, fluid therapy should be continued with 5% dextrose in 0.45% NaCl at a rate of 100–250 cm^3/h. Fluid therapy in general may be complicated by intravascular volume overload. Elderly patients and those with known cardiovascular disease, therefore, should have central venous or pulmonary artery and wedge pressures monitored with, when indicated, appropriate reductions in the rate of fluid administration.

In hypernatremic hyperosmolality, it is recommended that hypotonic solution, i.e. 0.45% NaCl, be used as initial therapy as soon as any accompanying shock or acidosis are corrected with volume expanders or sodium bicarbonate, respectively [4]. For these cases, the water deficit can be calculated using the formula

$$\text{Deficit} = (0.5 \times \text{body weight}) - \frac{140}{\text{actual}[Na^+]} \times (0.5 \times \text{body weight}),$$

where the body weight is the patient's weight in kilograms at the time of initial evaluation. The deficit should be replaced over 48 h with a goal of reducing serum osmolality by approximately 2 mosm/kg/h. Maintenance fluids, including urinary losses, should be given in addition to the replacement fluids [4]. As in NKHHC, it is important to avoid a rapid reduction in serum osmolality since brain osmolality, maintained by idiogenic osmoles, is relatively slow to equilibrate with changing extracellular osmolality. The development of seizures and cerebral edema have been associated with rapid correction of serum osmolality [4].

Insulin administration is best accomplished using the low-dose therapy protocols described for DKA. The advantages of low-dose therapy over conventional high-dose therapy are reviewed elsewhere [2, 12]. A priming dose of 10–20 U (approximately 0.15 U/kg normal body weight) of regular insulin given by intravenous bolus should be followed by 5–10 U/h (approximately 0.1 U/kg normal body weight) by continuous intravenous infusion. This usually results in a decline in plasma glucose concentration of about 100 mg/dl/h [2, 16]. When the blood glucose level reaches 250–300 mg/dl, dextrose-containing fluids should be started and the rate of fluid administration and insulin infusion adjusted to maintain the plasma glucose concentration in the 200 to 300 mg/dl range until the patient is able to eat or an appropriate maintenance nutritional protocol has been instituted.

Potassium replacement is critical and should follow the previously outlined guidelines for DKA. Phosphate replacement should be reserved for those patients who have documented hypophosphatemia on admission or develop hypophosphatemia during therapy. Prophylactic administration of phosphate has not been shown to alter the outcome of therapy for DKA or NKHHC [5, 11].

Intensive therapy should be continued until the patient has regained normal mental status. Most of the neurological signs will reverse with the improvement in serum osmolality, however, the reversal of some will be delayed a variable amount of time. Metabolic end-points of therapy are a serum glucose concentration of 200–250 mg/dl, serum osmolality of

300 mosm/kg or less, and normal serum potassium. The duration of fluid and insulin therapy needed to reach a plasma glucose concentration of 250 mg/dl will vary from 4 to 12 h [2, 20]. Any intensive therapy for concurrent medical conditions should be completed before the episode of NKHHC is considered stable. When the patient is able to eat or appropriate nutritional protocols are instituted, maintenance subcutaneous insulin administration should be begun. Some patients with specific isolated causes for NKHHC may be managed with diet alone or diet and oral hypoglycemic agents if the precipitating cause has been corrected. It is our opinion, however, that most patients who have an episode of NKHHC should have their diabetes managed chronically with insulin therapy.

References

1 Arieff, A.I.; Guisado, R.; Lazarowitz, V.C.: Pathophysiology of hyperosmolar states; in Andreoli, Grantham, Rector, Disturbances in body fluid osmolality, pp. 227–250 (American Physiological Society, Bethesda 1977).

2 Bendezu, R.; Wieland, R.G.; Furst, B.H.; Mandel, M.; Genuth, S.M.; Schumacher, O.P.: Experience with low-dose insulin infusion in diabetic ketoacidosis and diabetic hyperosmolarity. Archs intern. Med. *138:* 60–62 (1978).

3 Clements, R.S., Jr.; Vourganti, B.: Fatal diabetic ketoacidosis: major causes and approaches to their prevention. Diabetes Care *1:* 314–325 (1978).

4 Covey, C.M.; Arieff, A.I.: Disorders of sodium and water metabolism and their effects on the central nervous system; in Brenner, Stein, Contemporary issues in nephrology, vol. I: Sodium and water homeostasis, pp. 212–241 (Churchill Livingstone, London 1978).

5 Fisher, J.N.; Kitabchi, A.E.: A randomized study of phosphate therapy in the treatment of diabetic ketoacidosis. J. clin. Endocr. Metab. *57:* 177–180 (1983).

6 Fulop, M.; Rosenblatt, A.; Kreitzer, S.M.; Gerstenhaber, B.: Hyperosmolar nature of diabetic coma. Diabetes *24:* 594–599 (1975).

7 Gerich, J.E.; Martin, M.M.; Recant, L.: Clinical and metabolic characteristics of hyperosmolar nonketotic coma. Diabetes *20:* 228–238 (1971).

8 Gerich, J.; Penhos, J.C.; Gutman, R.A.; Recant, L.: Effect of dehydration and hyperosmolarity on glucose, free fatty acid and ketone body metabolism in the rat. Diabetes *22:* 264–271 (1973).

9 Joffe, B.I.; Seftel, H.C.; Goldberg, R.; Van As, M.; Krut, L.; Bersohn, I.: Factors in the pathogenesis of experimental nonketotic and ketoacidotic diabetic stupor. Diabetes *22:* 653–657 (1973).

10 Joffe, B.I.; Krut, L.H.; Goldberg, R.B.; Seftel, H.C.: Pathogenesis of nonketotic hyperosmolar diabetic coma. Lancet *i:* 1069–1071 (1975).

11 Keller, U.; Berger, W.: Prevention of hypophosphatemia by phosphate infusion during treatment of diabetic ketoacidosis and hyperosmolar coma. Diabetes *29:* 87–95 (1980).

12 Kitabchi, A.E.: Treatment of diabetic ketoacidosis with low dose insulin. Adv. internal Med. *23:* 115–135 (1978).
13 Knowles, H.C., Jr.: Editorial. Syrupy blood. Diabetes *15:* 760–761 (1966).
14 Lindsey, C.A.; Faloona, G.R.; Unger, R.H.: Plasma glucagon in nonketotic hyperosmolar coma. J. Am. med. Ass. *229:* 1771–1773 (1974).
15 Maccario, M.: Neurological dysfunction associated with nonketotic hyperglycemia. Archs Neurol. *19:* 525–534 (1968).
16 Matz, R.: Coma in the nonketotic diabetic [hyperosmolar nonketotic coma (HNKC) in the diabetic]; in Ellenberg, Rifkin, Diabetes mellitus theory and practice; 3rd ed., pp. 655–666 (Medical Examination Publishing Co., New York 1983).
17 Owen, O.E.; Licht, J.H.; Sapir, D.G.: Renal function and effects of partial rehydration during diabetic ketoacidosis. Diabetes *30:* 510–518 (1981).
18 Schade, D.S.; Eaton, R.P.: Pathogenesis of diabetic ketoacidosis: a reappraisal. Diabetes Care *2:* 296–306 (1979).
19 Turpin, B.P.; Duckworth, W.C.; Solomon, S.S.: Simulated hyperglycemic hyperosmolar syndrome. Impaired insulin and epinephrine effects upon lipolysis in the isolated rat fat cell. J. clin. Invest. *63:* 403–409 (1979).
20 Waldhäusl, W.; Kleinberger, G.; Korn, A.; Dudczak, R.; Bratusch-Marrain, P.; Nowotny, P.: Severe hyperglycemia: effects of rehydration on endocrine derangements and blood glucose concentration. Diabetes *28:* 577–584 (1979).

Charles R. Rost, MD, Assistant Professor of Medicine,
University of Oklahoma Health Sciences Center, Oklahoma City, OK 73106 (USA)

Prog. crit. Care Med., vol. 2, pp. 229–250 (Karger, Basel 1985)

Metabolic Acid-Base Problems

John A. Mitas, II

The University of Oklahoma Health Sciences Center, Oklahoma City, Okla., USA

Overview

In the maintenance of normal body functions, the body regulates acid-base balance within a relatively narrow range, frequently expressed in terms of pH as 7.38–7.44. This is accomplished through numerous buffer systems, and the modulation of the most important buffer system (the carbon dioxide-bicarbonate system) by the lungs (through CO_2 elimination) and the kidneys (through reclamation of filtered bicarbonate, generation of new bicarbonate and excretion of titrable acids).

Normal balance can be disrupted by a host of processes which alter pulmonary or renal function. Those disorders which do not primarily affect ventilation are considered metabolic disorders and may be characterized by the addition of acids, loss of bicarbonate, or addition of bicarbonate. In the critical care setting, these disorders may take on greater magnitude or become mixed in character. Through our actions we may create or aggravate existing metabolic disorders. Knowledge of these disorders and their sequelae, as well as the consequences of therapeutic intervention, will enhance patient care.

In the course of this discussion various terms will be used. Acidosis and alkalosis apply to the process of generating or removing hydrogen ion, respectively. The pH may be normal despite this process and mild disorders may not cause significant laboratory abnormalities. However, mixed disorders may result in essentially normal pH and should be considered. Acidemia will refer to a state of greater hydrogen ion concentration $[H^+]$ and thus a lower pH. Alkalemia will refer to a state of lower $[H^+]$ and thus greater pH. The term mixed disorders refers to two or more primary disorders and assumes that compensatory respiratory alterations are appropriate responses.

In the protection of the normal pH, a number of buffer symptoms are active, including cellular proteins, hemoglobin, plasma proteins, bicarbonate, phosphate, and sulfate. The relative contribution of each of these systems varies according to the clinical situation or the experimental model. However, the isohydric principle states that all buffer pairs in a homogeneous solution (e.g., plasma) are in equilibrium with the same $[H^+]$. Changes in one system should reflect changes in the other system, thus facilitating measurement and diagnostic considerations. Bicarbonate is unique in this setting for a number of reasons: (1) Quantitatively it is the major buffer system in solution and all of its components may be determined easily; (2) it has an open-ended respiratory outlet; (3) reclamation as well as regeneration is performed by the kidney.

$$H^+ + HCO_3^- \rightleftharpoons H_2CO_3 \rightleftharpoons H_2O + CO_2. \quad (1)$$

Although the Henderson-Hasselbalch equation (equation 2), describing the relationship of $[H^+]$ to various buffer components, is familiar to most clinicians, facility with its application is not.

$$pH = pK + \log \frac{[HCO_3^-]}{[H_2CO_3]}. \quad (2)$$

Of more practical usefulness in the assessment of acid-base disorders and the management of patients is the Henderson equation [1] as applied to the bicarbonate system (equation 3).

$$[H^+] = \frac{24\,(PCO_2)}{[HCO_3^-]}. \quad (3)$$

In this equation $[H^+]$ is expressed in n*M*/l, PCO_2 in mm Hg, and $[HCO_3^-]$ as bicarbonate concentration in mEq/l. This relationship emphasizes the fact that hydrogen ion concentration, and therefore pH, is dependent upon the ratio rather than absolute values for PCO_2 and $[HCO_3^-]$. The pH and PCO_2 are measured by electrodes from an arterial blood sample while $[HCO_3^-]$ is determined from a venous sample rather than derived from the Siggaard-Andersen curve nomogram after plotting pH and PCO_2. There are several reasons for an independent determination of bicarbonate: Errors may be made in reading the nomogram, it should be possible to check the accuracy of the pH and PCO_2 determinations, and reliable data must be available for calculations which aid in the diagnosis and assessment of acid-base disorders [1, 2].

Table I. Conversion of pH to H^+

pH	$[H^+]$, n*M*/l
Rapid estimation of $[H^+]$ for pH within the range 7.30–7.50	
7.38	42
7.39	41
7.40	40
7.41	39
7.42	38
Estimation of $[H^+]$ for pH within the range 6.80–7.70 [3]	
6.80	156
6.90	125
7.00	100
7.10	80
7.20	64
7.30	51
7.40	40
7.50	32
7.60	25
7.70	20

In order to use the Henderson equation, it is necessary to convert the pH to $[H^+]$. Within the narrow range of pH 7.30–7.50 this can be accomplished by using a baseline value for $[H^+]$ of 40 n*M*/l at pH = 7.40 and increasing $[H^+]$ by 1 n*M*/l for each 0.01 decrement in pH and decreasing $[H^+]$ by 1 n*M*/l for each 0.01 increment in pH. Because patients develop pH values beyond this range, it is necessary to estimate $[H^+]$ for these pH values. A reliable '80% method' has been proposed by *Fagan* [3] which multiplies a known $[H^+]$ value (for a given pH) by 0.8 to obtain the $[H^+]$ for a pH which is 0.10 higher than the known pH. This extends the rapid estimation of $[H^+]$ to a pH range of 6.8–7.7 with a minimum of errors (table I). Knowledge of the hydrogen ion concentration and the ability to determine its deviation from a baseline value of 40 n*M*/l at pH 7.40 permits one to evaluate certain expected relationships and detect the presence of acute or chronic respiratory disorders (acidosis or alkalosis) (table II).

Other useful relationships identify metabolic acidosis and the adequacy of ventilatory compensation or the presence of additional primary disorders. These determinations require the use of arterial blood gas values, serum electrolytes, and urinary electrolytes. The concept of the 'anion gap'

Table II. Useful relationships in assessing acid-base disorders

Respiratory acidosis		
Ratio $\frac{\Delta [H^+]}{\Delta PCO_2}$	acute = 0.8	chronic = 0.3
Respiratory alkalosis		
Ratio $\frac{\Delta [H^+]}{\Delta PCO_2}$	acute = 0.8	chronic = 0.17
Metabolic acidosis		
Ratio $\frac{\Delta PCO_2}{\Delta [HCO_3^-]}$	compensated acidosis	1.0–1.3
	mixed metabolic acidosis and respiratory acidosis ≤ 1.0	
	mixed metabolic acidosis and metabolic alkalosis > 1.3	
Anion gap: normal range 12 ± 2 mEq/l	$[Na^+] + UC = [HCO_3^-] + [Cl^-] + UA$	
	$[Na^+] - ([HCO_3^-] + [Cl^-]) = UA - UC$	
Metabolic alkalosis		
Urinary $[Cl^-]$	chloride-responsive alkalosis < 10 mEq/l	
	chloride-unresponsive alkalosis > 10–20 mEq/l	

Δ = Change; normal values from which deviation is measured are $[H^+]$ = 40 n*M*/l PCO_2 = 40 mm Hg, $[HCO_3^-]$ = 25 mEq/l. UC = Unmeasured cations; UA = unmeasured anions.

is important in the identification and assessment of metabolic acidosis. The anion gap represents the unmeasured anions and is usually expressed as the difference between serum sodium concentration and the sum of chloride and bicarbonate concentrations.

$$[Na^+] - ([Cl^-] + [HCO_3^-]) = \text{anion gap}. \quad (4)$$

However, the anion gap actually is the difference between the above electrolytes and is equal to the difference between unmeasured anions and unmeasured cations [4, 5]. The former consist of phosphate, sulfate, protein, and organic acids while the latter consist of potassium, calcium, magnesium, and IgG. Elevations or decrements of any of these ions may alter the anion gap from its normal value of 12 ± 2 mEq/l. The anion gap is most helpful in dividing metabolic acidosis between those where a fall in bicarbonate is replaced by an equal compensatory rise in chloride (the hyperchloremic acidoses = normal anion gap acidoses) and those where a fall in bicarbonate is replaced by anions other than chloride (elevated anion gap). Other conditions which affect the anion gap will be discussed below.

Metabolic alkalosis does not lend itself to the simple determinations of ratios between expected PCO_2 change in compensation for a rising $[HCO_3]$ because the increment in PCO_2 is highly variable and inconsistent. However, quite useful information may be found in the measurement of urinary electrolytes to categorize the disorder as chloride-responsive or chloride-resistant. Metabolic alkalosis is somewhat unique in the realm of acid-base disorders because inciting events may be quite distinct from factors which perpetuate the alkalosis unless they are corrected [1, 6–8].

Pathophysiology

Metabolic Acidosis

Metabolic activity involves the generation and consumption of hydrogen ions in a variety of biochemical reactions. In spite of the constant addition and removal of hydrogen ions, the pH (and thus hydrogen ion concentration) remains within a relatively narrow range. This is accomplished by (a) the multiple buffer systems which are present in great quantity, (b) the special properties of carbonic acid, H_2CO_3, from which carbon dioxide may be formed and equilibrated with the alveolar gas (equation 1), and (c) the activity of the kidney in the excretion of acid as well as the reclamation and generation of bicarbonate. In metabolic acid-base disorders the kidney plays a central role.

Normally the body produces 1.0–1.5 mEq of acid (apart from carbonic acid)/kg of body weight each day. This production is offset by daily renal input of an equal amount of bicarbonate, thus restoring the buffer systems and bicarbonate values to normal. At the proximal convoluted tubule, this is accomplished by reclamation of at least 75% of the filtered bicarbonate load. Because of evidence of acid disequilibrium pH within the tubular lumen, proton secretion is believed to be the primary mechanism for acidifying tubule fluid [9]. Secreted hydrogen ion titrates the filtered bicarbonate which is converted to carbonic acid and CO_2 and reabsorbed. Some of this bicarbonate reabsorption is dependent upon carbonic anhydrase activity at the luminal brush border as well as within the cell (to generate H_2CO_3 from the absorbed CO_2, which then dissociates into H^+, in turn secreted

Table III. Metabolic acidosis with elevated anion gap

Type of acidosis	Mechanism of acidosis
(I) Exogenous acid	
(A) HCl, NH_4Cl, arginine-HCl, lysine-HCl, hyperalimentation	acid load exceeding renal excretory capacity
(B) Salicylate ingestion	increased salicylic acid plus increased production of organic acids (including lactic acid)
(C) Ethylene glycol ingestion	oxalic acid, hippuric acid, glycoaldehyde; altered metabolism causing production of organic acids (including lactic acid)
(D) Methanol ingestion	formic acid plus formaldehyde lead to altered metabolism and organic acid production; lactic acids and keto acids may be increased
(E) Paraldehyde	metabolism to acetic acid plus increased organic acids; starvation ketosis may play a role
(F) Toluene inhalation	benzoic and hippuric acid formation; possible ketosis
(G) Isoniazid overdose	lactic acidosis
(II) Endogenous acid	
(A) Lactic acidosis	altered metabolism of pyruvate associated with hypoperfusion and reduced tissue oxygenation
(B) Ketoacidosis	diabetes – hypoinsulinism; accentuated production of keto acids alcoholism – altered redox state, lactic acid production starvation – hypoinsulinism and accentuated hepatic ketone production
(C) Uremia	normal protein metabolism and decreased renal acid excretion

into the lumen, and HCO_3^-, crossing the basolateral surface and entering the blood). At the distal nephron, protons are secreted at a rate sufficient to reclaim the small fraction of HCO_3^- escaping proximal reabsorption and to titrate HPO_4^{2-} and NH_3 in amounts to provide for net secretion of acid. Ammonia is secreted at proximal as well as distal nephron sites but the exact role in final urinary acidification is unknown. Overall 98% or more of the protons secreted are employed in recapture of bicarbonate.

Renal disease may lead to metabolic acidosis by virtue of a depressed net rate of hydrogen ion secretion. This may occur on the basis of decreased numbers of functioning nephrons as in uremic acidosis [10]. Increased distal delivery of bicarbonate due to inhibition of carbonic anhydrase activity, hyperkalemia, hyperparathyroidism, or hypophosphatemia may manifest itself as acidosis with decreased net proximal tubule hydrogen ion secretion [11, 12]. This is characteristic of a proximal (or type II) renal tubular acidosis. A distal renal tubular acidosis (type I or classic) may occur on the basis of an inability to secrete hydrogen ion or the failure to maintain a steep lumen-to-blood concentration gradient for [H^+] [11–14]. This may be seen in a variety of disorders causing interstitial renal disease, insufficient distal delivery of nonbicarbonate anions, impaired aldosterone secretion or responsiveness, or hyperkalemic states.

Metabolic acidosis also may occur due to extrarenal losses of bicarbonate as in gastrointestinal diseases (severe diarrhea, pancreatic fistulae and/or drainage, biliary drainage) or ureterosigmoid anastomosis. In the latter condition chloride is exchanged for bicarbonate by the enteric mucosa and bicarbonate is lost from the body.

The other conditions in which metabolic acidosis may arise are those in which exogenous acid is added to the body or endogenous acids such as keto acids or lactic acid are generated. Bicarbonate is utilized in buffering the acidosis and is frequently replaced by these exogenous or endogenous anions leading to an elevation of the anion gap. The proposed mechanisms involved with each of these disorders include production of acid or toxic metabolites and impaired cellular metabolism with production of organic acids (including lactic acid and keto acids) [4, 8, 15–21] (table III). Lactic acidosis is believed to be the most commonly encountered metabolic acidosis and may be subdivided into a type A due to tissue hypoperfusion or acute hypoxia and a type B due to toxins, ingestions (table III), or common disorders such as diabetes, renal failure, or liver disease [16, 21].

Metabolic Alkalosis

Metabolic alkalosis may be described as any process which causes a primary increase in bicarbonate concentration or a net loss of hydrogen ion. Because a major source of H^+ is the dissociation of H_2CO_3 to H^+ and HCO_3^-, any process involving loss of hydrogen ion may lead to increasing [HCO_3^-]. The absolute values are not as important as the ratio PCO_2/HCO_3^- which, when decreased, indicates a lower hydrogen concentration and an elevated pH.

Gain of HCO_3^- per se occurs in few situations: excessive bicarbonate administration or ingestion; metabolism of bicarbonate precursors such as citrate, acetate, or lactate; or in the posthypercapnic state when ventilatory abnormalities have been treated or corrected [1, 6–8, 16]. The other etiologies of metabolic alkalosis can best be categorized as chloride-responsive or chloride-unresponsive causes. This distinction addresses the maintenance factors of the alkalosis which may not be the same as the transient initiating factors.

The chloride-responsive group includes gastrointestinal as well as renal etiologies. Among the former are nasogastric suction, emesis, and chloride-wasting diarrhea (occasionally associated with a villous adenoma). In these settings H^+ is lost resulting in a quantitatively equal gain of bicarbonate. During continued emesis or nasogastric suction there is continued addition of HCO_3^- to plasma in exchange for chloride. If these conditions persist, extracellular fluid volume (ECV) decreases while bicarbonate content remains the same or increases. The decreased ECV stimulates aldosterone production with the result of increased sodium reabsorption distally as avid chloride reabsorption occurs. This leads to the distal nephron exchange of sodium for potassium and very low urinary chloride values in the face of sodium, potassium, and bicarbonate excretion [6–8, 16]. Chloride-containing diarrhea would result in similar consequences. Renal losses of chloride due to thiazide or loop diuretics use (or abuse) are not accompanied by bicarbonaturia. Instead, there is an acute volume contraction with an unchanged total body HCO_3^- content leading to an increased concentration. The PCO_2 does not change simultaneously, thus there is a shift in the ratio and a consequent alkalosis. Chronic diuretic usage occasionally may lead to volume contraction, however, there is increased distal nephron delivery of sodium with consequent sodium-hydrogen exchange and sodium-potassium exchange. Maintenance of the alkalosis occurs as a result of secondary hyperaldosteronism, potassium loss, and chloride loss due to continued use of diuretics.

Hypercalcemia (without increased parathyroid hormone) or hypoparathyroidism may cause enhanced renal bicarbonate reabsorption although the mechanisms are not fully understood [16]. Use of carbenicillin or penicillin may cause alkalemia as a result of their renal excretion as nonreabsorbable anions. This results in potassium secretion and hydrogen ion secretion (with bicarbonate generation) [27].

The chloride-unresponsive alkaloses are primarily due to adrenal or steroid-related disorders [1, 8, 16]. In these disorders hyperaldosteronism or Cushing's syndrome (of any cause) generate an alkalosis while a normal or expanded ECV is present. Hypokalemia results as distal nephron sodium reabsorption increases and expands the ECV. With an expanded ECV, distal sodium delivery is increased. Acid excretion is enhanced as a consequence of potassium depletion in the presence of aldosterone [16]. Excessive licorice ingestion or use of carbenoxalone may have an identical outcome due to mineralocorticoid-like effects. Because the stimuli are independent of ECV, chloride is excreted normally in the urine (i.e. $>$10–20 mEq/l) permitting distinction of these groups. Severe potassium deficits of 500–1,000 mEq alone may alter the renal handling of chloride resulting in chloride wasting with metabolic alkalosis [23]. When hypertension with metabolic alkalosis is present, in the absence of diuretics or chloride reabsorption, disorders such as hyperaldosteronism, Cushing's syndrome, or renin-mediated hypertension should be considered.

From the variety of disorders identified, it is clear that the factors involved in the initiation of metabolic alkalosis may be transient but result in common final pathways involving either volume (chloride) depletion or hypokalemia which in turn maintain the process until they are corrected.

Diagnosis

The patient with metabolic acidemia may exhibit symptoms as mild as anorexia, lethargy, and headache or as severe as stupor, seizures, tachycardia, and peripheral vasodilatation. The patient with alkalemia may be asymptomatic or may manifest increased neuromuscular irritability, possibly tetany, and with severe alkalemia will be at risk of serious cardiac arrhythmias and leftward shift of the oxyhemoglobin dissociation curve. Because many of these symptoms and findings are nonspecific, chemical determinations are required to assess and confirm the diagnosis.

Findings which should be assessed early are the arterial blood gas report (pH, PCO_2) and serum electrolytes. Urinary electrolytes and pH as well as tests for ketones and lactic acid are secondary determinations. A pH of 7.35 indicates acidemia while a pH of 7.45 indicates alkalemia. With any simple acid-base disorder the $[HCO_3^-]$ and PCO_2 values are expected to change in the same direction. Thus, a decrement in PCO_2 and $[HCO_3^-]$ from normal values could be caused by either respiratory alkalosis or metabolic acidosis. A pH determined concurrently should identify whether an acidemia or alkalemia is present. Similarly, a rise in $[HCO_3^-]$ and PCO_2 could represent either respiratory acidosis or metabolic alkalosis and the pH would distinguish between the choices. In the critical care setting considerations arise beyond the mere labeling of the type of disorder. For respiratory abnormalities it is desirable to know whether the change is acute or chronic. For metabolic acidosis, the degree or adequacy of ventilatory compensation helps identify the need for mechanical ventilation and the possibility of additional disorders such as concurrent metabolic alkalosis [1]. Calculation of the anion gap aids in categorization of the etiology and in the delivery of appropriate therapy [4, 5, 24]. A disparity between measured and calculated plasma osmolality often suggests specific substances causing an elevated anion gap. In metabolic alkalosis the identification of low urinary chloride (10 mEq/l) would identify a group of disorders responding to volume expansion rather than potassium administration.

Table II identifies relationships which are helpful in approaching acid-base disorders. Respiratory disorders are considered elsewhere in this text as well as in the review by *Narins and Emmett* [1]. When a metabolic acidosis is confirmed by a fall in [HCO_3^-] and acidemia a number of questions should be asked. Is the anion gap normal or elevated? If the anion gap is normal (i.e. 12 ± 2), representing a hyperchloremic acidosis, the acidosis is usually associated with one of the following disorders:

(1) Gastrointestinal loss of HCO_3^-
   (a) Pancreatic fistula, biliary drainage
   (b) Diarrhea
(2) Ureteral diverting procedures such as ileal bladder or ureterosigmoidostomy
(3) Carbonic anhydrase inhibitors (acetazolamide)
(4) Administration of HCl or NH_4Cl, arginine-HCl or lysine-HCl
(5) Renal tubular acidosis
   (a) Proximal
   (b) Distal, may be acquired [11–14]
   (c) Phosphate deficiency
   (d) Post-obstructive, type IV [25]
(6) Post-hypocapnea

These disorders should be distinguishable by examination of the patient, review of medication records, and by history. With the exception of a post-obstructive type IV renal tubular acidosis these entities should not have an elevated potassium concentration, [K^+].

If the anion gap is 15 or greater, other entities must be considered. The addition of exogenous acids via ingestion or administration includes salicylate intoxication, methanol, ethylene glycol, or paraldehyde ingestion [1, 16–18]. Salicylate intoxication should be suspected in young children, individuals suspected of suicide attempts, and patients with marked tinnitus, rapid respirations, and normochloremic metabolic acidemia. Measurement of the plasma salicylate level will confirm this diagnosis. Ethylene glycol may be ingested accidentally, as a substitute for alcohol, or in a suicide attempt. Central nervous system dysfunction appears within the first 12 h. Patients may appear drunk, comatose, or have seizures – all without ketones detectable on the breath. During the ensuing 12–24 h hypertension and congestive heart failure may predominate. Finally, oliguric acute renal failure develops [4, 17, 26]. The anion gap may exceed 25 and the urine may contain calcium oxalate and hippuric acid crystals [4]. Calculated plasma osmolality much lower than measured osmolality should suggest the presence of ethylene glycol or methanol.

Symptoms of methanol intoxication may occur 12– 18 h after ingestion. These include weakness, headache, nausea, epigastric pain, and blurred vision [27] and may be rapidly followed by blindness, coma, and cardiac arrest. As in ethylene glycol ingestion there is no odor of alcohol or acetone on the breath in a patient who may appear drunk. The optic discs are edematous on physical examination and scotomata are frequently detected if the patient is awake. The anion gap may exceed 25 and there may be an increase in plasma osmolality. Formic acid levels or methanol levels may be elevated. Paraldehyde intoxication has been described in 7 individuals who ingested large quantities. Abdominal pain of several days duration coupled with central nervous system depression in individuals with a history of acohol abuse and the characteristic odor of the drug should lead to the diagnosis [1, 4, 16]. Additional findings include marked leukocytosis without obvious cause and an increasingly positive nitroprusside test for ketones.

Endogenous acid generation may occur in combinations with the above disorders, with isoniazid intoxication (thought to be lactic acidosis) [16, 19], toluene or paint sniffing [20], and nalidixic acid overdose [28] with a consequent high anion gap. Patients with isoniazid overdose may have a severe acidosis, coma, and uncontrollable grand mal seizures. In the other disorders shock is not necessarily present and a thorough history is required to make the diagnosis.

Lactic acidosis may occur as a result of poor tissue perfusion due to shock or acute hypoxemia (type A) or as a concomitant of common disorders such as diabetes, renal or hepatic disease, ingestion of various substances, or following grand mal seizures (type B) [16, 21, 29]. The presence of an elevated anion gap acidosis associated with shock should lead to the diagnosis of type A lactic acidosis. A type B lactic acidosis should be considered in the presence of an elevated anion gap with a history of drug ingestion (phenformin, ethanol, methanol, salicylates, etc.), in diabetes mellitus and hepatic or renal dysfunction. Occasionally, an unexplained high anion gap metabolic acidosis is detected in association with Hodgkin's disease or a solid tumor [30, 31]. Plasma levels of *l*-lactic acid would identify this as a lactic acidosis. Special considerations should be given to the constellation of altered mental status, a history of small bowel resection, elevated anion gap with acidemia, and plasma lactate values, in the absence of an obvious explanation for the acidosis. Several reports have now identified abnormal gut flora in the short bowel syndrome producing *d*-lactic acid which is not detected by the usual assay [32].

Ketosis leading to acidemia may be found in diabetic patients with absolute or relative insulin deficiency, patients with severely restricted carbohydrate intake, and in alcoholics (in whom a major component may be inadequate dietary intake) [33–36]. These patients may be dehydrated, vomiting, obtunded, hyperpneic, and have acetone on the breath. Diagnostic studies should include arterial pH and blood gases which will demonstrate acidemia, serum electrolytes which frequently reveal an elevated anion gap, glucose determination, and serum and urine ketone determinations. A diagnosis of diabetic ketoacidosis is made if the urine has 4+ glucose and strong reactions for ketones (with Acetest tablet); hyperglycemia, blood pH less than 7.30 with decreased PCO_2, and strongly positive serum ketone reaction with undiluted serum. The Acetest tablet tests primarily for acetoacetate and slightly for acetone but not for β-hydroxybutyrate which may be the predominant ketoacid present [34]. In alcoholic or fasting ketosis the plasma glucose level is below 250 mg/dl and may be strikingly low [36]. The pathogenesis of ketosis has recently been reviewed by *Cahill* [35] and is beyond the scope of this discussion. Because there is no absolute relation between the initial serum [HCO_3^-] and the anion gap in diabetic ketoacidosis, a hyperchloremic metabolic acidosis should not exclude the diagnosis [37]. Renal insufficiency may lead to the greater retention of ketones, especially in diabetics with more severe volume depletion.

Metabolic acidosis may be detected in mild to moderate renal insufficiency when the serum creatinine is 2–4 mg/dl and hyperchloremia is present. With more severe renal insufficiency (creatinine greater than 4 mg/dl) the anion gap becomes elevated as the bicarbonate level falls [10].

This does not correlate with urinary volume. Additionally, when the initial serum creatinine is $\leqslant 1.5$ mg/dl it may be necessary to serially measure serum creatinine to detect a rise of 0.5–1.5 mg/dl/day which is indicative of acute renal failure (but does not distinguish prerenal, parenchymal, or obstructive etiologies).

When using the anion gap to assist in diagnosing metabolic acidosis, certain caveats are warranted. The anion gap may be elevated due to other disorders including dehydration, therapy with certain antibiotics (penicillin, carbenicillin), sodium salts of various acids (lactic acid, sulfates, phosphates), and occasionally with alkalosis (due to salicylates and respiratory stimulation). A positive nitroprusside test for ketones in the *absence* of an elevated anion gap should alert the physician to the presence of a high acetone level which may be due to ingested isopropyl alcohol [4, 5]. The anion gap may be elevated by deficiency of calcium, magnesium, and potassium which are unmeasured cations. Hypoalbuminemia may lower the anion gap as may increased IgG and the above normally present cations.

Use of the ratio of *change* from normal values

$$\frac{\Delta PCO_2}{\Delta [HCO_3^-]}$$

should fall within the expected range of 1.0–1.3 for a simple (compensated) metabolic acidosis. Values below this level indicate inadequate respiratory compensation and a possible need for mechanical ventilation. Values greater than 1.3, due to a higher-than-expected $[HCO_3^-]$, in the presence of an acidemia and elevated anion gap are indicative of an additional primary disorder – metabolic alkalosis [1].

Metabolic alkalosis should be considered in patients with volume depletion – especially gastrointestinal volume losses – and in patients recently treated with mechanical ventilation, those resuscitated after cardiac arrest, and in patients with hypokalemia or marked urinary potassium wasting. Refeeding of patients after nutritional deficiency may lead to alkalosis. The diagnosis of metabolic alkalosis may be made by finding a bicarbonate concentration greater than 27 mEq/l, an elevated PCO_2, and an alkalemic pH > 7.44. Urinary electrolytes are needed, particularly chloride values. If urinary chloride is less than 10 mEq/l, the patient is considered to have a chloride-responsive metabolic alkalosis. If the urinary chloride exceeds 10–20 mEq/l, a mineralocorticoid- or glucocorticoid-related problem should be suspected. The serum potassium should be reviewed in these latter individuals to assess for low values which may lead to dangerous cardiac arrhythmias. Finally, it should not be assumed that a patient presenting with ketosis, normal blood sugars, and history of alcoholism has an acidosis. In a series of 24 alcoholic ketosis patients reported by *Fulop and Hoberman* [36], 7 patients were alkalemic due to coexisting respiratory or metabolic alkalosis.

In the past, it was suggested that review of serum anions and potassium values would help distinguish alkalemic from acidemic patients. The former would be expected to have a low [K^+] while the latter would be hyperkalemic. This relationship was suggested from early reports [38, 39] of experimental acid-base changes. Subsequently, it has been recognized that potassium may be more dependent upon bicarbonate than blood pH [40], that hyperkalemia is infrequent in lactic acidosis and ketoacidosis [41, 42], and that if hyperkalemia is present with acidosis it is generally mild due to respiratory acidosis or elevated as a result of nonorganic acid administration [43]. The direction of potassium movement during acute acid-base disorders is not uniform among the various tissues and should not be relied upon in making the diagnosis of a particular acid-base disorder.

Treatment

The treatment of metabolic disorders includes group-specific therapy, discontinuation or removal of an offending agent, or patient-specific procedures and interventions.

Therapy of metabolic acidosis characterized by hyperchloremia and a normal anion gap generally requires replacement with bicarbonate. Although numerous formulae have been proposed to identify adequate replacement and the volume of distribution, therapy remains individualized to the disease process (e.g. requirements for renal tubular acidosis) and for the severity of the metabolic acidosis. *Garella* et al. [44] were able to demonstrate several years ago that the volume of distribution for bicarbonate may exceed 200% of an individual's body weight.

Pancreatic fistulae, biliary drainage, and diarrhea may require parenteral bicarbonate administration because of the route and volume of fluid loss as well as the need for volume support – particularly if deficits are in the 4- to 5-liter range. If calcium deficits coexist, acetate or lactate solutions may be employed to prevent precipitation of $CaCO_3$ in the replacement solutions. Bicarbonate is generally required only when pH is below 7.20 or falling toward this level, due to the hemodynamic consequences of acidemia. Cessation of biliary drainage or surgical repair of fistulae may be required.

Carbonic anhydratase inhibitors usually do not result in [HCO_3^-] less than 18–20 mEq/l and generally do not require discontinuation or administration of bicarbonate. Because of the respiratory alkalosis associated with these drugs, they may be of some benefit in treating metabolic alkalosis perpetuating hypercarbia [45, 46]. Metabolic acidosis is relatively uncommon with urinary diverting procedures to the ileum unless they become obstructed. Ureterosigmoidostomies are associated more frequently with exchange of Cl^- from urine for HCO_3^- and may require treatment with HCO_3^- as Shohl's solution which contains 1 mEq of alkali (as citrate)/ml, $NaHCO_3$ tablets, or parenteral bicarbonate.

Renal tubular acidosis (RTA) generally requires replacement of the bicarbonate deficit. In distal (type I) RTA, 1–3 mEq of bicarbonate (or citrate)/kg/day may be required to replace the HCO_3^- deficit. In the case of proximal (type II) RTA, the bicarbonate requirements are higher and may necessitate replacement with 2–10 mEq of HCO_3^- (or equivalent)/kg/day. The replacement dose may be reduced with concomitant use of hydrochlorothiazide. RTA associated with hyperkalemia (type IV) may be seen with diabetes, any preexisting renal disease, or after relief of urinary obstruction. This disorder may respond to mineralocorticoid administration in the form of fludrocortisone 0.2 mg/day or more [47, 48]. The hyperkalemia usually responds to therapy with lower doses (0.05–0.10 mg) although the acidosis may not. Volume contraction in this group of patients should be avoided because this would decrease distal delivery of sodium and further reduce potassium excretion.

Acidemia due to administration of HCl is treated by discontinuation of the infusion. Parenteral hyperalimentation solutions no longer contain high concentrations of arginine or lysine hydrochloride, but acidosis with hyperalimentation solutions may be due to relative insulin deficiency. Hypocapnea-induced metabolic acidosis is usually of brief duration and does not require treatment.

Patients who demonstrate an elevated anion gap require vigorous diagnostic and therapeutic efforts. The report by *Gabow* et al. [24] showed that an anion gap exceeding 30 mEq/l was usually due to identifiable organic acidosis (lactic acidosis or ketoacidosis). However, 29% of the patients in this report with an anion gap $\leq$29 mEq/l had no organic acidosis. The etiology of metabolic acidosis in this patient population is more diverse, more serious, and therapy is more varied.

Drugs such as salicylate, isoniazid, etc. may result in acidosis and merely require a forced alkaline diuresis. However, if the salicylate level exceeds 75 mg/dl, hemodialysis should be considered. Isoniazid overdose resulting in acidemia and intractable seizures will require pyridoxine 1 mg parenterally for each milligram isoniazid ingested to arrest seizure activity [19, 49, 50], but bicarbonate administration and hemodialysis may still be required. An excellent review of drugs which respond to dialysis and hemoperfusion was compiled by *Winchester* et al. [51].

Ethylene glycol or methanol intoxication may result in severe acidosis. Therapy should consist of bicarbonate administration, ethanol infusion to competitively block formation of the toxic metabolites, and hemodialysis [17, 18, 26, 27, 52]. Even with early dialysis and the combined administration of ethanol and bicarbonate, therapy is not uniformly successful.

Paraldehyde ingestion leading to metabolic acidosis with an elevated anion gap is rare [1, 4]. Intravenous alkali therapy to maintain [HCO_3^-] at 15–18 mEq/l may be the only therapy required. However, due to the possibility that this may be a masked alcoholic ketoacidosis (with predominant β-hydroxybutyrate), the provision of adequate carbohydrate calories is warranted. In alcoholic ketoacidosis intravenous glucose and NaCl solutions rapidly lead to resolution of the ketosis indicating that starvation may be an important factor [36]. Insulin is not required with this form of ketosis and may be dangerous.

Diabetic ketoacidosis is usually accompanied by volume contraction; urinary bicarbonate, phosphate, and potassium loss, and hyperglycemia. Therapy is multifaceted and consists of adequate rehydration with NaCl, repletion of potassium and phosphate, bicarbonate administration to reverse markedly low pH, and insulin administration. Bicarbonate requirements may exceed 150 mEq in the severely acidotic patient. Hyperglycemia and ketoacidosis may be safely and expeditiously reversed by low-dose insulin administered as continuous intravenous infusion or intramuscular injection [53]. There is no disadvantage to using less than 100 U of regular insulin (cumulative) in this manner and there is the real advantage of avoiding hypoglycemia. This topic is discussed elsewhere in this volume.

Lactic acidosis may be the most commonly encountered metabolic acidosis, but therapy for this condition varies markedly depending on the underlying pathogenesis. Therapy is directed at reversal of the acidemia via bicarbonate administration as well as removal of the inciting condition or drug. Type B lactic acidosis will require sufficient bicarbonate to maintain the serum [HCO_3^-] at or above 15 mEq/l. Forced alkaline diuresis may be employed to remove an offending agent. At the same time dialysis may be required to remove an offending toxin, to treat underlying renal insufficiency, and to give a bicarbonate equivalent. Some authors [54] suggest that insulin may be useful in the treatment of type B lactic acidosis due to its inhibition of amino acid release and possible stimulation of lactate utilization.

Type A lactic acidosis is due to poor tissue perfusion, shock, or marked hypoxemia. Therapy in this more severe form must include early bicarbonate administration – often of hundreds of milliequivalents [44] and treatment of the underlying sepsis or ineffective arterial volume (volume depletion or congestive heart failure). In sepsis with shock, use of naloxone should be considered. Vasodilator therapy with sodium nitroprusside [55] may improve systemic perfusion despite a fall in cardiac output. Careful regulation of the dose administered should preclude a fall in blood pressure. In some patients this therapy is not feasible. Because of the poor prognosis associated with severe lactic acidosis, bicarbonate-buffered peritoneal dialysis should be considered and initiated early in conjunction with other therapy [56]. This therapy is not uniformly successful but has significant advantages among which are (a) avoidance or treatment of hypervolemia, (b) prevention of therapy-induced hypernatremia, and (c) provision of large quantities of physiologic buffer via the dialysate. Additionally, this form of therapy is useful when cardiac performance is compromised. The choice of fluids for intravenous volume expansion is debatable. Some concern has been expressed regarding the use of lactated Ringer's solution (RL) or D_5RL in this condition due to the impaired metabolic function of the liver and kidney in the face of severe acidosis – the two major sites of conversion of lactate to bicarbonate [21]. Others note a fall in lactate levels and reversal of the acidemia with volume expansion following administration of these solutions. If the cardiac output makes hemodialysis feasible, only bicarbonate dialysate (rather than acetate) should be employed due to the instability of these patients and the potential for myocardial depressant effect of sodium acetate [57–59].

Acidosis associated with renal failure may be treated with either hemodialysis or peritoneal dialysis. Even though lactic acid may accumulate with renal insufficiency alone, the use of bicarbonate dialysis is not critical unless another organ dysfunction is present [60].

Therapy of metabolic alkalosis is directed at alleviation of the maintenance factors which perpetuate the alkalosis. This is accomplished by replacing any extracellular fluid deficiency with saline. If hypotension is present, volume expansion should be vigorous. Potassium losses should be anticipated (even though serum potassium may be within the normal range) due to the hyperaldosteronism which accompanies volume depletion. Usually oral potassium repletion is sufficient. However, if the deficit is severe – as suggested by low serum values and urinary excretion of 5–10 mEq/day –, intravenous replacement at a rate of 5–10 mEq/h may be used to supplement oral potassium administration.

If the precipitating factors are still present, they should be addressed. Whenever possible, nasogastric suction should be discontinued. When this is not possible, cimetidine may be given intravenously – 300 mg every 6 h in patients with normal renal function or every 12 h in those with renal insufficiency [61, 62]. Diuretic use infrequently causes severe metabolic alkalosis but should be curtailed to permit retention of chloride as volume expansion is undertaken. Alkali administered as bicarbonate, lactate, or citrate may be replaced with other solutions.

Chloride-unresponsive alkalosis requires administration of potassium and interruption of the mineralocorticoid effects or potassium wasting [8, 54]. Potassium wasting may be stopped with specific hormone antagonists such as spironolactone or more rapidly with amiloride or triamterene. Evaluation and definitive correction of a hypermineralocorticoid state or Cushing's syndrome should be performed as soon as possible. Patients with Bartter's syndrome may not respond to any of these potassium-sparing agents or potassium repletion alone and may require indomethacin or other prostaglandin synthetase inhibitors [63, 64]. Potassium-sparing agents and prostaglandin synthetase inhibitors may pose a grave risk in patients with coexistent insufficiency or renal failure. These patients exhibit an impaired ability to secrete bicarbonate and potassium as well as acid. Such patients may benefit from the use of intravenous hydrochloric acid [65] or by hemodialysis with specialized high-chloride, low-acetate dialysate of varying compositions [66, 67]. A portable dialysis system using the Redy machine and frequent dialysate replacement has been advocated for treatment of metabolic alkalosis in patients with renal failure [68], but the Sorb 42 cartridge needed for this procedure is no longer available. A modified low-acetate, high-chloride dialysate for the Redy system may be used with currently available cartridges and may be employed as often as needed [69]. Patients whose cardiovascular status or lack of vascular access preclude hemodialysis may be treated by peritoneal dialysis with a modified saline solution as dialysate to correct a metabolic alkalosis [70].

References

1 Narins, R.G.; Emmett, M.: Simple and mixed acid-base disorders: a practical approach. Medicine, Baltimore *59:* 161–187 (1980).
2 Hood, I.; Campbell, E.L.M.: Is pK ok? New Engl. J. Med. *306:* 864–866 (1982).
3 Fagan, T.J.: Estimation of hydrogen ion concentration. New Engl. J. Med. *288:* 915 (1973).
4 Emmett, M.; Narins, R.G.: Clinical use of the anion gap. Medicine, Baltimore *56:* 38–54 (1977).
5 Oh, M.S.; Carroll, H.J.: Current concepts: the anion gap. New Engl. J. Med. *297:* 814–817 (1977).
6 Schwartz, W.B.; Van Ypersele De Strihou, C.; Kassirer, J.P.: Role of anions in metabolic alkalosis and potassium deficiency. New Engl. J. Med. *279:* 630–639 (1968).
7 Seldin, D.W.; Rector, F.C.: The generation and maintenance of metabolic alkalosis. Kidney int. *1:* 306–321 (1972).
8 Arruda, J.A.L.; Kurtzman, N.A.: Metabolic acidosis and alkalosis. Clin. Nephrol. *7:* 201–215 (1977).
9 Warnock, D.G.; Rector, F.C.: Renal acidification mechanisms; in Brenner, Rector, The kidney; 2nd ed. (Saunders, Philadelphia 1981).
10 Widmer, B.; Gerhardt, R.E.; Harrington, J.T.; Cohen, J.J.: Serum electrolyte and acid-base composition: the influence of graded degrees of chronic renal failure. Archs intern. Med. *139:* 1099–1102 (1979).
11 Sebastian, A.; Morris, R.C.: Renal tubular acidosis. Clin. Nephrol. *7:* 216–230 (1977).
12 Gennari, F.J.; Cohen, J.J.: Renal tubular acidosis. Annu. Rev. Med. *29:* 521–541 (1978).
13 Batlle, D.C.; Sehy, J.T.; Roseman, M.K.; Arruda, J.A.L.; Kurtzman, N.A.: Clinical and pathophysiologic spectrum of acquired distal renal tubular acidosis. Kidney int. *20:* 389–396 (1981).
14 Stinebaugh B.J.; Scholoeder, F.X.; Tam, S.C.; Goldstein, M.B.; Halperin, M.L.: Pathogenesis of distal renal tubular acidosis. Kidney int. *19:* 1–7 (1981).
15 Heird, W.D.; Dell, R.B.; Driscoll, J.M.; Grebin, B.; Winters, R.W.: Metabolic acidosis resulting from intravenous alimentation mixtures containing synthetic amino acids. New Engl. J. Med. *287:* 943–948 (1972).
16 Cogan, M.C.; Rector, F.C.; Seldin, D.W.: Acid-base disorders; in Brenner, Rector, The kidney; 2nd ed. (Saunders, Philadelphia 1981).
17 Scully, R.E.; Galdabini, J.J.; McNeely, B.U.: Weekly clinicopathological exercises. New Engl. J. Med. *301:* 650–657 (1979).
18 McMartin, K.E.; Ambre, J.J.; Tephly, T.R.: Methanol poisoning in human subjects; role for formic acid accumulation in the metabolic acidosis. Am. J. Med. *68:* 414–418 (1980).
19 Brown, C.V.: Acute isoniazid poisoning. Am. Rev. resp. Dis. *105:* 206–216 (1972).
20 Fischman, C.M.; Oster, J.R.: Toxic effects of toluene: a new cause of high anion gap metabolic acidosis. J. Am. med. Ass. *241:* 1713–1715 (1979).
21 Kreisberg, R.A.: Lactate homeostasis and lactic acidosis. Ann. intern. Med. *92:* 227–237 (1980).
22 Zager, J.; Tjandramaga, T.B.; Cucinell, S.A.; Dayton, P.G.: Letters. Ann. intern. Med. *78:* 774–776 (1973).

23 Garella, S.; Chazan, J.A.; Cohen, J.J.: Saline-resistant metabolic alkalosis or 'chloride-wasting nephropathy'. Ann. intern. Med. *73:* 31–38 (1970).

24 Gabow, P.A.; Kaehny, W.D.; Fennessey, P.V.; Goodman, S.I.; Gross, P.A.; Schrier, R.W.: Diagnostic importance of an increased serum anion gap. New Engl. J. Med. *303:* 854–858 (1980).

25 Battle, D.C.; Arruda, J.A.L.; Kurtzman, N.A.: Hyperkalemic distal renal tubular acidosis associated with obstructive uropathy. New Engl. J. Med. *304:* 373–380 (1981).

26 Peterson, C.D.; Collins, A.J.; Himes, J.M.; Bulock, M.L.; Keane, W.F.: Ethylene glycol poisoning: pharmacokinetics during therapy with ethanol and hemodialysis. New Engl. J. Med. *304:* 21–23 (1981).

27 Gonda, A.; Gault, H.; Churchill, D.; Hollomby, D.: Hemodialysis for methanol intoxication. Am. J. Med. *64:* 749–758 (1978).

28 Dash, H.; Mills, J.: Severe metabolic acidosis associated with nalidixic acid overdose. Ann. intern. Med. *84:* 570–572 (1976).

29 Orringer, C.E.; Eustace, J.C.; Wunsch, C.D.; Gardner, L.B.: Natural history of lactic acidosis after grand-mal seizures: a model for the study of an anion-gap acidosis not associated with hyperkalemia. New Engl. J. Med. *297:* 796–799 (1977).

30 Nadiminti, Y.; Wang, J.C.; Chou, S.; Pineles, E.; Tobin, M.S.: Lactic acidosis associated with Hodgkin's disease. New Engl. J. Med. *303:* 15–17 (1980).

31 Fraley, D.S.; Adler, S.; Bruns, F.J.; Zeit, B.: Stimulation of lactate production by administration of bicarbonate in a patient with a solid neoplasm and lactic acidosis. New Engl. J. Med. *303:* 1100–1102 (1980).

32 Stolberg, L.; Rolfe, R.; Gitlin, N.; Merritt, J.; Mann, L.; Linder, J.; Sinegold, S.: *D*-Lactic acidosis due to abnormal gut flora: diagnosis and treatment of two cases. New Engl. J. Med. *306:* 1344–1348 (1982).

33 Felig, P.: Combating diabetic ketoacidosis and other hyperglycemic-ketoacidotic syndromes. Postgrad. Med. *59:* 150–153 (1976).

34 Schade, D.S.; Eaton, R.P.: Differential diagnosis and therapy of hyperketonemic state. J. Am. med. Ass. *241:* 2064–2065 (1979).

35 Cahill, G.F.; Ketosis. Kidney int. *20:* 416–425 (1981).

36 Fulop, M.; Hoberman, H.D.: Alcoholic ketosis. Diabetes *24:* 785–790 (1975).

37 Adrogue, H.J.; Wilson, H.; Boyd, A.E.; Suki, W.N.; Eknoyan, G.: Plasma acid-base patterns in diabetic ketoacidosis. New Engl. J. Med. *307:* 1603–1610 (1982).

38 Abrams, W.B.; Lewis, D.W.; Bellet, S.: The effect of acidosis and alkalosis on the plasma potassium concentration and the electrocardiogram of normal and potassium depleted dogs. Am. J. med. Sci. *222:* 506–515 (1951).

39 Burnell, J.M.; Villamil, M.F.; Uyeno, B.T.; Scribner, B.H.: The effect in humans of extracellular pH change on the relationship between serum potassium concentration and intracellular potassium. J. clin. Invest. *35:* 935–939 (1956).

40 Fraley, D.S.; Adler, S.: Correction of hyperkalemia by bicarbonate despite constant blood pH. Kidney int. *12:* 354–360 (1977).

41 Fulop, M.: Serum potassium in lactic acidosis and ketoacidosis. New Engl. J. Med. *300:* 1987–1089 (1979).

42 Sterns, R.H.; Cox, M.; Feig, P.U.; Singer, I.: Internal potassium balance and the control of the plasma potassium concentration. Medicine, Baltimore *60:* 339–354 (1981).

43 Adrogue, H.J.; Madias, N.E.: Changes in plasma potassium concentration during acute acid-base disturbances. Am. J. Med. *71:* 456–466 (1981).

44 Garella, S.; Dana, C.L.; Chazan, J.A.: Severity of metabolic acidosis as a determinant of bicarbonate requirements. New Engl. J. Med. *289:* 121–126 (1973).

45 Miller, P.D.; Berns, A.S.: Acute metabolic alkalosis perpetuating hypercarbia: a role for acetazolamide in chronic obstructive pulmonary disease. J. Am. med. Ass. *238:* 2400–2401 (1977).

46 Bear, R.; Goldstein, M.; Phillipson, E.; Ho, M.; Hammeke, M.; Feldman, R.; Handelsman, S.; Halperin, M.: Effect of metabolic alkalosis on respiratory function in patients with chronic obstructive lung disease. Can. med. Ass. J. *117:* 900–903 (1977).

47 Sebastian, A.; Schambelan, M.; Lindedeld, S.; Morris, R.C.: Amelioration of metabolic acidosis with fludrocortisone therapy in hyporeninemic hypoaldosteronism. New Engl. Med. *297:* 576–582 (1977).

48 DeFronzo, R.A.: Hyperkalemia and hyporeninemic hypoaldosteronism. Kidney int. *17:* 118–134 (1980).

49 Wason, S.; Lacouture, P.G.; Lovejoy, F.H.: Single high-dose pyridoxine treatment for isoniazid overdose. J. Am. med. Ass. *246:* 1102–1104 (1981).

50 Sievers, M.L.; Chin, L.: Treatment of isoniazid overdose. J. Am. med. Ass. *247:* 583–584 (1982).

51 Winchester, J.F.; Gelfand, M.C.; Knepshield, J.H.; Schreiner, G.E.: Dialysis and hemoperfusion of poisons and drugs – update. Trans. Am. Soc. artif. internal Organs *23:* 762–842 (1977).

52 McCoy, H.G.; Cipolle, R.J.; Ehlers, S.M.; Sawchuk, R.J.; Zaske, D.E.: Severe methanol poisoning: application of a pharmacokinetic model for ethanol therapy and hemodialysis. Am. J. Med. *67:* 804–807 (1979).

53 Kleeman, C.R.; Narins, R.G.: Diabetic acidosis and coma; in Maxwell, Kleeman, Clinical disorders of fluid and electrolyte metabolism; 3rd ed. (McGraw-Hill, Maidenhead 1980).

54 Narins, R.G.; Gardner, L.B.: Simple acid-base disturbances; in Beck, The medical clinics of North America, vol. 65, No. 2 (Saunders, Philadelphia 1981).

55 Taradash, M.R.; Jacobson, L.B.: Vasodilator therapy of idiopathic lactic acidosis. New Engl. J. Med. *293:* 468–471 (1975).

56 Vaziri, N.D.; Ness, R.; Wellikson, L.; Barton, C.; Greep, N.: Bicarbonate-buffered peritoneal dialysis: an effective adjunct in the treatment of lactic acidosis. Am. J. Med. *67:* 392–396 (1979).

57 Aizawa, Y.; Ohmori, T.; Imai, K.; Nara, Y.; Matsuoka, M.; Hirasawa, Y.: Depressant action of acetate upon the human cardiovascular system. Clin. Nephrol. *8:* 477–480 (1977).

58 Kirkendol, P.L.; Pearson, J.E.; Bower, J.D.; Holbert, R.D.: Myocardial depressant effects of sodium acetate. Cardiovasc. Res. *12:* 127–136 (1978).

59 Vincent, J.L.; Vanherweghem, J.L.; Degaute, J.P.; Berré, J.; Dufaye, P.; Kahn, R.J.: Acetate-induced myocardial depression during hemodialysis for acute renal failure. Kidney int. *22:* 653–657 (1982).

60 Borges, H.F.; Fryd, D.S.; Rosa, A.A.; Kjellstrand, C.M.: Hypotension during acetate and bicarbonate dialysis in patients with acute renal failure. Am. J. Nephrol. *1:* 24–30 (1981).

61 Vaziri, N.D.; Barton, C.H.; Ness, R.; Mirahmadi, K.: Special uses of cimetidine. Ann. intern. Med. *88:* 266 (1978).
62 Aronoff, G.R.; Hamburger, R.J.: Special uses of cimetidine. Ann. intern. Med. *88:* 266–267 (1978).
63 Mitas, J.A.; Frank, L.R.; Rabetoy, G.M.; Steinberg, S.M.: Treatment of Bartter's syndrome with naproxen. Kidney int. *16:* 933 (1979).
64 Dunn, M.J.: Prostaglandins and Bartter's syndrome. Kidney int. *19:* 86–102 (1981).
65 Shavelle, H.S.; Parke, R.: Postoperative metabolic alkalosis and acute renal failure: rationale for the use of hydrochloric acid. Surgery, St. Louis *78:* 439–445 (1975).
66 Swartz, R.D.; Rubin, J.E.; Brown, R.S.; Yager, H.M.; Steinman, T.I.; Frazier, H.S.: Correction of postoperative metabolic alkalosis and renal failure by hemodialysis. Ann. intern. Med. *86:* 52–55 (1977).
67 Ayus, J.C.; Olivero, J.J.; Adrogue, H.J.: Alkalemia associated with renal failure: correction by hemodialysis with low-bicarbonate dialysate. Archs intern. Med. *140:* 513–515 (1980).
68 Meislin, H.; Lerner, S.A.: Modified dialysis for metabolic alkalosis. Ann. intern. Med. *88:* 432 (1978).
69 Custom dialysis primer. Monograph, Organon Teknika Corporation, Oklahoma City 1982.
70 Vilbar, R.M.; Ing, T.S.; Shin, K.D.; Gandhi, V.C.; Viol, G.W.; Chen, W.T.; Geis, W.P.; Hano, J.E.: Treatment of metabolic alkalosis with peritoneal dialysis in a patient with renal failure. Artif. Organs *2:* 421–422 (1978).

J.A. Mitas, II, MD, The University of Oklahoma Health Sciences Center,
Oklahoma City, OK 73106 (USA)

Prog. crit. Care Med., vol. 2, pp. 251–261 (Karger, Basel 1985)

Diabetic Ketoacidosis and Coma

Charles R. Rost, David C. Kem

Endocrinology, Metabolism and Hypertension Section, University of Oklahoma Health Sciences Center, Oklahoma City, Okla., USA

Overview

Diabetic ketoacidosis (DKA) is a severe metabolic derangement characterized by volume depletion, hyperosmolarity, and metabolic acidosis. Untreated, it will result in hypovolemic shock, mental obtundation, coma, and death.

Approximately 14% of all hospitalizations of diabetic patients in the United States are due to DKA. The reported mortality rate ranges from close to 0 to almost 20% [7, 11]. Many, if not all, of the fatalities are probably avoidable [2]. Critical care decisions of the physician with meticulous attention to the clinical course can be the single most important factor in successful recovery while inappropriate therapeutic maneuvers may produce hypokalemia, hypoglycemia, tissue hypoxia, cerebral edema, and death.

Pathophysiology

Hormonal Abnormalities

The hallmark of DKA is a deficiency of insulin. Despite considerable debate as to the importance of other hormones, especially glucagon, it is fairly well established that a relative or absolute deficiency of insulin must exist for DKA to develop. When pretreatment serum or plasma insulin concentrations in 106 patients with DKA were examined, they were found to be comparable to plasma insulin concentrations in normal persons following an overnight fast, 10 ± 4 μU/ml [11]. However, the patients had serum glucose concentrations greater than 250 mg/dl compared to 90 mg/dl for the normal subjects. An appropriate plasma insulin concentration for a serum glucose over 250 mg/dl is greater than 50 μU/ml. Since no patient with DKA was observed to have comparable pretreatment plasma insulin values, a relative insulin deficiency was present.

Although insulin deficiency is necessary for development of DKA, other hormones contribute to the metabolic abnormalities. The counterregulatory or stress hormones, including glucagon, catecholamines, cortisol, and growth hormone have been reported to be increased in the plasma of untreated patients with DKA [11]. Concentrations of these hormones may be 2–7 times greater than normal. When insulin-dependent diabetics have their exogenous insulin withdrawn under controlled conditions, the acute administration of glucagon or epinephrine or the subacute administration of glucocorticoid or growth hormone produces a significant increase in blood glucose and ketone body concentrations [4, 11]. The increased concentrations of the stress hormones coupled with the relative deficiency of insulin results in accelerated ketogenesis and gluconeogenesis.

Ketogenesis

There are two major points of metabolic control of ketogenesis [8, 9]. The first is in the adipose tissue where hormone-sensitive lipase cleaves intracellular triglycerides releasing free fatty acids (FFA) into the circulation. Catecholamines, glucagon, and glucocorticoids stimulate hormone-sensitive lipase while insulin markedly suppresses it. The degree of lipolytic activity suppression by insulin is greatest when the enzyme has been previously stimulated by one of the stress hormones. In normal people, when hormone-sensitive lipase is stimulated by the stress hormones, endogenously secreted insulin will limit the enzymatic activity and control FFA release. In the diabetic with reduced endogenous insulin secretion, stress hormone-stimulated lipolysis will continue until exogenous insulin is administered. Plasma insulin concentrations of 40 μU/ml, easily achieved with small doses of insulin, will maximally inhibit stimulated hormone-sensitive lipase activity [2].

Hepatic metabolism of fatty acid (FA) is the second metabolic control point in ketogenesis [8]. When insulin concentrations are adequate, FFA taken up from the circulation and FA synthesized from glucose are assimilated into triglycerides and phospholipids. Under conditions of insulin deficiency FA is transported into the mitochondria, oxidized, and the acetyl-coenzyme A produced is condensed into acetoacetic acid. The ambient

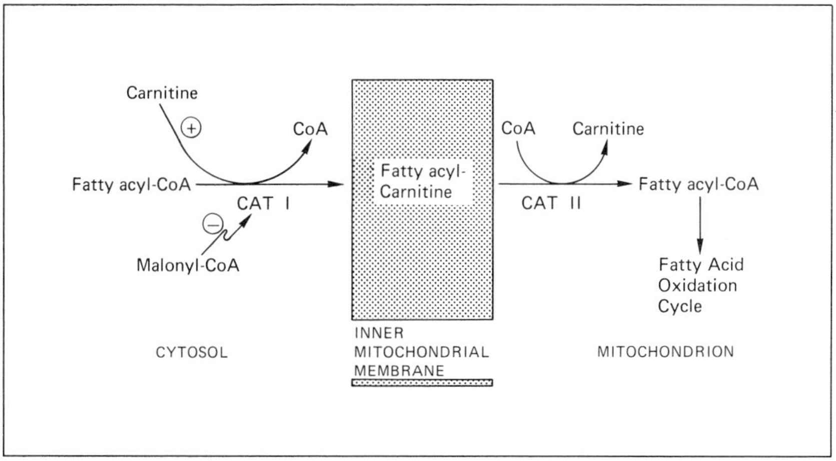

Fig. 1. Regulation of the transport of fatty acids into the hepatic mitochondrion for oxidative metabolism [adapted from ref. 8].

concentration of glucagon helps determine the hepatic fate of FA. Increased glucagon, with deficient insulin, favors the oxidative pathway and predisposes for ketogenesis.

Beta-oxidation of FA is an intramitochondrial process. FA complexed to coenzyme A (CoA) to form fatty acyl-CoA in the cytoplasm must be translocated across the mitochondrial membrane to enter the oxidation pathway (fig. 1). The predominantly medium chain fatty acyl-CoA molecules cannot freely diffuse into the mitochondrion. The enzyme carnitine acyltransferase (CAT) I, located on the outer surface of the inner mitochondrial membrane, replaces the CoA portion of fatty acyl-CoA with carnitine. Fatty acyl-carnitine can diffuse across the membrane. Inside the mitochondrion CAT II replaces the carnitine with CoA, allowing fatty acyl-CoA to enter the oxidation pathway. The enzymatic activity of CAT I is the rate-limiting step in FA oxidation.

CAT I activity is regulated by intracellular concentrations of carnitine and malonyl-CoA. Carnitine levels appear to be inversely related to insulin concentrations and hepatic glycogen stores. The mechanisms responsible are not fully understood. However, insulin deficiency and glycogen depletion are associated with increased intracellular carnitine levels and increased CAT I activity. Increased glucagon concentrations are also associated with increased intracellular carnitine levels. Malonyl-CoA, the first committed intermediate in the FA synthesis pathway, directly inhibits CAT I activity. When insulin is present, FA synthesis is active and malonyl-CoA levels are high. Glucagon inhibits pyruvate kinase, preventing the flow of glucose carbon atoms into the FA synthesis pathway, and also inhibits acetyl-CoA carboxylase, the enzyme which converts acetyl-CoA to malonyl-CoA. Thus, insulin deficiency and glucagon excess lead to increased intracellular carnitine and decreased intracellular malonyl-CoA levels. These changes allow maximal activity of CAT I, favoring the entrance of FA into the oxidation pathway. In other words, a high glucagon to insulin ratio increases the production of ketones by the liver.

Hyperglycemia

Serum glucose concentrations are a balance between glucose production, intestinal absorption, and disposal. In DKA the major source of blood glucose is hepatic gluconeogenesis. By this process glycerol, lactate, and alanine are converted into glucose by a reversal of glycolysis.

There are three irreversible enzymatic steps in the glycolytic pathway to assure unidirectional flow of substrate to pyruvate. Four key enzymes permit flow of carbon around these steps during gluconeo-genesis. These enzymes, pyruvate carboxylase, phosphoenolpyruvate carboxykinase, fructose 1,6-diphosphatase, and glucose 6-phosphatase, are stimulated by glucagon and glucocorticoids. Their activity is suppressed by insulin. In DKA, with insulin deficiency and increased circulating concentrations of glycerol, lactate, and alanine, elevated levels of glucagon and glucocorticoids provide maximal activity of the gluconeogenesis pathway.

In addition, catecholamines and glucagon activate liver phosphorylase and, thus, stimulate glycogenolysis. Glucose 6-phosphate produced by glycogenolysis is converted to free glucose by glucose 6-phosphatase, which is activated by glucagon and glucocorticoids and suppressed by insulin. The combined effects of glycogenolysis and gluconeogenesis result in massive hepatic output of glucose. A plasma insulin concentration of about 40 μU/ml will inhibit hepatic gluconeogenesis [2].

When the blood glucose concentration exceeds the renal threshold for glucose, glycosuria will develop. As long as renal function is good and renal perfusion remains adequate, the blood glucose concentration will not increase far above the threshold concentration. However, the subsequent osmotic diuresis produces substantial water and electrolyte losses. In addition, insulin deficiency and glucagon excess may directly cause natriuresis.

If water and electrolyte intake is not adequate, intravascular volume depletion results. Reduced renal perfusion causes reduced glucose and ketone excretion with greater hyperglycemia. The intravascular volume depletion further stimulates stress hormone secretion resulting in increased hepatic glucose production.

Coincident with the development of ketosis and hyperglycemia, several other important metabolic changes occur. The ketone bodies produced by FA oxidation are strong organic acids. They have a pK = 3.8 and, therefore, completely dissociate at body pH [7]. Hydrogen ions generated are buffered by the bicarbonate system. Normally, ketone bodies are metabolized by peripheral tissues and bicarbonate is regenerated. However, in DKA, the combination of insulin deficiency and volume depletion reduce ketone body utilization. As acidosis develops and the body's bicarbonate buffering system is depleted, more hydrogen ions are buffered by intracellular anions. With hydrogen ion influx there is potassium ion efflux. Intravascular volume depletion stimulates the renin-angiotensin-aldosterone system promoting a distal tubular excretion of potassium. The resultant kaliuresis is so intense that 70% of an administered potassium load will be excreted, despite severe total body potassium depletion.

Diagnosis

History

Some patients will present in DKA with a clear history of discontinuing their insulin administrations. Others may have DKA as the initial manifestation of diabetes mellitus. Often, a patient will present with DKA despite continued administration of insulin. In these cases, a physiologic stress, such as infection or myocardial infarction, produces increased secretion of stress hormones. A fixed dose of exogenous insulin may be insufficient to inhibit stress hormone-induced lipolysis, ketogenesis, and gluconeogenesis. Also, these patients frequently have decreased their insulin dosage coincident with the onset of the physiologic stress. Occasionally it will be impossible to determine a cause of the DKA.

Physical Examination

The physical examination may be relatively unremarkable or markedly abnormal. Mental status ranges from normal to comatose. Vital signs reflect the intravascular volume depletion. Fever is usually absent even when infection is present. Classic Kussmaul breathing results from respiratory compensation for the metabolic acidosis. It is usually present at a pH less than 7.2 but with severe acidosis (pH < 7.0), the respiratory rate may decrease due to brain stem depression. The cardiovascular examination may indicate underlying pathology which could play a role in precipitating DKA or alter therapeutic plans. Abdominal pain is common in DKA. Careful examination and guarded observation are often necessary to rule out acute pancreatitis or a surgically acute abdomen. A complete and careful search for any infection is mandatory.

Laboratory

Laboratory findings in DKA can be predicted from an understanding of the pathophysiology. The degree of hyperglycemia is variable. With minimal volume depletion and good renal function, blood glucose concentrations may be near normal. However, with increasing volume depletion or impaired renal function, it is possible to find blood glucose concentrations ranging to 800 mg/dl or higher. The level of hyperglycemia may be used to estimate the severity of volume depletion and/or renal dysfunction. Serum ketone levels are elevated and a strongly positive nitroprusside reaction can confirm the diagnosis. However, the internal milieu of the patient with DKA is in a reduced state with a high NADH:NAD ratio. Increased concentrations of NADH shift the equilibrium of the ketone bodies from acetoacetate to betahydroxybutyrate. The molar ratio of betahydroxybutyrate to acetoacetate ranges from 3:1 to 30:1. Since betahydroxybutyrate reacts weakly with nitroprusside, this test may give a misleadingly low titer despite high concentrations of ketones.

Arterial blood demonstrates a low pH with a low P_{CO_2}. The P_{O_2} should be high, with a low P_{O_2} indicating underlying pulmonary pathology. Serum osmolality is usually elevated. The osmolality can be measured or calculated by the formula:

$$\text{Osmolality} = 2\,[\text{Na} + \text{K}] + \frac{[\text{glucose}]}{18} + \frac{[\text{BUN}]}{2.8}.$$

The serum sodium concentration may be low, normal, or high. Despite total body potassium depletion, plasma potassium levels are usually normal or elevated due to the acidosis-mediated shift of the ion to the extracellular space. Hypokalemia at diagnosis indicates a critical potassium deficiency. The plasma bicarbonate concentration is suppressed to a degree appropriate for the degree of acidosis. Serum phosphate is usually normal or elevated at diagnosis. Urine analysis, electrocardiogram, and chest X-ray are useful tests for diagnosing causes of physiologic stress and for monitoring therapy.

Differential Diagnosis

In addition to DKA, the patient with diabetes mellitus can have an altered sensorium from hypoglycemia, nonketotic hyperglycemic hyperosmolar coma, intracranial pathology, poisoning, drug overdose, and anything else which could cause coma in the nondiabetic patient. Metabolic acidosis, associated with an increased anion gap, may also be caused by alcoholic ketoacidosis, lactic acidosis, uremia, and poisoning. Most of the time the diagnosis of DKA can be differentiated from these other disorders at the time of initial evaluation.

A specifically directed history and physical examination can help rule out intracranial pathology, drug overdose, poisoning, and some other diagnoses. A normal arterial pH and a negative serum ketone test will differentiate DKA from nonketotic hyperglycemic hyperosmolar coma. A positive nitroprusside reaction will confirm ketoacidosis and an elevated blood sugar concentration will differentiate DKA from alcoholic ketoacidosis and hypoglycemia. Because of the urgent nature for diagnosing hypoglycemia when present, any person with diabetes mellitus who is comatose or has altered mental function should have immediate determination of the blood glucose concentration. With the availability of reagent-coated strips, this determination can be made within a few minutes.

Therapy

Treatment of the patient with DKA in the intensive care unit is directed to specific goals. There is no single protocol which has superiority over other protocols for achieving these goals. Therapy must be individualized for each patient. Close observation by the physician with meticulous attention to the clinical course is the single most important factor determining successful treatment.

The specific goals of therapy are: (1) Replenish and maintain intravascular volume. (2) Inhibit hepatic gluconeogenesis and ketogenesis. (3) Prevent the development of hypokalemia and hypoglycemia. (4) Discover and treat any associated diseases.

The accomplishment of these goals requires a balance of fluid, insulin, and potassium administration, the judicious use of antibiotics and other supportive measures, and frequent assessments of progress. Mental status, blood pressure, and pulse should be monitored frequently. During the first 12–24 h of therapy, blood glucose, serum electrolytes, BUN, arterial pH, urine output, and calculated serum osmolality should be monitored every 1–2 h.

Fluid therapy is directed to replenish and maintain intravascular volume. Unless a contraindication is present, normal saline is preferred. Restoration of adequate tissue perfusion is necessary to prevent tissue hypoxia, ischemic complications, and lactic acidosis. Correction of the hyperosmolarity and water deficits are of a less urgent nature and take place over several hours of therapy. Repletion of intravascular volume increases renal perfusion resulting in increased glycosuria and a decline in serum glucose concentration, independent of insulin effect [10, 12].

Initial administration of 0.9% NaCl at 1,000 cm^3/h is indicated in the adult patient. This rate should be maintained until a brisk urine output is established. Then, 0.9% NaCl at a rate of 500 cm^3/h is recommended. When the blood glucose concentration declines to 250–300 mg/dl, the intravenous infusion should be changed to 5% dextrose in 0.45% NaCl and administered at a rate of 250 cm^3/h. The rate of fluid administration should be adjusted to maintain adequate intravascular volume. The rates of administration of dextrose and insulin should be adjusted to keep the blood glucose around 250 mg/dl until the acidosis has corrected and the patient has begun oral intake and maintenance insulin administration. Further reduction of blood glucose can be attempted then. The too rapid decline in blood glucose concentration and the administration of hypotonic fluids can result in cerebral edema [3].

As discussed previously, stress hormone-induced adipose tissue lipolysis, hepatic ketogenesis, and hepatic gluconeogenesis can be inhibited by physiologic circulating levels of insulin. Plasma insulin concentrations of 40 μU/ml will give the desired results. Substantially higher concentrations are required to increase peripheral glucose disposal. In the past, high doses of insulin, e.g. 100 U/h, were used to treat DKA. The rationale for this practice was a suspected insulin resistance in patients with acute DKA. However, recent experience with low-dose, e.g. 5–10 U/h, insulin therapy has demonstrated good therapeutic efficacy with insulin resistance rarely observed [1, 6]. There is similarity between low-dose and high-dose therapy in the duration of treatment needed to achieve target values of blood glucose concentration, arterial pH, serum bicarbonate concentration, and clearing of serum acetone. In addition, the suppression of cortisol and glucagon concentrations occur over similar time courses with the two forms of therapy. The major difference appears to be an increased incidence of hypoglycemia (glucose $<$ 200 mg/dl) and hypokalemia (K $<$ 3.0 mEq/l) when high-dose therapy is employed [1]. Although there appears to be no difference in the time course of response to therapy between intravenous, intramuscular, and subcutaneous routes for low-dose administration [6], the intravenous route is preferred when intravascular volume depletion is severe.

A priming dose of 10–20 U (approximately 0.15 U/kg normal body weight) of regular insulin given by intravenous bolus should be followed by 5–10 U/h (approximately 0.1 U/kg normal body weight) continuous intravenous infusion. If a 10% decrease in blood glucose concentration is not observed in the first hour of therapy, one should repeat the priming dose or double the infusion rate. When the blood glucose level reaches 250–300 mg/dl, glucose-containing fluids should be infused so as to maintain the blood glucose in the 250 mg/dl range until the acidosis is completely resolved. The insulin infusion should be maintained until the acidosis has resolved and the patient is eating. It is advisable to continue the insulin infusion until 1–2 h after maintenance subcutaneous insulin administration has been initiated.

Almost all patients in DKA are severely potassium depleted. This is primarily a combined effect of intracellular hydrogen ion buffering causing potassium ion efflux and mineralocorticoid action causing excessive kaliuresis. However, because of the extracellular shift of potassium and volume depletion, most patients at admission have normal or high plasma potassium concentrations. As the acidosis and hypovolemia are corrected, there is a precipitous fall in plasma potassium levels. If the patient is eukalemic of hyperkalemic on admission, one should wait until urine output is adequate and then begin KCl infusion at a rate of 20–40 mEq/h. Should the patient be hypokalemic on initial evaluation, KCl administration is begun immediately at a rate of 20 mEq/h until urine output is established. The nadir in plasma potassium is seen 1–4 h after initiation of fluid and insulin therapy. In most cases, 80–160 mEq of KCl are needed over the first 8–12 h. Since up to 70% of the administered potassium will be lost in the urine and total body potassium depletion is severe, it is advised to continue potassium replacement with oral KCl for 7–10 days after recovery from DKA.

Phosphate depletion is also present in almost all patients with DKA. As with potassium, the serum phosphate concentration will decline with appropriate fluid and insulin therapy. However, unlike hypokalemia, correction of the hypophosphatemia has not been shown to alter the outcome of DKA [5, 13]. Severe hypophosphatemia may delay the generation of erythrocyte 2,3-DPG, cause rhabdomyolysis, and produce hemolytic anemia. The reduced erythrocyte 2,3-DPG will cause an increased affinity of hemoglobin for oxygen, potentially decreasing oxygen delivery to tissues. However, this is offset by a decrease in hemoglobin-oxygen affinity caused by the acidosis. The administration of phosphate can result in hypocalcemia, hypomagnesemia, and transient hypoparathyroidism. Thus, phosphate administration is recommended only in cases where hypophosphatemia of 1.5 mg/dl or lower is documented on admission or during the course of therapy. It may be conveniently administered as potassium phosphate, at a rate of 20 mEq/h, with appropriate reduction of potassium chloride dosage. The serum calcium and magnesium concentrations should be monitored in all patients treated with phosphate.

There is no place for *routine* bicarbonate administration in the treatment of DKA. Intravenous bicarbonate infusion will cause an efflux of hydrogen ions from the intracellular space with associated influx of potassium and may worsen hypokalemia. As discussed previously, the acidosis produces a change in hemoglobin-oxygen affinity which counters the change produced by 2,3-DPG deficiency. A rapid correction of the acidosis removes this effect and contributes to tissue hypoxia. Therefore, bicarbonate therapy is only recommended in cases with an arterial pH of 7.1 or less. Sufficient bicarbonate should be given to return the pH to the 7.1–7.2 range.

Intensive therapy should be continued until the arterial pH is 7.35 or greater, serum bicarbonate is 15 mEq/l or more, and the patient is able to resume a diabetic diet. At this time, the patient can be transferred to a general medical ward and an appropriate subcutaneous insulin regimen begun. Usually the pre-DKA regimen will suffice. If the patient was not previously taking insulin, a daily dose equal to the total number of units administered over the preceeding 24 h can be used. The daily dose is divided, with two thirds given before breakfast and one third prior to the evening meal. The morning insulin should be divided between intermediate and short acting (e.g. NPH and regular) in a 2:1 ratio with the evening insulin given in a 1:1 ratio. Further adjustment of the insulin regimen to attain desired diabetes control is usually necessary. The insulin infusion should be continued until 1–2 h after the first dose of maintenance subcutaneous insulin is given. Appropriate therapy for any associated conditions and potassium replacement should be continued after the transfer. Early and frequent communication between the intensive care staff and the ward physicians will facilitate the chronic management of the patient with DKA.

References

1 Burghen, G.A.; Etteldorf, J.N.; Fisher, J.N.; Kitabchi, A.E.: Comparison of high-dose and low-dose insulin by continuous intravenous infusion in the treatment of diabetic ketoacidosis in children. Diabetes Care *3:* 15–20 (1980).

2 Clements, R.S.; Vourganti, B.: Fatal diabetic ketoacidosis: major causes and approaches to their prevention. Diabetes Care *1:* 314–325 (1978).

3 Duck, S.C.; Weldon, V.V.; Pagliara, A.S.; Haymond, M.W.: Cerebral edema complicating therapy for diabetic ketoacidosis. Diabetes *25:* 111–115 (1976).

4 Gerich, J.E.; Lorenzi, M.; Bier, D.M.; Schneider, V.; Tsalikian, E.; Karam, J.H.; Forsham, P.H.: Prevention of human ketoacidosis by somatostatin. Evidence for an essential role of glucagon. New Engl. J. Med. *292:* 985–989 (1975).

5 Keller, U.; Berger, W.: Prevention of hypophosphatemia by phosphate infusion during treatment of diabetic ketoacidosis and hyperosmolar coma. Diabetes *29:* 87–95 (1980).

6 Kitabchi, A.E.: Treatment of diabetic ketoacidosis with low dose insulin. Adv. internal Med. *23:* 115–135 (1978).

7 Kreisberg, R.A.: Diabetic ketoacidosis: new concepts and trends in pathologenesis and treatment. Ann. intern. Med. *88:* 681–695 (1978).

8 McGarry, J.D.; Foster, D.W.: Hormonal control of ketogenesis. Biochemical considerations. Archs intern. Med. *137:* 495–501 (1977).

9 McGarry, J.D.: Banting lecture. New perspectives in the regulation of ketogenesis. Diabetes *28:* 517–523 (1979).

10 Owen, O.E.; Licht, J.H.; Sapir, D.G.: Renal function and effects of partial rehydration during diabetic ketoacidosis. Diabetes *30:* 510–518 (1981).

11 Schade, D.S.; Eaton, R.P.: Pathogenesis of diabetic ketoacidosis: a reappraisal. Diabetes Care *2:* 296–306 (1979).

12 Waldhäusl, W.; Kleinberger, G.; Korn, A.; Dudczak, R.; Bratusch-Marrain, P.; Nowotny, P.: Severe hyperglycemia: effects of rehydration on endocrine derangements and blood glucose concentration. Diabetes *28:* 577–584 (1979).

13 Wilson, H.K.; Kever, S.P.; Lea, A.S.; Boyd, A.E., III; Eknoyan, G.: Phosphate therapy in diabetic ketoacidosis. Archs intern. Med. *142:* 517–520 (1982).

Charles R. Rost, MD, Assistant Professor of Medicine,
University of Oklahoma Health Sciences Center, Oklahoma City, OK 73106 (USA)

Prog. crit. Care Med., vol. 2, pp. 262–272 (Karger, Basel 1985)

Thyroid and Adrenal Disorders in Critically Ill Patients

John R. Higgins

Veterans Administration Medical Center and University of Oklahoma Health Sciences Center, Oklahoma City, Okla., USA

Overview

Endocrine emergencies including those of the thyroid and adrenal gland usually present as an exaggerated form of the underlying disease. However, sometimes disturbances of the hormone in question have disproportionate effects on one organ system, and it is easy to focus attention on that organ system and fail to recognize the underlying endocrine problem. On the other hand, endocrine emergencies are frequently precipitated by factors such as infection, and we must be vigilant in our search for these precipitating factors if treatment of endocrine emergencies is to have a successful outcome. Patients with endocrine emergencies are usually severely ill and may face a high risk of death. A decision to treat and to treat aggressively must often be made on clinical grounds before the result of confirming laboratory test become known. However, the treatment of endocrine emergencies can be most gratifying. Early diagnosis and effective treatment can often rescue a patient from the brink of death and lead to the restoration of full health within a short time.

Thyroid Storm

Pathophysiology

Graves' disease is the most common type of hyperthyroidism associated with thyroid storm although occasionally a toxic multinodular goiter can lead to thyroid storm. Most other causes of hyperthyroidism are associated with a milder form of the disease and rarely progress to thyroid storm. In the past, thyroid surgery as a means to treat hyperthyroidism was a common event leading to thyroid storm. However, with proper selection of surgical candidates and with proper preparation of the patient prior to surgery, it is now possible to minimize this particular risk. Infection is such a common precipitating factor that its presence should be considered in all cases of thyroid storm. Other precipitating factors include the use of drugs which displace thyroid hormones from their binding sites to plasma proteins, the withdrawal of antithyroid drugs with a rebound effect on thyroid hormone secretion, and the increase in thyroid hormone secretion which may occur 2–3 weeks after treatment of hyperthyroidism with radioactive iodine.

Diagnosis of Thyroid Storm

The clinical picture of thyroid storm includes fever, marked tachycardia, some degree to obtundation, and congestive heart failure. Classically the full picture of thyroid storm is preceded by a period of heightened activity which gives way to obtundation, coma, circulatory collapse, and death, often within 24–48 h. However, elderly patients with apathetic hyperthyroidism may lapse quietly into coma and death without a preceding period of heightened activity. The presence of fever and tachycardia often suggest that infection may be a precipitating factor. It is sometimes very difficult to determine whether or not a given patient has the coexistence of hyperthyroidism and infection, whether the patient has thyroid storm precipitated by infection, or whether the patient has thyroid storm with signs and symptoms mimicking infection. In uncertain situations, it is usually advisable to obtain appropriate cultures and other diagnostic studies, and to treat with antibiotics while at the same time treating for thyroid storm. In younger individuals and in those without underlying heart disease, the rapid heart rate is usually due to sinus tachycardia. In older individuals and in those with underlying heart disease, tachycardia is often associated with atrial fibrillation and occasionally with atrial flutter. High output congestive heart failure, tachycardia, arrhythmias, and systolic hypertension with a wide pulse pressure result from a high oxygen demand, vascular shunting, direct cardiac stimulation by thyroid hormones, and a synergistic effect of thyroid hormones and catecholamines. Fever results from accelerated metabolism and excessive heat generation. The severity of the clinical picture of thyroid storm has a poor correlation with the circulating levels of thyroid hormones. Because of this and because even a few hours delay in treatment can be associated with a lethal outcome, the decision to treat for thyroid storm must be based on the clinical picture.

Therapy of Thyroid Storm

There are four general objectives in the treatment of thyroid storm: (1) precipitating factors and underlying illnesses must be recognized and treated; (2) general support must be provided; (3) the production and secretion of thyroid hormones must be reduced; and (4) the metabolic effects of circulating thyroid hormones must be diminished.

Patients with severe hyperthyroidism are usually in poor nutritional status because of protein catabolism, accelerated consumption of water-soluble vitamins, fever with loss of fluids and electrolytes, and a preceding period of poor oral intake. Replacement of fluids and electrolytes should be vigorous, but tempered by the possibility of provoking or worsening underlying congestive heart failure. Because of depletion of glycogen stores and decreased gluconeogenesis, blood glucose levels should be added to the IV fluid. Multivitamins including those of the B complex should also be added to the IV fluid and efforts to provide supplemental calories should be made when the patient's condition permits oral feeding.

Congestive heart failure should be treated in the usual manner with diuretics, digitalis, and oxygen, but it must be realized that while these measures are beneficial, complete resolution of congestive heart failure may only result from effective treatment of the underlying hyperthyroidism. The continued presence of the factors in hyperthyroidism which lead to congestive heart failure may diminish the effectiveness of the digitalis preparations and may create a state where the difference between therapeutic doses and toxic doses is relatively small. Accordingly, one must be alert for the presence of digitalis toxicity.

High fever should be controlled with cooling blankets and with acetaminophen. High doses of aspirin should be avoided because aspirin may lead to further increases in metabolic rate and because aspirin in high doses is capable of displacing thyroid hormone from its plasma protein binding sites. The incidence of acute adrenal insufficiency concurrent with thyroid storm is difficult to assess. Disturbances in fluids and electrolytes including hyponatremia, hyperkalemia, and volume depletion may suggest the presence of adrenal insufficiency. Furthermore, hyperthyroidism is accompanied by alterations in steroid metabolism in addition to the disturbances which always accompany severe forms of stress. Because formal testing for adrenal insufficiency is difficult and time consuming in these circumstances, it is often advisable to administer 200–500 mg/day of hydrocortisone in divided doses, or the equivalent dose of another glucocorticoid.

The more specific therapy of thyroid storm includes a reduction of thyroid hormone synthesis, a reduction in the release of preformed thyroid hormone, and a reduction in the effect of thyroid hormone already in the circulation. Antithyroid drugs inhibit the oxidation and organic binding of iodine within 1 h. They also inhibit the coupling of iodotyrosines. In emergency situations, PTU is superior to methimazole because PTU also blocks the peripheral conversion of T_4 to T_3. Hydrocortisone and propranolol have similar effects that might account for their beneficial activity in the treatment of thyroid storm. Often the circulating level of T_3 is reduced by 50% within the first 24 h of PTU therapy. This relatively rapid decrease in T_3 may account for the rapid clinical improvement that is observed before measurable falls of T_4 occur. The initial dose of PTU should be in the range of 600–1,000 mg. If the patient is obtunded, the PTU tablets can be crushed and delivered through a nasogastric tube. Subsequent doses need to be adjusted according to the clinical response, but doses in the range of 100–200 mg every 4–6 h can be tried initially. If methimazole is used, the dose should be approximately one-tenth that of PTU.

Iodide leads to a prompt and dramatic slowing of thyroid secretion by somewhat obscure mechanisms which seem to involve inhibition of colloid resorption that initiates the secretion of T_4 and T_3. Iodide also inhibits thyroid hormone synthesis (Wolff-Chaikoff effect) but this effect is probably of little clinical importance. Because iodide is a substrate for further hormone synthesis, its administration should be delayed for an hour or two until PTU has been allowed to exert its effect on blocking thyroid hormone synthesis. Iodide can be administered in the form of Lugol's solution or SSKI, 10 drops of either preparation every 8 h. Alternatively, sodium iodide may be administered intravenously, 1 g by slow IV push every 8 h.

While the duration of effect of T_3 is much shorter, T_4 has a plasma half-life of approximately 1 week and provides a constant reservoir for further T_3 production. Hence, it is important to control the effects of thyroid hormones already in circulation. Reserpine and guanethidine have been employed for this purpose, but both have a relatively slow onset of action, and reserpine can cause central nervous system depression, cutaneous flushing and diarrhea. The beta-blocker, propranolol, controls cardiac and psychomotor manifestations within 2–10 min when given intravenously at a rate of 1 mg/min for a total dose of 2–10 mg. The effect of a single dose lasts 3–4 h. Oral propranolol in doses of 20–120 mg is effective in 1 h and the effect may last 4–8 h.

Myxedema Coma

Pathophysiology

Hypothalamic or pituitary disease may lead to hypothyroidism through inadequate TSH stimulation, but disease of the thyroid gland itself is the most common cause of hypothyroidism. Chronic thyroiditis, or Hashimotos disease, heads a long list of thyroid disorders. Radioactive iodine and surgical treatment of hyperthyroidism are important iatrogenic causes of hypothyroidism. The disorders causing hypothyroidism are more common in women than in men, and hypothyroidism must be present for many years before true myxedema develops. Hence, myxedema coma is a disease most commonly affecting older women. Myxedema coma often appears during the winter months and is often precipitated by infection, particularly pneumococcal pneumonia.

Diagnosis of Myxedema Coma

Like the other diseases dealt with in this chapter, the diagnosis of myxedema coma should be based on the clinical picture and treatment must often begin before laboratory confirmation becomes available. When a typical history and physical findings are present, establishing a diagnosis is not difficult. However, patients are often obtunded and signs and symptoms of one organ system may be so prominent that the complete picture of myxedema coma may be apparent only to those with a high index of suspicion.

Central nervous system findings are among the cardinal features of myxedema coma. By the time the patient presents, preceding personality changes have often given way to progressive lethargy, obtundation and coma. However, many patients do not lapse into coma until after hospital admission. Failure to recognize and treat hypothyroidism contributes to this problem as does the exquisite sensitivity of hypothyroid patients to sedatives. Other factors contributing to coma include hypothermia, fluid and electrolyte imbalances, carbon dioxide retention and cerebral anoxia. Seizures, often in association with hyponatremia, occur in about one quarter of patients. CSF protein concentration tends to be elevated and cerebellar signs of ataxia, intention tremor and nystagmus may suggest the presence of a posterior fossa tumor. A slowed relaxation phase of the deep tendon reflexes is one of the hallmarks of hypothyroidism, but neurological functions in myxedema coma may be so depressed that deep tendon reflexes cannot be elicited.

Some degree of hypothermia is often present and is a bad prognostic sign if severe. The magnitude of hypothermia can be underestimated by those who are used to searching for fever and who do not shake the thermometer down completely. In fact, clinical thermometers may not register low enough to record the actual body temperature. On the other hand, a normal temperature may actually represent fever in a myxedematous patient. Other abnormalities of vital signs include hypotension and bradycardia.

Hyponatremia occurs in half of the patients. Although inappropriate levels of ADH have been reported, most feel that the principal mechanism is related to tubular dysfunction. When accompanied by hypokalemia and hypochloremia, the hyponatremia is usually dilutional in nature with the total body sodium being high. The hyponatremia does not respond to steroids, but usually corrects promptly with thyroid hormone replacement. Because of the fragile cardiovascular status of most patients, vigorous saline replacement should be avoided unless seizures are present or the serum sodium is less than 115 mEq/l.

Pulmonary abnormalities include alveolar hypoventilation, CO_2 narcosis, and respiratory acidosis. Aspiration during seizures may lead to rapid worsening of pulmonary function and clinicians should be prepared to provide early ventilatory support. At least one other component of the clinical picture deserves special emphasis. Bowel hypomotility can be severe enough to suggest obstruction or other intra-abdominal emergencies. Failure to recognize this situation could result in tragic results if the patient was taken to surgery.

Therapy of Myxedema Coma

Treatment of myxedema coma is relatively straightforward. After a single IV bolus of 500 mg of *L*-thyroxine, vital signs can be expected to improve within 6 h and consciousness to be restored within 24–36 h. Failure to observe this rapid improvement may imply incorrect diagnosis or the influence of other disease processes. Because *L*-thyroxine has a plasma half-life of nearly 1 week, no further treatment may be necessary for several days.

Some maintain that triiodothyronine is superior to *L*-thyroxine because T_3 is more active and more rapid in onset. However, T_3 has the disadvantages of a more variable therapeutic response, greater risk for cardiac toxicity, and a lack of a stable preparation for parenteral administration.

Hydrocortisone 100 mg IV every 6 h is often used empirically, but there may be a good rationale for its use. Hypothyroidism may be only one component of pituitary deficiency and even with primary hypothyroidism relative adrenal insufficiency can exist. The secretion, turnover and metabolism of steroids are all slowed in myxedema. Rapid restoration of a euthyroid state may evoke relative adrenal insufficiency. However, serum cortisol levels are usually normal as is the cortisol response to ACTH administration. Some of the concern about concomitant adrenal insufficiency is a hold-over from older studies that relied on urinary metlabolites to estimate steroid levels. The urinary 17-OH-corticosteroid and 17-ketosteroids are often low because of the decreased degradation rates of circulating steroids.

As mentioned above early ventilatory support may be required. Passive rewarming with blankets and room temperature control is usually preferred to more active measures in order to prevent circulatory collapse.

Acute Adrenal Insufficiency

Pathophysiology

Adrenal insufficiency may result from disease of the adrenal glands or from a lack of stimulation by ACTH as a consequence of hypothalamic or pituitary disease. At one time, tuberculosis was the most common cause of adrenal disease, but with better therapy available the incidence of this form of adrenal insufficiency has decreased markedly. Various forms of cancer metastasize to the adrenal glands more often than one might expect, but because of the enormous reserve function of the adrenal glands, adrenal insufficiency is a fairly uncommon sequela. Other infiltrative processes include histoplasmosis and amyloidosis. Adrenal insufficiency often accompanies surgical procedures involving the adrenal glands. This is an obvious situation when bilateral adrenalectomies are performed for Cushing's disease or for pheochromocytoma, but may be less obvious in other situations. For example, in a patient with Cushing's syndrome caused by a unilateral adrenal adenoma, removal of the involved gland may be followed by a prolonged state of adrenal insufficiency. In this situation the autonomous overproduction of cortisol by the adenoma suppresses hypothalamic and pituitary functions, and the prolonged low levels of ACTH are accompanied by atrophy of the remaining adrenal tissue. Probably the most common cause of adrenal insufficiency now is the idiopathic variety that is thought to be associated with autoimmune phenomena in a high percentage of cases.

Another type of adrenal insufficiency is that associated with deficiencies of enzymes necessary for steroid biosynthesis. The general feature of these adrenogenital syndromes includes a partial block in steroid synthesis before the production of cortisol, low cortisol production and blood levels, a compensatory rise in ACTH production, a partial or complete restoration in cortisol production, and a rise in the production levels of all steroids proximal to the block. Naturally, the clinical expression of these disorders depends on which enzyme is deficient and where the block occurs. In the most common example, 21-hydroxylase deficiency, only virilism is present if the enzyme deficiency is mild. The virilism occurs because the adrenal androgens do not require the placement of a hydroxyl group at ^{21}C and because their production is increased by chronic overstimulation by ACTH. However, the mineralocorticoids 11-deoxycorticosterone and aldosterone do include a hydroxyl group at position 21, and in more severe forms of 21-hydroxylase deficiency salt losing may be a very prominent feature. With 11β-hydroxylase deficiency both virilism and hypertension occur. In this situation the hypertension is caused by excessive levels of 11-deoxycorticosterone, one of the steroids formed immediately prior to the 11β-hydroxylase step in the synthesis of both cortisol and aldosterone. Other enzyme deficiencies are less common and their clinical picture depends on where the deficiency occurs in the biosynthetic pathway.

Acute adrenal insufficiency often occurs in patients with unrecognized adrenal insufficiency or partial adrenal insufficiency. Because of the insidious nature of chronic adrenal insufficiency there is often a delay in establishing the diagnosis. When some form of stress, such as surgery, infection, or trauma intervenes, the patient with unrecognized adrenal insufficiency or partial adrenal insufficiency may deteriorate very rapidly. Another common cause of acute adrenal insufficiency is the withdrawal of exogenous steroids. When patients are treated with a dose of steroid equivalent to a full replacement dose of cortisol for a month or more, the chances of suppression of the adrenal-pituitary-hypothalamic axis are great, and the patient must be presumed to have adrenal insufficiency until otherwise proved. Sudden and dramatic causes of acute adrenal insufficiency include pituitary apoplexy, adrenal destruction accompanying overwhelming sepsis such as the Waterhouse-Friderichsen syndrome, and hemorrhage into the adrenal glands during anticoagulant therapy.

Diagnosis of Adrenal Insufficiency

The diagnosis of acute adrenal insufficiency must be based on anticipating clinical settings in which it can occur and on recognizing the clinical picture. Nausea, vomiting, diarrhea, and abdominal pain are common and lead to hypovolemia and hypotension, especially orthostatic hypotension. Particularly when there is mineralocorticoid deficiency as well as glucocorticoid deficiency, hyponatremia and hyperkalemia occur. Other features include prerenal azotemia, hypoglycemia because of loss of glucocorticoid activity, and hypercalcemia. When the acute adrenal insufficiency results from adrenal disease of a chronic nature, hyperpigmentation may be present. Fever may be a prominent sign, and may cause confusion. Because acute adrenal insufficiency is often precipitated by severe infection and because many of the clinical features of acute adrenal insufficiency are reminiscent of the clinical picture of a patient with overwhelming sepsis, it is easy to miss the diagnosis unless one maintains a high index of suspicion.

It is worth re-emphasizing that a presumptive diagnosis must be based of the clinical picture and that therapy should be begun immediately when acute adrenal insufficiency is suspected. Laboratory confirmation must be a second priority and is usually rather simple. In the highly stressed patient suspected of having acute adrenal insufficiency, obtaining a single blood measurement for cortisol may be adequate. If time permits, a Cortrosyn stimulation test may be performed. This test involves obtaining blood for a baseline cortisol determination, administering 25 units of Cortrosyn intramuscularly and repeating blood levels for cortisol 30 and 60 min later. A normal response is for the serum cortisol to rise by at least 7 μg/dl and to a value over 20 μg/dl. In situations where the diagnosis of acute adrenal insufficiency is relatively certain, but the cause – pituitary versus adrenal – is unknown, one of several protocols for prolonged ACTH stimulation may be followed. In general, these involve the administration of ACTH for several successive days. A normal person will show a prompt and near maximal rise of cortisol during the first day of ACTH administration. A patient with primary adrenal disease will have a severely blunted cortisol response which will persist despite several days of ACTH stimulation. A person with hypothalamic or pituitary disease and atrophic adrenal gland will initially show a blunted response, but after several days of ACTH stimulation the cortisol production rate will eventually rise to normal or near normal levels. The prolonged ACTH stimulation test may be undertaken while the patient is taking a synthetic glucocorticoid such as dexamethasone.

Therapy of Adrenal Insufficiency

The four principles of treating acute adrenal insufficiency include restoration of normal steroid levels, correction of fluid and electrolyte abnormalities, search for precipitating causes, and prevention of similar episodes in the future. The normal adrenal glands are capable for producing 200–400 mg of hydrocortisone daily during periods of maximum stress, and the goal of steroid therapy should be to emulate this condition. 100 mg of hydrocortisone should be given immediately by IV push. Many protocols have been described for subsequent therapy, but the simplest is to give another 200–300 mg of hydrocortisone over the next 24 h by continuous IV infusion. After 2 or 3 days of high dose treatment, or after the precipitating stress factors have been identified and treated, the dose may be reduced fairly rapidly to about twice maintenance level. Hydrocortisone is the most commonly employed glucocorticoid, but equivalent doses of other glucocorticoids are also effective. During high dose therapy of glucocorticoids, mineralocorticoids are usually not necessary. As the dose of glucocorticoid is tapered one should watch for the appearance of orthostatic hypotension, hyponatremia, and hyperkalemia. If any of these occur, the addition of mineralocorticoid, such as 9α-flurocortisol should be considered. Fluid should be administered rapidly until the blood pressure rises to satisfactory levels; usually 2–3 liters or more are required over the first 24 h. The administration of glucocorticoid and fluids almost always is accompanied by a rapid rise in the blood pressure and vasopressors are rarely indicated. Similarly, the simultaneous administration of fluids, electrolyes and glucocorticoids almost always leads to rapid correction of hyperkalemia. Other maneuvers such as insulin administration should be avoided. By using high doses of steroids and by presenting the kidneys with a high sodium load, hypokalemia may occur after several hours of therapy.

When fever is part of the clinical picture, a careful search for infections should be conducted, and often the administration of broad-spectrum antibiotics is desirable after appropriate cultures and other studies have been obtained.

Patient education is of paramount importance because the patients are usually vulnerable to repeated attacks of acute adrenal insufficiency if adequate prevention is not undertaken. Patients should be thoroughly knowledgeable about the clinical settings in which adrenal crisis may occur, the early symptoms and signs of adrenal crisis, and on the management of their steroid doses. All patients with adrenal insufficiency should wear a device to alert medical personnel of their condition such as a Medic-alert bracelet and carry clinical information at all times.

Because many patients develop acute adrenal insufficiency after withdrawal of exogenous steroids, this topic deserves special emphasis. The principles to be stressed include avoiding the use of steroids as therapeutic agents whenever possible, using as small a dose as possible and limiting the duration of therapy. When it has been necessary to use steroids for a month or more, each patient must be presumed to have adrenal insufficiency. To wean a patient off steroids involves a considerable time commitment. First, the patient should be switched to a short-acting steroid such as hydrocortisone. Then the dose should be decreased to approximately twice maintenance levels (50 mg hydrocortisone/day). Thereafter, the patient should be gradually converted to receiving steroids every other day. This is usually done by gradually increasing the dose on one day and reducing the dose by the same increment the following day. For example, if one is on 50 mg hydrocrotisone/day, one would begin the change to an alternate day dosing by alternating 60 and 40 mg, then 70 and 30 mg, finally achieving 100 and 0 mg. Then the every other day dose of the steroid should be decreased. Periodically, blood levels of cortisol may be obtained in the early morning just prior to the steroid dose. When the serum cortisol is above 10 µg/dl, it is safe to assume that at least partial recovery of the adrenal-pituitary-hypothalamic axis has occurred. This can be confirmed by a normal response during a Cortrosyn stimulation test. However, a normal response to the Cortrosyn stimulation test does not rule out the persistence of a partial ACTH deficiency. After the patient has been off steroids for a month or more, a metyrapone stimulation test or insulin-induced hypoglycemia may be employed to test pituitary function. If either of these tests is less than normal, or if neither has been performed, steroid coverage should be employed during stressful events for many months after withdrawal of steroid therapy.

References

1 Liddle, G.W.: The adrenals; in Williams, Textbook of endocrinology; 6th ed., pp. 281–290 (Saunders, Philadelphia 1981).

2 Mackin, J.F.; Canary, J.J.; Pittman, C.S.: Thyroid storm and its management. New Engl. J. Med. *291:* 1396–1398 (1974).

3 Senior, R.M.; Birge, S.J.; Wessler, S.; Avoili, L.V.: The recognition and management of myxedema coma. J. Am. med. Ass. *217:* 61–65 (1971).

John R. Higgins, MD, Veterans Administration Medical Center and University of Oklahoma Health Sciences Center, Oklahoma City, OK 73106 (USA)

Infections

Prog. crit. Care Med., vol. 2, pp. 273–279 (Karger, Basel 1985)

The Problem of Sepsis

R. Timothy Coussons

Department of Medicine, University of Oklahoma Health Sciences Center, Oklahoma City, Okla., USA

Overview

For patients requiring intensive care unit (ICU) support, infection is a major risk with sepsis representing its most life-threatening form. Sepsis can be defined as the clinical condition associated with the presence of pathogenic microorganisms or their byproducts in the bloodstream. The burden of these infections as measured by mortality, morbidity, and hospital cost is staggering [6].

Recent prospective studies reveal that nosocomial infections involve 12–18% of ICU patients compared to only 5–6% of general hospital patients. Sepsis accounts for 22–29% of the ICU infections with mortality as high as 50% in some situations. Colonization and infection rate increase as duration of stay in the ICU lengthens [2, 3].

The clinical setting is key in the identification of septic patients. These patients tend to share characteristics hauntingly familiar to personnel involved in infection control and include: prolonged hospital stay with frequent invasive treatment and procedures, major underlying disease, multiple and prolonged antibiotic therapy, extremes of age (both newborn and elderly), compromised host defenses, and exposure to an environment in the ICU rich in potential infectious agents. Each of these elements alone or in combination increases the infection risk and should heighten our suspicion of sepsis [3].

Pathophysiology

The pathophysiology of sepsis and its major complication, shock, has been the focus of innumerable human and animal studies. To date a unifying reasonably accepted understanding of the abnormal physiology remains elusive. Highlights from this wealth of information will be reviewed.

The major determinants of infections in ICU patients are the microorganism (usually a bacteria) and the host defense mechanisms, both local and systemic. Both endogenous and exogenous bacterial flora are involved, but as the patient's stay in the ICU lengthens, the endogenous flora is progressively replaced by colonization with organisms from the hospital environment. Hospital-acquired bacteria are often more pathogenic and antibiotic-resistant. The problem of transfer of resistance between organisms increases with high antibiotic usage in the ICU.

Organisms may enter the bloodstream from multiple sources and result in sepsis. Classically, the sites of origin of sepsis, in decreasing order of occurrence, have been the urinary tract, 'spontaneous' (no site identified), the gastrointestinal (GI) tract, the respiratory tract, vascular (usually intravenous) sites, and burns. In surgical patients, wound infections are also common sources. Recently, invasive devices including venous catheters, arterial lines, Swan-Ganz catheters, urinary catheters, and respiratory endotracheal tubes have been increasingly implicated [10].

The biological effects of endotoxin seem adequate to explain many of the clinical symptoms and signs of sepsis. Lipid A, a portion of the bacterial cell wall outer membrane, is a prime candidate as the active element. Past literature has suggested a significant difference in the pathophysiologic response to gram-negative versus gram-positive sepsis. A recent study of 59 patients with 70 septic episodes measured multiple physiologic parameters and revealed no significant difference between gram-positive and gram-negative organisms or between specific organisms. Leukocytosis, febrile response, and acid-base status were similar [12]. With adequate volume replacement, all patients showed a hyperdynamic cardiovascular response with abnormal vascular tone and some element of myocardial depression. While the precise pathogenesis of sepsis remains undefined, the response seems host- not organism-dependent.

Data on the immunology of sepsis are accumulating from animal and human studies. Abnormalities, including both humoral and cellular immunity, seem well established. They are often associated with underlying disease (cancer, diabetes, cirrhosis, renal failure, or trauma), surgery, malnutrition, or drug treatment (cytotoxic or anti-inflammatory). Recent studies have shown that patients with early sepsis and minimal hemodynamic problems have normal or increased immunoglobulin and complement levels with circulating immune complexes (CIC) being demonstrated in their blood. Patients with advanced septic shock show decreased immunoglobulin and complement levels with the absence of CIC. The disappearance of CIC with evidence of complement activation may suggest a possible role in the pathogenesis of shock [4]. Differences in complement levels in patients with gram-negative versus gram-positive shock have not been consistently demonstrated [9].

Other alterations in immunologic parameters may also compromise host defense against sepsis. Depression of delayed hypersensitivity skin test reactivity has been demonstrated in acutely ill patients and correlates with increased mortality due to sepsis. Prospective testing for anergy may help to identify patients at high risk for sepsis [1]. Clearance of bacteria and endotoxin require intact polymorphonuclear leukocytes (PMN) and reticuloendothelial system (RES) function. 'Natural antibodies' formed against digestive tract bacteria as well as complement provide some bactericidal activity against many gram-negative bacilli. Hepatic RES clearance of bacteria, while not requiring specific antibody, is enhanced by its presence. Adequate PMN function seems to require opsonizing antibody. Recent studies have demonstrated the importance of antibody to somatic O or core glycolipid (anti-Re) antigens of gram-negative bacilli (GNB) in improved outcome in GNB sepsis. A strong correlation exists between higher levels of anti-O IgG antibody and improved survival with GNB sepsis [1]. Possible therapeutic implications are discussed under therapy.

Diagnosis

The diagnosis of sepsis classically depends on positive blood cultures combined with an appropriate clinical presentation. Problems include when and how to draw blood cultures and whether 'sepsis' is a tenable diagnosis despite negative blood cultures. Clinical manifestations of sepsis indicating the need for blood cultures include unexplained fever, tachycardia, hypotension, tachypnea, altered mental state, hypoxia, respiratory alkalosis, metabolic acidosis, thrombocytopenia, renal failure, bilirubinemia or GI bleeding [10].

Recent interest in geriatric medicine has led to the recognition of afebrile bacteremia in older patients. In one prospective study [5], 25 patients representing 13% of all elderly patients (65 or older) with bacteremia had no fever. Only 4% of the patients under 65 had afebrile bacteremia. Clinical clues including unexplained leukocytosis or changes in mental status were once again demonstrated to be good guides to performing blood cultures. Afebrile bacteremia when associated with an indwelling intravenous catheter or underlying malignant disease was invariably fatal.

Blood cultures should be obtained when clinical suspicion of sepsis arises. Many bacteremias are intermittent in nature and involve small numbers of organisms in the circulation. This information indicates the need for proper timing of cultures and the importance of sample size. Studies have demonstrated close to 100% recovery with three separately collected blood cultures compared to 75% recovery if a single sample is taken. Controlled evaluations have shown greater recovery of bacteria with increases in the volume of blood sampled, but obvious practical limitations apply [11]. Good aseptic technique should reduce the number of contaminants which usually represent approximately 1% of all cultures taken. The 'true' recovery rate is usually 6–7% [13]. Each set of blood cultures should consist of two vacuum bottles containing media appropriate for the organism suspected and inoculated with the largest practical volume of blood (at least 10 ml for adults). One bottle usually remains unvented (relatively anaerobic) while the other is transiently vented. Precise recommendations regarding venting, media used, and atmosphere of incubation are difficult and should be determined by the local laboratory's capability and expertise [11].

Is 'non-bacteremic' clinical sepsis an entity? Several authors [7, 10] have raised this question. Their 6-month prospective study of 153 patients admitted to a surgical ICU identified 56 episodes of 'clinical' sepsis based on underlying disease process, clinical and laboratory findings, 'signs' of occult sepsis (hypoxia, bilirubinemia, renal failure, thrombocytopenia, abnormal mentation, gastric bleeding, and transient hypotension) and clinical course. 28 episodes of 'clinical' sepsis occurred in 22 patients with positive blood cultures. 28 clinically similar episodes occurred in 25 patients with negative cultures. Antibiotic use was similar in both groups. Clinical parameters including leukocytosis, anemia, bleeding, azotemia, jaundice, confusion, hypoxia and respiratory failure (including ventilator requirements) were comparable. Death rate (approximately 40%), 'the duration of sepsis', and identification of a 'septic focus' at autopsy or surgery were similar. The data suggest that we should be more aware of the possibility of 'non-bacteremic sepsis' and execute a vigilant search for possible infected foci even in patients with negative blood cultures.

Newer techniques for the detection of sepsis, such as accelerated organism recovery and analysis of blood samples for antigens or byproducts of microorganisms seem promising, but are not yet clinically established.

Therapy

Successful intervention in the natural course of sepsis remains a difficult problem with many unresolved issues. Prompt recognition on clinical grounds and initiation of therapy, usually involving two antibiotics, should be started after clinical suspicion has led to collection of blood cultures and perhaps specimens of urine, sputum, or wound drainage that might indicate the source of the bacteremia. Knowledge of the expected organisms and their sensitivities based on the literature as well as personal hospital experience is essential to facilitate an appropriate initial empirical antibiotic selection.

It has been difficult to establish what represents optimum antibiotic therapy in the septic patient because of the multiple factors influencing outcome. Several studies have demonstrated the strong role of the patient's host defense mechanism as modified by the severity of underlying disease. Patients have been categorized by their underlying disease into those with illnesses that are rapidly fatal (usually acute leukemias), ultimately fatal (commonly including solid tumors) and nonfatal. *Kreger* et al. [8], in a comprehensive review of 612 patients with gram-negative bacteremia studied over a 10-year period, clearly established improved patient survival when initial antibiotic therapy is appropriate for the organisms that are later recovered. This improvement occurs in each of the underlying host disease categories. The survival for patients receiving appropriate therapy is twice that of patients who receive ineffective therapy. Initial appropriate antimicrobial therapy also reduces the frequency of shock by twofold in all patients although there is variation between patients in disease categories. Even after shock has developed, appropriate antimicrobial therapy increases survival with differing levels of significance among the different groups of patients.

GNB usually represent 50–60% of the organisms recovered, with *Escherichia coli, Klebsiella, Pseudomonas, Serratia, Enterobacter,* and *Proteus* predominating. The gram-positive organisms including *Staph. aureus, Staph. epidermidis* (may be a contaminant but should not be routinely discarded as such), *Streptococci, Pneumococci, and Enterococci* occur in 35–40% of blood isolates with fungi being less than 5% [2, 13]. Knowledge of the organisms recovered from septic patients in your hospital as well as their sensitivities should be routinely available from the clinical laboratory and should influence initial antibiotic selection. Broad gram-positive and gram-negative coverage such as provided by combination of a cephalosporin and an aminoglycoside is reasonable.

Extended spectrum cephalosporins of the 'third generation' (moxalactam, cefotaxime, and cefoperazone) and 'newer penicillins' (mezlocillin, piperacillin, and azlocillin), which have recently become clinically available, show promise but should not lead to abandonment of tested combinations until more data are available. Single antibiotic coverage is not adequate initially, but may be justified when culture results are available. Dosage should be adjusted for age and weight, as well as for renal and hepatic function, and, in selected patients, from monitoring of antimicrobial levels.

Drainage of a septic focus or removal of a possible entry site for organisms (intravenous catheter, urinary catheter, etc.) should be aggressively pursued and promptly accomplished. Volume monitoring and replacement, pharmacologic interventions, and general supportive care appropriate for septic patients with possible shock are covered elsewhere in this volume. More recent therapeutic developments for the septic patient include possible manipulation of the inflammatory response by newer drugs through complement, PMN, kallikrein and prostaglandin mechanisms.

Of major significance is a recent report [14] on the first prospective controlled clinical trial of immunotherapy in gram-negative sepsis (GNS). This study demonstrates the protective effect of antibody to core lipopolysaccharide (LPS) made by vaccinating healthy men with heat-killed *E. coli* J5. This organism lacks the LPS oligosaccharide side chain thereby allowing antibody to form to the exposed underlying core. Death in septic patients fell from 39% in controls to 22% in recipients of the serum. In those with severe shock, mortality was reduced from 77–44%. While not yet clinically available, this application of knowledge of the immunology and pathophysiology of GNS to clinical situations is encouraging and holds considerable promise.

References

1 Clumeck, N.; George, C.: Immunological aspects of severe bacterial sepsis. Intensive Care Med. *7:* 109–114 (1981).
2 Daschner, F.D.; Frey, P.; Wolff, G.; Baumann, P.C.; Suter, P.: Nosocomial infections in intensive care wards: a multicenter prospective study. Intensive Care Med. *8:* 5–9 (1982).
3 Donowitz, L.G.; Wenzel, R.P.; Hoyt, J.W.: High risk of hospital-acquired infection in the ICU patient. Crit. Care Med. *10:* 355–357 (1982).
4 George, C.; Carlet, J.; Sobel, A.; Intrator, L.; Robin, M.; Sabatier, C.; Prevot, D.; Rapin, M.: Circulating immune complexes in patients with gram-negative septic shock. Intensive Care Med. *6:* 123–127 (1980).
5 Gleckman, R.; Hibert, D.: Afebrile bacteremia: a phenomenon in geriatric patients. J. Am. med. Ass. *248:* 1478–1481 (1982).
6 Haley, R.W.; Schaberg, D.R.; Crossley, K.B.; Von Allmen, S.D.; McGowan, J.E., Jr.: Extra charges and prolongation of stay attributable to nosocomial infections: a prospective interhospital comparison. Am. J. Med. *70:* 51–58 (1980).
7 Koliner, C.; Boulanger, M.; McLean, A.P.H.; Meakins, J.L.: Nonbacteremic clinical sepsis: an entity? Crit. Care Med. *8:* 230 (1980).
8 Kreger, B.E.; Craven, D.E.; McCabe, W.R.: Gram-negative bacteremia. IV. Re-evaluation of clinical features and treatment in 612 patients. Am. J. Med. *68:* 344–355 (1980).
9 Leon, C.; Rodrigo, M.J.; Tomasa, A.; Gallart, M.T.; Latorre, F.J.; Rius, J.; Brugues, J.: Complement activation in septic shock due to gram-negative and gram-positive bacteria. Crit. Care Med. *10:* 308–315 (1982).
10 Meakins, J.L.; Wicklund, B.; Forse, R.A.; McLean, A.P.H.: The surgical intensive care unit: Current concepts in infection. Surg. Clins N. Am. *60:* 117–132 (1980).
11 Tenney, J.H.; Reller, L.B.; Mirrett, S.; Wang, W.L.; Weinstein, M.P.: Controlled evaluation of the volume of blood cultured in detection of bacteremia and fungemia. J. clin. Microbiol. *15:* 558–561 (1982).
12 Wiles, J.B.; Cerra, F.B.; Siegel, J.H.; Border, J.R.: The systemic septic response: does the organism matter? Crit. Care Med. *8:* 55–60 (1980).
13 Young, L.S.; Martin, W.J.; Meyer, R.D.; Weinstein, R.J.; Anderson, E.T.: Gram-negative rod bacteremia: microbiologic, immunologic, and therapeutic considerations. Ann. intern. Med. *86:* 456–471 (1977).
14 Ziegler, E.J.; McCutchan, J.A.; Fierer, J.; Glauser, M.P.; Sadoff, J.C.; Douglas, H.; Braude, A.I.: Treatment of gram-negative bacteremia and shock with human antiserum to a mutant *Escherichia coli.* New Engl. J. Med. *307:* 1225–1268 (1982).

R.T. Coussons, MD, Department of Medicine, University of Oklahoma Health Sciences Center, Oklahoma City, OK 73104 (USA)

Prog. crit. Care Med., vol. 2, pp. 280–290 (Karger, Basel 1985)

Antimicrobial Selection in the Intensive Care Unit

Douglas P. Fine, Ronald A. Greenfield

Department of Medicine, University of Oklahoma Health Sciences Center and Veterans Administration Medical Center, Oklahoma City, Okla., USA

Introduction

The intensive care unit is an environment in which infections commonly occur. Antimicrobial therapy is often required and the proper selection and administration of antimicrobials is both especially important and especially difficult. In seriously ill patients, the normal antibiotic-susceptible flora may soon be displaced by more generally resistant microbes, usually gram-negative enteric bacilli; administration of antimicrobial agents probably hastens this process [1, 2]. In such a setting, it becomes important to avoid unnecessary antimicrobial therapy and to choose antimicrobials with as narrow a spectrum as possible. Practically, however, one is often faced with a need to administer antimicrobials to a critically ill patient who is colonized with many relatively resistant organisms and in whom the precise site of infection or the precise agent of infection may not be immediately determinable.

This chapter will review antimicrobial agents commonly used in an intensive care setting. Space does not permit complete pharmacological reviews, which are readily available in standard textbooks. The focus will be on intensive-care uses and on newer agents.

Penicillins

Penicillin G, ampicillin: although penicillins remain a mainstay of antimicrobial therapy in all types of practice, usefulness of older penicillins in an ICU is limited by prominence of resistant staphylococci and gram-negative bacilli. Nonetheless, penicillin G remains the drug of choice for most infections caused by streptococci (including the pneumococcus), *Neisseria* and *Clostridia.* Ampicillin in combination with an aminoglycoside is optimum therapy for enterococcal infections. Aspiration pneumonia, bacterial lung abscess and meningitis in an adult provide indications for both agents. In addition, the limited gram-negative spectrum of ampicillin permits its use in certain circumstances based on in vitro susceptibility testing.

Carbenicillin, ticarcillin: in general, these agents have a spectrum similar to ampicillin but with better activity against some gram-negative bacilli, particularly *Pseudomonas* species. Their primary indication is treatment of suspected or established *Pseudomonas* infections, in which case they should be used in combination with an aminoglycoside.

Piperacillin, mezlocillin, azlocillin: these new agents [3] are similar to carbenicillin and ticarcillin but with a greater gram-negative spectrum. Their gram-positive and anaerobic activity is similar to that of penicillin G. They are active against most gram-negative bacilli, including most strains of *Klebsiella pneumoniae, Serratia* and *Pseudomonas.*

In general, azlocillin and piperacillin are most effective against *Pseudomonas aeruginosa,* mezlocillin and piperacillin against Enterobacteriaceae. Thus, piperacillin has the broadest spectrum, azlocillin is somewhat specific for *P. aeruginosa,* and mezlocillin represents a more modest advance over carbenicillin or ticarcillin.

Piperacillin or mezlocillin could be used as single-agent therapy for hospital-acquired infections, particularly pneumonias or skin infections. Such therapy would not treat most *Staphylococcus aureus* infections and gram-negative bacilli may be resistant. Furthermore, resistance can emerge during therapy. For established *Pseudomonas* infections, piperacillin or azlocillin should be used in combination with an aminoglycoside [3].

Nafcillin, oxacillin, methicillin: these agents remain drugs of choice for *S. aureus* infections. However, in recent years, primarily in intensive care units, *S. aureus* resistant to these antibiotics (methicillin-resistant *S. aureus*) have emerged as serious pathogens [4, 5]. In general, unless methicillin-resistant *S. aureus* infection has been a problem in a particular intensive-care unit, nafcillin (or one of the other agents) may still be used to treat *S. aureus* infections, pending in vitro susceptibility studies.

With high doses and prolonged use, nafcillin may produce serious but reversible neutropenia. Oxacillin is potentially hepatotoxic. Because of nephrotoxicity, an immunologically mediated interstitial nephritis, methicillin is less commonly used in recent years.

Cephalosporins

The cephalosporins are commonly subdivided into three generations. They offer several advantages in intensive-care settings (e.g., relative lack of toxicity, broad spectrum) but are seldom the drug of first choice for any specific infection and they are expensive. In recent years, many new cephalosporins have been introduced although their clinical role is not as yet fully defined.

First-generation cephalosporins: these agents were introduced primarily for therapy of infections due to gram-positive aerobic cocci and remain an alternative therapy for these infections, excluding those due to enterococci and methicillin-resistant *S. aureus* [5] or *S. epidermidis.* They have good activity against many anaerobes, but many *Clostridia* and *Bacteroides fragilis* are typically resistant. Among the gram-negative bacilli, their activity is limited to some *Escherichia coli, Proteus mirabilis* and *K. pneumoniae.* Currently available first-generation cephalosporins (cephalothin, cefazolin, cephapirin, and cephradine) are essentially interchangable and choice can be made on the basis of cost.

Cephalosporins are commonly used in combination with an aminoglycoside for initial broad-spectrum therapy of etiologically undefined infection or septicemia. *Barza* [6] has reviewed the evidence that this combination may be more nephrotoxic than either agent administered alone. Data are contradictory but do not clearly support the concept of synergistic nephrotoxicity.

Second-generation cephalosporins: cefamandole has an expanded gram-negative spectrum, particularly for *Haemophilus influenzae* and several Enterobacteriaceae, at the expense of somewhat diminished effectiveness against *S. aureus* and other gram-positive cocci [7]. Resistance to cefamandole may rapidly emerge during therapy, especially among Enterobacteriaceae, apparently as a result of induction of β-lactamase synthesis [8]. This resistance can be clinically important and can extend to other antimicrobials as well [8].

In the treatment of infections due to gram-negative bacilli, cefamandole is inferior to other agents now available. Effectiveness against gram-positive cocci is less than that of first-generation cephalosporins. Thus, in combination with an aminoglycoside, a first-generation cephalosporin or a penicillin is preferable to cefamandole. Alone, the newer penicillins or third-generation cephalosporins provide better therapy.

Cefoxitin, the other parenteral second-generation cephalosporin, appears to be more stable to gram-negative β-lactamases, but is also capable of inducing enzyme synthesis [9]. In general, cefoxitin is somewhat less effective than cefamandole in vitro against gram-positive cocci and some Enterobacteriaceae, more effective against other Enterobacteriaceae [10].

Cefoxitin is the most effective cephalosporin against most anaerobes, including *B. fragilis* [11]. In some circumstances, primarily community-acquired gynecological [12] and abdominal [13] surgical infections, this spectrum may permit the use of cefoxitin as single-agent therapy, although this use is highly controversial and probably not relevant to an intensive-care situation.

Third-generation cephalosporins: the third-generation cephalosporins share the property of greater β-lactamase stability and therefore a much expanded gram-negative spectrum. The durability of this enhanced spectrum has yet to be established. In one study [14] of moxalactam therapy of adults infected with cephalothin-resistant bacteria (*Klebsiella, E. coli, Serratia, Pseudomonas,* etc.), the overall success rate was 76%, rather good for this group of difficult infections. All but 7 of the 33 infecting organisms (21%) became resistant to moxalactam during therapy. *Pseudomonas* resistance is already common, even though *Pseudomonas* was a primary target when the third-generation cephalosporins were introduced [15]. In addition, the expanded gram-negative spectrum has brought a lessened effectiveness against gram-positive organisms, including staphylococci and streptococci [15].

Third-generation cephalosporins attain therapeutic concentrations in cerebrospinal fluid [16]. In experimental [17] and human [18] infections, responses have been encouraging. They may well be important drugs in the management of some meningitides, primarily those due to *H. influenzae* and many Enterobacteriaceae [15, 19]. However, recent anecdotal reports of treatment failures in pneumococcal [20], streptococcal [21], and *Klebsiella* [22] meningitis should make one wary.

The third-generation cephalosporins share some side effects novel for cephalosporins. Many of them have a disulfiram-like effect [23]. Prolongation of the prothrombin time and interference with platelet function can be associated with clinically important bleeding [24, 25]. All patients on these agents, especially moxalactam, should probably receive vitamin K. Suppression of normal enteric anaerobes and Enterobacteriaceae can be profound [26]. The resulting microbiological vacuum is filled by resistant *Pseudomonas,* staphylococci, *Candida* [26], *Clostridia* including *C. difficile* [15], and enterococci [27].

Unlike the first-generation cephalosporins, these third-generation cephalosporins are not interchangeable. Thus, in vitro susceptibility testing with the specific agent under consideration needs to be evaluated. Additionally, there are major pharmacokinetic differences among these agents, as has recently been reviewed [15].

Cefotaxime: this agent retains greatest effectiveness against staphylococci, streptococci, and *Neisseria.* Against gram-negative bacilli, cefotaxime is similar to or slightly less efficacious than moxalactam but superior to cefoperazone. Activity against *B. fragilis,* generally the most drug-resistant of anaerobes, is relatively poor [15].

Moxalactam: this agent is similar to, or slightly better than cefotaxime against gram-negative rods. Gram-positive cocci tend to be considerably more resistant to moxalactam than to other available third-generation agents. Moxalactam exhibits good activity against *B. fragilis* and other anaerobes, except *Clostridia,* against which no cephalosporin is active [15]. Cerebrospinal fluid penetration is good [28].

Cefoperazone: cefoperazone is similar to cefotaxime in activity against streptococci and staphylococci but is in general less effective against most other organisms [15]. In contrast to cefotaxime and moxalactam, cefoperazone is cleared primarily through the liver; thus, dosage alteration in renal failure is not necessary [29].

Clindamycin

Clindamycin remains a drug of choice for serious abdominal and pelvic anaerobic infections. Most anaerobes, including almost all strains of *B. fragilis,* are susceptible to clindamycin. Notable exceptions are some *Clostridia,* including *Clostridium perfringens* and *Clostridium difficile* [30]. Most aerobic gram-positive cocci are sensitive as well, including most *S. aureus* strains. Gram-negative bacilli are generally resistant.

The major use for clindamycin is treatment of serious infections in which anaerobes, particularly *B. fragilis,* play an important role. Alternatives to clindamycin include chloramphenicol, metronidazole, cefoxitin, and moxalactam. Concomitant administration of an aminoglycoside is usually necessary for treatment of coinfecting aerobes.

Diarrhea, and in some cases pseudomembranous colitis, is the principal toxicity of clindamycin [30]. This syndrome reflects overgrowth of clindamycin-resistant, toxin-producing *C. difficile* [31]. Treatment is with oral vancomycin, 1–2 g daily for at least 7 days [32].

Chloramphenicol

Chloramphenicol remains a mainstay in the management of abdominal anaerobic infections and the drug of choice for the treatment of anaerobic brain abscesses. Because of its generally good central nervous system penetration, it has had a prominent role in the management of meningitis. The spectrum of chloramphenicol includes most aerobic gram-positive cocci, *Neisseria meningitidis*, most anaerobes, *H. influenzae*, and a number of Enterobacteriaceae. Recent studies, however, have made it clear that failure rates with chloramphenicol in the treatment of gram-negative bacillary meningitis are unacceptably high, presumably because chloramphenicol, in doses achievable in spinal fluid, is bacteriostatic at best [33–35]. In contrast, bactericidal levels are usually achieved in spinal fluid against *H. influenzae, N. meningitidis,* and *S. pneumoniae;* for these organisms chloramphenicol remains a good alternative to penicillins.

Vancomycin

Vancomycin was introduced clinically in 1958, primarily for the treatment of infections caused by penicillin-resistant *S. aureus.* Toxicity of the drug (local irritative phenomena, ototoxicity, nephrotoxicity) made vancomycin noncompetitive when methicillin was introduced in about 1960. Newer formulations are much less toxic, and in recent years vancomycin has reemerged as an important antimicrobial agent [36, 37].

Vancomycin is an intravenously administered bactericidal agent whose spectrum of antimicrobial activity includes staphylococci, streptococci, pneumococci, *Corynebacteria,* and *Clostridia.* It inhibits but does not itself kill enterococci; nevertheless, it can be used effectively in therapy of enterococcal infections [36]. Vancomycin is the drug of choice in the treatment of infections due to methicillin-resistant *S. aureus* and *S. epidermidis* and a good alternative to penicillinase-resistant penicillins or cephalosporins for severe staphylococcal infections of any kind [38].

Excretion of vancomycin is renal; the drug is not dialyzed [39]. Therefore, vancomycin is uniquely convenient for the therapy of infections due to susceptible organisms in anephric or anuric patients. In such situations, the dosage is 1 g followed by 500–1,000 mg every 5–10 days with monitoring of serum levels. In patients with impaired renal function, nomograms for dosage adjustment have been published [40].

Aminoglycosides

The aminoglycosides are the ‘gold standard’ in therapy of gram-negative bacilli [41]. Three major factors limit their clinical usefulness. First, they have a narrow therapeutic index. This necessitates close monitoring of serum levels and prevents attainment of blood levels manyfold in excess of minimum inhibitory concentrations. Secondly, all aminoglycosides are nephrotoxic and ototoxic. Thirdly, resistance to aminoglycosides, especially gentamicin and tobramycin, has been an increasing clinical problem, especially in hospitals dealing with large numbers of immunosuppressed and critically ill patients.

The major aminoglycosides in current practice are gentamicin, tobramycin, and amikacin. The choice of agent in a given patient is based on many considerations. There seems to be little *clinical* relevance to demonstrated differences in ototoxicity or nephrotoxicity [41]. With all agents, serum concentrations and renal function must be frequently monitored and dosage adjusted as necessary [42]. In some hospitals, gentamicin/tobramycin resistance is widespread among gram-negative bacteria, and there amikacin would reasonably be the first-line aminoglycoside. If gentamicin/tobramycin resistance is uncommon, there is no great advantage to routine use of amikacin, which can then be kept in reserve [43].

In one situation, amikacin may be clearly preferable [44]. In patients with renal failure, including those on chronic hemodialysis, carbenicillin and other penicillins can interact with gentamicin or tobramycin with resultant inactivation of both agents. Amikacin appears to be resistant to this phenomenon [44] and thus would be preferred in such patients.

Trimethoprim-Sulfamethoxazole

This fixed combination agent has been available for some time in oral form but only recently in the United States for intravenous usage [45, 46]. The intravenous form is currently used primarily for therapy of *Pneumocystis carinii* infections or urinary tract infections when oral therapy is not possible. It has been suggested in patients with serious systemic infections, especially granulocytopenic or otherwise immunocompromised patients, because of a broad spectrum, including both gram-positive and gram-negative, aerobic bacteria (specifically excluding *Pseudomonas),* but the exact role in such situations remains to be established [45, 47, 48].

Metronidazole

Metronidazole, long recognized as effective for some protozoal agents, is also effective against most anaerobic bacteria, including *B. fragilis* [49]. The intravenous form has recently been introduced in the USA. The drug can be considered a good alternative to clindamycin in the treatment of anaerobic infections [49, 50]. Metronidazole, unlike clindamycin, has no activity against aerobic or facultative bacteria.

References

1 Johanson, W.; Pierce, A.; Sanford, J.; Thomas, G.: Nosocomial respiratory infections with gram-negative bacilli. The significance of colonization of the respiratory tract. Ann. intern. Med. *77:* 701–706 (1972).
2 Schwartz, S.; Dowling, J.; Benkovic, C.; De Quittner-Buchanan, M.; Prostko, T.; Yee, R.: Sources of gram-negative bacilli colonizing the tracheae of intubated patients. J. infect. Dis. *138:* 227–231 (1978).
3 Eliopoulos, G.; Moellering, R., Jr.: Azlocillin, mezlocillin, and piperacillin: new broad-spectrum penicillins. Ann. intern. Med. *97:* 755–760 (1982).
4 Crossley, K.; Loesch, D.; Landesman, B.; Mead, K.; Chern, M.; Strate, R.: An outbreak of infections caused by strains of *Staphylococcus aureus* resistant to methicillin and aminoglycosides. I. Clinical studies. J. infect. Dis. *139:* 273–279 (1979).
5 Wenzel, R.: The emergence of methicillin-resistant *Staphylococcus aureus.* Ann. intern. Med. *97:* 440–442 (1982).
6 Barza, M.: The nephrotoxicity of cephalosporins: an overview. J. infect. Dis. *137:* S60–S73 (1978).

7 Mandell, G.; Sande, M.: Penicillins and cephalosporins; in Gilman, Goodman, Gilman, The pharmacological basis of therapeutics; 6th ed., pp. 1126–1161 (Macmillan, New York 1980).
8 Sanders, C.; Moellering, R., Jr.; Martin, R.; Perkins, R.; Strike, D.; Gootz, T.; Sanders, W., Jr.: Resistance to cefamandole: a collaborative study of emerging clinical problems. J. infect. Dis. *145:* 118–125 (1982).
9 Gootz, T.; Sanders, C.; Goering, R.: Resistance to cefamandole: derepression of β-lactamases by cefotoxin and mutation in *Enterobacter cloacae*. J. infect. Dis. *146:* 34–42 (1982).
10 Eickhoff, T.; Ehret, J.L.: In vitro comparison of cefoxitin, cefamandole, cephalexin, and cephalothin. Antimicrob. Agents Chemother. *9:* 994–999 (1976).
11 Chuchural, G.; Jacobus, N.; Gorbach, S.; Tally, F.: A summary of *Bacteroides* susceptibility in the US. J. Antimicrob. Chemother. *8:* suppl. D, pp. 27–31 (1981).
12 Sweet, R.; Ledger, W.: Cefoxitin: single-agent treatment of mixed aerobic-anaerobic pelvic infections. Obstet. Gynec. *54:* 193–198 (1979).
13 Tally, F.; McGowan, K.; Kellum, J.; Gorbach, S.; O'Donnell, T.: A randomized comparison of cefoxitin with or without amikacin and clindamycin plus amikacin in surgical sepsis. Ann. Surg. *193:* 318–323 (1981).
14 Platt, R.; Ehrlich, S.; Afarian, J.; O'Brien, T.; Pennington, J.; Kass, E.: Moxalactam therapy of infections caused by cephalothin-resistant bacteria: influence of serum inhibitory activity on clinical response and acquisition of antibiotic resistance during therapy. Antimicrob. Agents Chemother. *20:* 351–355 (1981).
15 Neu, H.: The new beta-lactamase-stable cephalosporins. Ann. intern. Med. *97:* 408–419 (1982).
16 Modai, J.; Wolff, M.; Lebas, J.; Meulemans, A.; Manuel, C.: Moxalactam penetration into cerebrospinal fluid in patients with bacterial meningitis. Antimicrob. Agents Chemother. *21:* 551–553 (1982).
17 Sheld, W.; Brodeur, J.; Sande, M.; Alliegro, G.: Comparison of cefoperazone with penicillin, ampicillin, gentamicin, and chloramphenicol in the therapy of experimental meningitis. Antimicrob. Agents Chemother. *22:* 652–656 (1982).
18 Olson, D.; Hoeprich, P.; Nolan, S.; Goldstein, E.: Successful treatment of gram-negative bacillary meningitis with moxalactam. Ann. intern. Med. *95:* 302–305 (1981).
19 Landesman, S.; Corrado, M.; Shah, P.; Armengaud, M.; Barza, M.; Cherubin, C.: Past and current roles for cephalosporin antibiotics in treatment of meningitis. Emphasis on use in gram-negative bacillary meningitis. Am. J. Med. *71:* 693–703 (1981).
20 Perlino, C.: Moxalactam therapy for bacterial pneumonia. Rev. infect. Dis. *4:* S617–S622 (1982).
21 Iannini, P.; Kunkel, M.: Cefotaxime failure in group A streptococcal meningitis. J. Am. med. Ass. *248:* 1878 (1982).
22 Bradsher, R.: Relapse of gram-negative bacillary meningitis after cefotaxime therapy. J. Am. med. Ass. *248:* 1214–1215 (1982).
23 Neu, H.; Prince, A.: Interaction between moxalactam and alcohol. Lancet *i:* 1422 (1980).
24 Bang, N.; Tessler, S.; Heidenreich, R.; Marks, C.; Mattler, L.: Effects of moxalactam on blood coagulation and platelet function. Rev. infect. Dis. *4:* S546–S554 (1982).

25 Weitekamp, M.; Aber, R.: Prolonged bleeding times and bleeding diathesis associated with moxalactam administration. J. Am. med. Ass. *249:* 69–71 (1983).
26 Mulligan, M.; Citron, D.; McNamara, B.; Finegold, S.: Impact of cefoperazone therapy on fecal flora. Antimicrob. Agents Chemother. *22:* 226–230 (1982).
27 Yu, V.: Enterococcal superinfection and colonization after therapy with moxalactam, a new broad-spectrum antibiotic. Ann. intern. Med. *94:* 784–785 (1981).
28 Landesman, S.; Corrado, M.; Cherubin, C.; Gombert, M.; Cleri, D.: Diffusion of a new beta-lactam (LY127935) into cerebrospinal fluid. Am. J. Med. *69:* 92–98 (1980).
29 Greenfield, R.; Gerber, A.; Craig, W.: Pharmacokinetics of cefoperazone in patients with normal and with impaired hepatic and renal function. Rev. infect. Dis. (in press).
30 LeFrock, J.; Molavi, A.; Prince, R.: Clindamycin. Med. Clins N. Am. *66:* 103–120 (1982).
31 Bartlett, J.; Chang, T.; Gurwith, M.; Gorbach, S.; Onderdonk, A.: Antibiotic-associated pseudomembranous colitis due to toxin-producing clostridia. New Engl. J. Med. *298:* 531–534 (1978).
32 Silva, J.; Bates, D.; Fekety, R.; Plouffe, J.; Rifkin, G.; Baird, I.: Treatment of *Clostridium difficile* colitis and diarrhea with vancomycin. Am. J. Med. *71:* 815–822 (1981).
33 Cherubin, C.; Marr, J.; Sierra, M.; Becker, S.: Listeria and gram-negative bacillary meningitis in New York City, 1972–1979. Am. J. Med. *71:* 199–209 (1981).
34 Sande, M.: Antibiotic therapy of bacterial meningitis: lessons we've learned. Am. J. Med. *71:* 507–510 (1981).
35 Rahal, J.; Simberkoff, M.: Host defense and antimicrobial therapy in adult gram-negative bacillary meningitis. Ann. intern. Med. *96:* 468–474 (1982).
36 Cook, F.; Farrar, W., Jr.: Vancomycin revisited. Ann. intern. Med. *88:* 813–818 (1978).
37 Griffith, R.: Introduction to vancomycin. Rev. infect. Dis. *3:* S200–S204 (1981).
38 Kirby, W.: Vancomycin therapy in severe staphylococcal infections. Rev. infect. Dis. *3:* S236–S239 (1981).
39 Cunha, B.; Quintiliani, R.; Deglin, J.; Izard, M.; Nightingale, C.: Pharmacokinetics of vancomycin in anuria. Rev. infect. Dis. *3:* S269–S272 (1981).
40 Moellering, R., Jr.; Krogstad, D.; Greenblatt, D.: Vancomycin therapy in patients with impaired renal function: a nomogram for dosage. Ann. intern. Med. *94:* 343–346 (1981).
41 Ristuccia, A.; Cunha, B.: The aminoglycosides. Med. Clins N. Am. *66:* 303–312 (1982).
42 Bennett, W.; Muther, R.; Parker, R.; Feig, P.; Morrison, G.; Golper, T.; Singer, I.: Drug therapy in renal failure: dosing guidelines for adults. I. Antimicrobial agents, analgesics. Ann. intern. Med. *93:* 62–89 (1980).
43 Meyer, R.: Amikacin. Ann. intern. Med. *95:* 328–332 (1981).
44 Blair, D.; Duggan, D.; Schroeder, E.: Inactivation of amikacin and gentamicin by carbenicillin in patients with end-stage renal failure. Antimicrob. Agents Chemother. *22:* 376–379 (1982).
45 Salter, A.: Trimethoprim-sulfamethoxazole: an assessment of more than 12 years of use. Rev. infect. Dis. *4:* 196–236 (1982).

46 Spicehandler, J.; Pollock, A.; Simberkoff, M.; Rahal, J., Jr.: Intravenous pharmacokinetics and in vitro bactericidal activity of trimethoprim-sulfamethoxazole. Rev. infect. Dis. *4:* 562–565 (1982).
47 Bodey, G.; Grose, W.; Keating, M.: Use of trimethoprim-sulfamethoxazole for treatment of infections in patients with cancer. Rev. infect. Dis. *4:* 579–585 (1982).
48 Braine, H.; Stuart, R.; Saral, R.; Lietman, P.: Parenteral trimethoprim-sulfamethoxazole and carbenicillin as empiric therapy for neutropenic patients with cancer. Rev. infect. Dis. *4:* 586–592 (1982).
49 Molavi, A.; LeFrock, J.; Prince, R.: Metronidazole. Med. Clins N. Am. *66:* 121–133 (1982).
50 George, W.; Kirby, B.; Sutter, V.; Wheeler, L.; Mulligan, M.; Finegold, S.: Intravenous metronidazole for treatment of infections involving anaerobic bacteria. Antimicrob. Agents Chemother. *21:* 441–449 (1982).

D.P. Fine, MD, Department of Medicine, University of Oklahoma Health Sciences Center and Veterans Administration Medical Center, Oklahoma City, OK 73106 (USA)

Prog. crit. Care Med., vol. 2, pp. 291–303 (Karger, Basel 1985)

The Problem of Nosocomial Infections

Daniel Sexton

University of Oklahoma Health Sciences Center and Oklahoma City Clinic, Oklahoma City, Okla., USA

Introduction

Patients in critical care units are not only the sickest in the hospital, but also tend to be at the extremes of age, subject to the most invasive procedures, and often crowded together. They frequently require intensive antibiotic use and prolonged hospital stays. It is therefore not surprising that they acquire nosocomial infections at rates 3–4 times higher than other hospitalized patients [1]. Not only are patients in critical care units regularly exposed to the routine risks of infection related to surgical, bladder, and venous catheters, they frequently face an array of special risks including arterial catheters and endotracheal tubes. In one 700-bed university hospital, approximately 40% of all nosocomial bacteremias occurred among intensive care unit patients who occupied only 8% of hospital beds [2]. Patients in this hospital's surgical intensive care unit had an 8-fold higher rate of nosocomial bacteremia than did patients on general wards.

The economic costs and human suffering induced by nosocomial infections, when viewed on a national level, are indeed staggering. For instance, more than 6 million hospital days in the United States are attributable annually to prolongation of stay for the treatment of nosocomial infections [3]. Over 2 million nosocomial infections are acquired each year in this country. Despite these huge numbers, it is easy to overlook the significance of individual nosocomial infections on a day-to-day basis. More importantly, strict adherence to preventive techniques – especially hand washing – is often 'lost in the shuffle' of a busy, crowded intensive care unit.

Basic Principles

By definition, a nosocomial infection is neither present nor incubating at the time of admission and usually does not become apparent in the first 48–72 h after admission. Occasionally, nosocomial infections may not become manifest until after transfer from the critical care unit or even after discharge from the hospital. The epidemiology of nosocomial infections has been extensively studied. Basic epidemiologic principles derived from these studies apply equally to ward patients as to patients in intensive care units. As a rule of thumb, approximately one-half of all nosocomial infections arise from the urinary tract, one-fourth from surgical wounds, one-eighth from the lower respiratory tract and one-sixteenth are bacteremias. Nosocomial bacteremias and lower respiratory tract infections occur at a substantially higher rate in intensive care patients and are frequently lethal [1]. Approximately one-half of all nosocomial infections are preventable using currently available techniques and procedures [4]. Aerobic gram-negative rods account for 60–70% of all hospital-acquired infections.

The metaphor of a 'chain of infection' is central to most infection control strategies. Three 'links' comprise this chain: a virulent agent, a susceptible host, and a mode of acquisition or transmission by which the host acquires the agent [5]. Breaking any one of these links will interrupt the nosocomial spread of disease.

Most nosocomial infections are transmitted directly by the hands of hospital personnel. Patients and staff (the animate environment) are in constant contact with the inanimate environment and people frequently exchange microorganisms with the surrounding inanimate world. But this exchange is far less important than transfer of microorganisms via direct human contact. In order to cause disease, microbes in the inanimate environment must first be transmitted to humans either by direct contact or indirectly via aerosols, contaminated solutions or other vectors. This transfer can frequently be interrupted by simple measures including hand washing, good nursing technique and standard infection control policies.

Many nosocomial infections arise endogenously from an individual patient's own flora. Alterations in normal bacterial flora without disease (colonization) often precede the appearance of a nosocomial infection. Many patients are colonized without disease. In others, long time delays between colonization with a nosocomial microbe and its appearance as a true pathogen make recognition of the actual cause of an individual nosocomial infection difficult or impossible. Complicating matters even further, 8–15% of patients admitted to hospitals have an established infection [3, 4]. These patients represent an important reservoir for transmission to other patients.

Urinary Tract Infections

40–50% of all nosocomial infections are related to the urinary tract. Almost 75% of nosocomial urinary tract infections occur in patients who have undergone some form of urologic instrumentation [4]. Indwelling urinary catheters are the single most important predisposing cause for nosocomial urinary tract infections. Between 10 and 15% of patients admitted to a general hospital ward and an even higher percentage of patients in intensive care units have an indwelling urinary catheter inserted during their hospitalization. It is axiomatic that the longer a urinary catheter is left in place the greater the risk of infection, and removing a urinary catheter greatly lowers this risk. Nonetheless, urinary catheters are frequently left in place longer than medically necessary. Surveys of urinary catheter use in hospitalized patients indicate that over one-third may have a urinary catheter without definite medical indication [6]. The risk of bacteriuria in a catheterized patient is remarkably constant at about 5% per day. After 11 days of continuous urinary catheter use, approximately 50% of women will have bacteriuria and after 13 days of catheterization, 50% of men will be bacteriuric [4]. Most catheterized bacteriuric patients are asymptomatic, but nosocomial urinary tract infections are the most common cause of secondary bacteremia in hospitalized patients. Between 1 and 3% of patients with catheter-related urinary tract infections develop secondary bacteremia. Approximately 30% of these bacteremic patients will die [7]. Nonbacteremic catheter-related infections occasionally prolong hospital stays and may greatly increase hospital costs [8, 9].

Bacteria that gain access to either the inner lumen or outer surface of urinary collection tubing can ascend into the bladder. Nosocomial pathogens on the unwashed hands of hospital personnel can first colonize the outer surface of catheter tubing and appear in the bladder or blood of a patient a few days later. Contaminated urinary collection devices and contaminated antiseptic or irrigation solutions have led to outbreaks of nosocomial urinary tract infection in intensive care units. Daily meatal care for catheterized patients is not effective and may be harmful in selected patient populations [10]. Neomycin-polymyxin irrigants used in catheterized patients are also ineffective [11].

Meticulous technique concerning catheter insertion, maintenance of a closed collection system, good hand washing and prompt removal of urinary catheters are all important and effective preventive measures. Collection systems should be well secured to prevent urethral trauma and positioned to prevent retrograde flow of urine. The use of these simple techniques can reduce the incidence of bacteriuria during the first few days of catheterization, but after 1 week the incidence of bacteriuria rises rapidly despite currently available preventive methods [4]. The use of intermittent catheterization is sometimes a reasonable alternative to an indwelling urinary catheter and may lower the risk of infection. Most importantly, indwelling urinary catheters should be inserted only when abolutely necessary and removed as quickly as is feasible.

Wound Infections

Patients in intensive care units frequently have either traumatic or surgical wounds. Although *Staphylococcus aureus* is the most common cause of surgical wound infection, it is responsible for less than 50% of all nosocomial wound infections. Most staphylococcal wound infections occur within 10 days of surgery and probably are acquired in the operating room [4]. Many wound infections are polymicrobic and include gram-negative enteric bacilli. These infections often have a complex epidemiology including both exogenous factors (e.g. the hands of hospital personnel) and endogenous factors (e.g. normal and abnormal endogenous flora). Streptococcal wound infections are infrequent, but when they do occur they are capable of high morbidity and occasional mortality. They usually arise from a human source and have short incubation periods. Streptococci may gain access to a wound directly (via hands) or indirectly (via aerosols).

The risk of a surgical wound infection is directly related to the type of surgery and indirectly related to the skill of the surgeon. For instance, class I (clean) surgical procedures have a surgical wound infection rate of approximately 1% whereas class IV (dirty) surgical procedures have postoperative wound infection rates of 25–40%. Prevention of surgical wound infections is primarily based upon good surgical technique including the proper use of prophylactic antibiotics [12]. Standard isolation procedures including strict hand washing is the cornerstone of prevention of cross-infection from infected surgical wounds in the intensive care unit.

Lower Respiratory Tract Infection

Patients in intensive care units are almost 5 times as likely to acquire nosocomial pneumonia than patients admitted to other hospital wards [1]. Recognition of a nosocomial pneumonia may be difficult. The appearance of a new pulmonary infiltrate, fever and purulent sputum is sufficient to classify a patient as having nosocomial pneumonia. However, drug- or immune-induced pulmonary disease, pulmonary emboli or heart failure frequently lead to diagnostic confusion.

Nosocomial pneumonias are usually due to gram-negative bacilli and often are fatal. Pneumonia is the most lethal nosocomial infection [13]. Between 40 and 60% of patients with hospital-acquired lower respiratory tract infections die. This high fatality rate undoubtedly is in part due to the severity of their underlying diseases [14, 15].

Up to three-fourths of nosocomial pneumonias occur in postoperative patients, particularly in patients undergoing thoracic or abdominal surgery. The risk of pneumonia is increased up to 14-fold in patients undergoing thoracic surgery, 3-fold in patients undergoing abdominal surgery and 38-fold in those with combined thoracicoabdominal procedures [12]. Pathogens can reach the lower respiratory tract by aspiration, via contaminated aerosols or hematogenously. The first of these three routes is by far the most frequent. Colonization of the respiratory tract with gram-negative bacilli is common (up to 22% by the 1st intensive care unit day) and may at times be unavoidable because of such factors as intubation, leukopenia or antimicrobial therapy [15]. Colonization with gram-negative bacilli predictably precedes gram-negative pneumonia.

Respiratory equipment has been implicated in numerous outbreaks of nosocomial pneumonia. However, with current disinfection procedures, respiratory equipment has become a less common reservoir of infection. Rather, patients are the principal reservoirs of infection and the hands of hospital personnel are the chief source of contamination. An endotracheal tube is a major risk factor for acquiring a nosocomial infection in a critical care unit [16].

Although it is often impossible to completely prevent oropharyngeal colonization with gram-negative bacilli, it is practical to try to prevent aspiration of these bacilli, which is the next critical step in the pathogenesis of most nosocomial pneumonias. Proper use of sedatives, the state of hydration, suctioning technique, prudent anitmicrobial use, the proper inflation of endotracheal tube cuffs and proper positioning are all important preventive measures [12]. Preoperative instruction concerning cough and incentive spirometry and evaluation of high-risk surgical patients should be done whenever possible [14].

Bacteremias

Hospital-acquired bacteremias are classified as either primary or secondary to a definable infection in a body site such as the lung, skin or urinary tract. Between 40 and 50% of nosocomial bacteremias are secondary. In actual fact many 'primary bacteremias' arise from intravascular catheters and their true source is often overlooked. Many of these catheter-related bacteremias can be identified using semiquantitative catheter culture techniques [17]. The most common pathogens causing hospital-acquired bacteremia are *Escherichia coli, Staphylococcus epidermidis* and *S. aureus.*

Although relatively infrequent, nosocomial bacteremias are often lethal or greatly increase hospital morbidity [18, 19]. Mortality of patients with nosocomial bacteremia is over 10 times greater than that of matched controls with the same primary diagnosis. Patients surviving an episode of nosocomial bacteremia stay in the hospital an average of 1 month longer than matched controls [20]. Although many hospital-acquired bacteremias are not preventable, a substantial percentage of catheter-related bacteremias can be prevented by prompt removal of all peripheral venous catheters after 72 h and by use of proper insertion techniques and maintenance of other catheters.

Occasionally epidemics of pseudobacteremia (positive blood cultures due to reasons other than bacteremia) have occurred. 11% of 181 nosocomial epidemics investigated by the Centers for Disease Control from 1956 to 1971 were pseudoepidemics [22]. Pseudobacteremia can lead to much clinical confusion and unnecessary antibiotic use. Most instances of pseudobacteremia can be traced to errors in specimen processing or contaminated materials used to collect blood cultures. Contaminated povidone-iodine used in collecting blood culture specimens has led to the misdiagnosis of *Pseudomonas cepacia* bacteremia [23].

Device- or Procedure-Related Infection

Medical devices such as pressure transducers and monitors are commonplace in all modern critical care units. Many of these diagnostic or therapeutic devices act as foreign bodies placed temporarily or semipermanently into a patient's tissues. These devices are capable of causing both endemic and epidemic nosocomial infections. Many of the estimated 850,000 device-related nosocomial infections that occur annually in the United States are preventable. Patients in intensive care units usually have at least one invasive device and many have two, three, or more [2]. The risk of nosocomial infection is directly related to the type and number of devices or invasive procedures a patient encounters [16]. Of all outbreaks of nosocomial device-related infections investigated by the Centers for Disease Control from 1970 to 1975, 83% were linked to in-hospital contamination rather than manufacturer-related contamination. The hands of hospital personnel were the most common source from which devices became contaminated [4].

Intravascular Infections

A vascular catheter is a hollow tube directly linking a patient's blood stream with the outside world's abundant bacterial and fungal flora. Infections related to intravenous therapy may arise from either the administered fluid or an intravascular catheter and its tubing. Infusate-related infections are uncommon, tend to cause epidemics and are usually due to a member of the tribe *Klebsiella (Enterobacter, Klebsiella* or *Serratia), P. cepacia,* or *Citrobacter freundii.* In contrast, intravascular catheter-related infections are common endemic problems and are most frequently due to *S. aureus* or *S. epidermidis.* Intravascular catheter-related infections are in a large part preventable by careful and proper insertion technique, proper catheter care, and most importantly, by prompt removal. If all peripheral venous cannulae were routinely removed after 72 h of use (even if they are functioning perfectly), a large number of bacteremias and catheter-related local infections could be prevented [20]. Using the semiquantitative catheter-culture technique, it has been repeatedly shown that the risk of local infection and bacteremia rises rapidly after a peripheral venous catheter has been in place for more than 72 h [17]. Although the presence of phlebitis indicates an 18-fold increased risk of related sepsis, approximately one-half of all patients with intravascular catheter-related bacteremia have no visible signs of phlebitis [21]. This fact underscores the need to remove peripheral catheters after 72 h of use. Intravascular catheters placed under emergency conditions should be changed within 24 h.

Arterial catheters, pulmonary artery catheters, and central venous catheters all increase the risk of nosocomial bacteremia. Arterial catheters and arterial pressure monitoring devices have been associated with numerous nosocomial epidemics as well as chronic endemic problems with bacteremia. Intra-arterial catheters should be placed percutaneously using strict aseptic technique and removed or rotated within 4 days. Pressure monitoring devices should be gas-sterilized or chemically disinfected between use [20]. If disposable domes are used in pressure monitoring transducers, it is important to realize that they do not prevent reflux of bacteria from the transducer head or its connections directly into the patient [24]. Improper sterilization or disinfection procedures of reusable pressure transducers has caused numerous epidemics of nosocomial sepsis in critical care units [20].

Parenteral Hyperalimentation

Because of improved intravascular catheters and the technique of their insertion and maintenance, the rate of infection due to hyperalimentation has decreased over the past decade [25]. However, parenteral hyperalimentation is still a substantial risk factor for acquiring a nosocomial infection. Patients receiving parenteral hyperalimentation face all the risks of routine intravenous therapy and have three additional special problems. Unlike most other intravenous fluids, hyperalimentation fluid is an excellent medium for bacterial and fungal growth. Hyperalimentation catheters are usually left in place for long periods of time. Finally, patients receiving parenteral hyperalimentation are usually immunocompromised. Rates of sepsis due to parenteral hyperalimentation are inversely related to the degree of meticulous adherence to standard protocols or guidelines [20].

Special Problems

Outbreaks of nosocomial infection have been traced to contaminated inanimate objects and substances including tube feedings, antiseptic solutions, antibiotic ointments and hand lotions. Most outbreaks due to contaminated articles are due to cross-contamination from the hands of hospital personnel rather than contamination at the time of manufacture or commercial packaging.

Room air 'humidifiers' which use a spinning disk to nebulize water frequently become contaminated with gram-negative bacteria, especially *Pseudomonas* species. These appliances cannot be reliably disinfected and should not be used in hospitals. If moist air is needed it is better supplied with a face mask [12].

Nosocomial sinusitis is an occasional, newly appreciated and sometimes obscure cause of prolonged fever in the intensive care patient [26]. The presence of nasogastric and nasotracheal tubes in the nasal airway may lead to obstruction of sinus ostia and secondary infection, usually with gram-negative aerobic bacilli. Infections are frequently polymicrobic.

Outbreaks of hospital-acquired infections caused by methicillin-resistant *S. aureus* have become an important problem in the United States. Two-thirds of outbreaks have originated or centered in intensive care units [27]. Both infected and colonized patients become the institutional reservoir, and transient carriage on the hands of hospital personnel is the most important mechanism of serial patient-to-patient transmission. Hospital-wide outbreaks of methicillin-resistant *S. aureus* have been initiated by spread from a single case in an intensive care unit [28]. In over 85% of hospitals into which they have been introduced, these staphylococci have become established as endemic nosocomial pathogens [27]. The most important control measure in outbreaks of methicillin-resistant staphylococci is the isolation of patients who are either colonized or infected with resistant staphylococci.

Principles of Infection Prevention in the Intensive Care Unit

An estimated one-half of all nosocomial infections are preventable with currently available methods and techniques. However, these preventive methods are often overlooked, forgotten or discounted as impractical or inconvenient. Just as there is a metaphorical chain of infection in hospitals, programs to prevent the infection can also be thought of as a chain with three links [5]. The first link is the epidemiological characterization of a disease problem. The second is a strategy to control or prevent disease. The third link (often the hardest) is the actual implementation of a prevention or control program. Each link is crucial. Understanding nosocomial infections (link one) and knowing how to prevent them (link two) are of little benefit unless the knowledge and understanding are translated into practice (the third link).

Because rates of nosocomial infection are highest in critical care units and because many patients are transferred from a critical care unit at the time they are incubating a nosocomial infection, special efforts to identify and prevent infections should logically focus in this section of the hospital. Surveillance is necessary to identify *where* and *when* infections occur so that it can be deduced *why* they occurred and *how* they can be prevented. Regular surveillance is the best way to determine a reliable baseline or 'normal' rate of infection in a particular unit or area of the hospital. This baseline provides an invaluable clue to the presence of an outbreak or insidious increase in the occurrence of a particular infection or pathogen. Regular surveillance activities also provide an important opportunity for the infection control practitioner to identify potential nosocomial problems and educate medical and paramedical personnel about sound infection control practices and policies.

The single most important method to prevent cross-infection in intensive care units is hand washing. This fact has been known for over a century, yet it is common knowledge that hand washing before and after patient contact is widely ignored or forgotten by medical and paramedical personnel [29]. Strict adherence to hand washing should be enforced in all critical care units. Even trivial patient contact such as positioning a patient in bed, taking vital signs and shaking hands can result in transfer of nosocomial pathogens between patient and staff [30]. Proper design of critical care units should include adequate numbers and easy availability of wash sinks and physical barriers to avoid cross-contamination between patients. Ideally, sinks should be placed at the entrances (not in corners) of intensive care unit rooms [2]. Sufficient space should be provided around each patient for equipment and personnel. Proper guidelines for aseptic technique should be developed and followed for all invasive procedures. Recognition and prevention of device-related infections may be facilitated by the use of individual 'flow sheets' indicating all devices used, their dates of insertion and the need for continuation [2]. Rigid cleaning policies should be formulated and followed by the housekeeping department [31]. Visitor restrictions should be enforced.

Low nurse-to-patient ratios may reduce the risk of cross-contamination. Nursing procedures should include standard isolation precautions and policies that are enforced. Patients colonized or infected with multiple-resistant bacteria sometimes need to be physically separated from noninfected patients or isolated with barrier precautions including gowns and gloves. Strategies for prevention and control of multiple drug-resistant nosocomial infections are not completely effective and remain controversial [32]. Microbiological monitoring of intensive care unit environments is generally futile and a waste of money unless epidemiologic data point to a suspected source or reservoir as a cause of the nosocomial infection.

Even though the hospital environment may be heavily contaminated with potentially pathogenic organisms, contaminated objects usually do not cause disease unless they are touched or placed into the body or unless body fluids flow through them. Thus, cleaning, disinfection and sterilization policies should focus on patient care supplies and adhere strictly to published guidelines [33].

Conclusions

The control of hospital-acquired infection is a process still very much in evolution. The introduction of antiseptics and aseptic techniques by *Lister* and *Semmelweis* had an immense effect on public health. The widespread use of sterilization further lowered rates of hospital-acquired infection. The introduction of antibiotics greatly lowered mortality but caused a new set of problems, in particular, microbial resistance. National accreditation regulations led to a new standard of care, including regular surveillance activities and the recognition of new problems related to new technologies. Major challenges remain to determine what is and what is not medically and cost effective in infection control activities. As the standards and techniques of medical care for critical care patients become more complicated and sophisticated, basic aseptic techniques become more and more important. It does no good to save a patient using complicated technology if he ultimately succumbs to a preventable nosocomial infection secondary to that technology.

References

1 Donowitz, L.G.; Wenzel, R.P.; Hoyt, J.W.: High risk of hospital-acquired infection in the ICU patient. Crit. Care Med. *10:* 355–357 (1982).

2 Wenzel, R.P.; Osterman, C.A.; Donowitz, L.G.; Hoyt, J.W.; Sande, M.A.; Martone, W.J.; Peacock, J.E.; Levine, J.I.; Miller, G.B.: Identification of procedure-related nosocomial infections in high risk patients. Rev. infect. Dis. *3:* 701–707 (1981).

3 Dixon, R.E.: Effect of infections on hospital care. Ann. intern. Med. *89:* 749–753 (1978).

4 Stamm, W.E.: Nosocomial infections: etiologic changes, therapeutic challenges. Hosp. Pract. *16(8):* 75–88 (1981).

5 Dixon, R.E.: Forging the missing link in infection control. Am. J. Med. *70:* 976–978 (1981).

6 Hartstein, A.I.; Garber, S.B.; Ward, T.T.; Jones, S.R.; Morthland, V.H.: Nosocomial urinary tract infection: a prospective evaluation of 108 catheterized patients. Infection Control *2:* 380–386 (1981).

7 Stamm, W.E.: Infections related to medical devices. Ann. intern. Med. *89:* 764–769 (1978).

8 Haley, R.W.; Schaberg, D.R.; Crossley, K.B.; Von Allmen, S.D.; McGowan, J.E.: Extra charges and prolongation of stay attributable to nosocomial infections: a prospective interhospital comparison. Am. J. Med. *70:* 51–58 (1981).

9 Givens, C.P.; Wenzel, R.P.: Catheter-associated urinary tract infections in surgical patients: a controlled study on the excess morbidity and costs. J. Urol. *124:* 646–648 (1980).

10 Burke, J.P.; Garibaldi, R.A.; Britt, M.R.; Jacobson, J.A.; Conti, M.; Alling, D.W.: Prevention of catheter-associated urinary tract infections. Efficacy of daily care regimens. Am. J. Med. *70:* 155–658 (1981).

11 Warren, J.W.; Platt, R.; Thomas, R.J.; Rosner, B.; Kass, E.H.: Antibiotic irrigation and catheter-associated urinary tract infections. New Engl. J. Med. *299:* 570–573 (1978).

12 Simmons, B.P.; Wong, E.S.: Guidelines for prevention of surgical wound infections. Infection Control *3:* 327–333 (1982).

13 Gross, P.A.; Neu, H.G.; Aswapokee, P.; Antwerperpen, C.A.; Aswapokee, N.: Deaths from nosocomial infections: experience in a university hospital and a community hospital. Am. J. Med. *18:* 219–223 (1980).

14 Britt, M.R.; Schleupher, C.J.; Matsumiya, S.: Severity of underlying disease as a predictor of nosocomial infection. Utility in the control of nosocomial infection. J. Am. med. Ass. *239:* 1047–1051 (1978).

15 Johanson, W.G.; Pierce, A.K.; Sanford, J.P.; Thomas, G.D.: Nosocomial respiratory infections with gram-negative bacilli. The significance of colonization of respiratory tract. Ann. intern. Med. *77:* 701–706 (1972).

16 Freeman, J.; McGowan, J.E.: Risk factors for nosocomial infection. J. infect. Dis. *138:* 811–819 (1978).

17 Maki, D.G.; Weise, C.E.; Sarafin, H.W.: A semiquantitative culture method for identifying intravenous-catheter-related infection. New Engl. J. Med. *296:* 1305–1309 (1977).

18 Rose, R.; Hunting, K.J.; Townsend, T.R.; Wenzel, R.P.: Morbidity/mortality and economics of hospital-acquired blood stream infections: a controlled study. Sth med. J. *70:* 1267–1269 (1977).
19 Spengler, R.F.; Greenough, W.B.: Hospital costs and mortality attributed to nosocomial bacteremias. J. Am. med. Ass. *240:* 2455–2458 (1978).
20 Simmons, B.P.; Hooton, T.M.; Wong, E.S.; Allen, J.R.: Guidelines for prevention of intravascular infections. Infection Control *2:* 61–72 (1981).
21 Maki, D.G.: Preventing infection in intravenous therapy. Hosp. Pract. *11:* 95–104 (1976).
22 Weinstein, R.A.; Stamm, W.E.: Pseudoepidemics in hospital. Lancet *ii:* 862–864 (1977).
23 Berkelman, R.L.; Lewin, S.; Allen, J.R.; Anderson, R.L.; Budnick, L.O.; Shapiro, S.; Friedman, S.M.; Nicholas, P.; Holzman, R.S.; Haley, R.W.: Pseudobacteremia attributed to contamination of povidone-iodine with *Pseudomonas cepacia.* Ann. intern. Med. *95:* 32–36 (1981).
24 Buxton, A.E.; Anderson, R.L.; Klimek, J.; Quintiliani, R.: Failure of disposable domes to prevent septicemia acquired from contaminated pressure transducers. Chest *74:* 508–513 (1978).
25 Schwartz-Fulton, J.; Valanis, B.: Sepsis related to intravenous and hyperalimentation catheters. A summary of recent research findings. Natn. intravenous Ther. Ass. *4:* 248–255 (1981).
26 Caplan, E.S.; Hoyt, N.J.: Nosocomial sinusitis. J. Am. med. Ass. *247:* 639–641 (1982).
27 Thompson, R.L.; Cabezudo, I.; Wenzel, R.P.: Epidemiology of nosocomial infections caused by methicillin-resistant *Staphylococcus aureus.* Ann. intern. Med. *97:* 309–317 (1982).
28 Peacock, J.E., Jr.; Marsik, F.J.; Wenzel, R.P.: Methicillin-resistant *Staphylococcus aureus:* introduction and spread within a hospital. Ann. intern. Med. *93:* 526–532 (1980).
29 Albert, R.K.; Condie, F.: Hand washing patterns in medical intensive care units. New Engl. J. Med. *304:* 1465–1466 (1981).
30 Casewell, M.; Phillips, I.: Hands as route of transmission for Klebsiella species. Br. med. J. *ii:* 1315–1317 (1977).
31 Simmons, B.P.; Hooton, T.M.; Mallison, G.F.: Guidelines for hospital environmental control. Infection control *3:* 53–60 (1982).
32 Weinstein, R.A.; Kabins, S.A.: Stretegies for prevention and control of multiple drug-resistant nosocomial infections. Am. J. Med. *70:* 449–454 (1981).
33 Simmons, B.P.; Hooton, T.M.; Mallison, G.F.: Guidelines for hospital environmental control. Infection Control *2:* 131–146 (1981).

Daniel Sexton, MD, Clinical Assistant Professor of Medicine,
University of Oklahoma Health Sciences Center and Oklahoma City Clinic,
Oklahoma City, OK 73106 (USA)

Pharmacology and Poisoning

Prog. crit. Care Med., vol. 2, pp. 304–315 (Karger, Basel 1985)

Determination of Drug Dose in the Critically Ill Patient

Thomas L. Whitsett, Agatha Gibney

Clinical Pharmacology Program, Veterans Administration Hospital, Oklahoma City, Okla., USA; Critical Care Satellite Pharmacy, Oklahoma Memorial Hospital, Oklahoma City, Okla., USA

Achievement of an optimal therapeutic response without undue toxicity is a special challenge in the critically ill patient. Serious problems afford little time between admission and therapeutic intervention, thus the appropriate drug and adequate dose is important at the onset. Avoidance of adverse reactions is especially important, since these patients may lack the ability to compensate for overzealous drug administration. Further, compromised cardiac, hepatic, and renal function may retard drug metabolism and excretion and predispose to adverse reactions.

Critically ill patients frequently require complex therapeutic regimens; however, the effects of these drugs on each other, on laboratory results, and other treatment modalities are often unknown or unrecognized. Impaired nutrition, especially with hypoalbuminemia, can significantly alter serum levels of highly protein-bound drugs. Consequently, the free fraction (active form) may increase and enhance both the desired and undesired effects. Also, the malnourished patient may not respond as well to drugs because of impaired end organ or effector cell responsiveness.

The purpose of this article is to discuss the various pharmacokinetic principles that influence drug effect and identify selected drugs used in the critical care setting that are affected by these phenomena.

Pharmacokinetics

Pharmacokinetics deal with rate processes of drug absorption, distribution, metabolism, and excretion. There are numerous factors that may influence these processes and in turn alter a drug's clinical effectiveness or toxicity (table I).

Table I. Factors that influence pharmacokinetics

Dosage form	Congestive heart failure
Route of administration	Protein binding
Compliance	Hypoalbuminemia
Duration of therapy	Accuracy of drug assay
Serum level relative to dose	Concurrent drug therapy
Renal function	Systemic and urinary pH
Hepatic function	

Absorption

Drug absorption is influenced by the dosage form and route of administration. An oral or nasogastric formulation must disintegrate and solubilize prior to absorption which primarily occurs in the small bowel. Delayed gastric emptying or hypermotility may decrease the rate and extent of absorption. Many drugs are associated with incomplete absorption, e.g., digoxin tablets exhibit 50–75% gastrointestinal absorption in healthy volunteers. Further variation in absorption may occur in critically ill patients and influence the overall effect.

Orally administered drugs are often subjected to first-pass metabolism by the liver. Because this is so pronounced in certain drugs, e.g., lidocaine, parenteral administration is required.

Interestingly, patients with portal hypertension and extensive collateral circulation may bypass the liver, thus increasing the amount of drug absorbed. Also in these patients, drugs that decrease hepatic blood flow (beta-adrenergic and H_2 receptor blockers) may facilitate ammonia absorption by flow through the collateral circuit.

In general, the intravenous route of administration is preferred for the critically ill patient, since the absorptive phase is eliminated. The faster onset of action allows the clinician to expeditiously judge the adequacy of therapy and make any necessary adjustments. In patients with vasoconstriction (secondary to hypovolemia, etc.), the onset of action and peak drug effect for subcutaneous and intramuscular administration is delayed.

Distribution

Protein binding, lipid solubility, and molecular size affect a drug's distribution phase. The unbound (active) drug is in equilibrium with that bound to serum proteins (inactive). If binding is greater than 80%, factors that reduce this can substantially increase the unbound fraction. Table II lists several commonly used drugs that are highly bound. In patients with decreased plasma proteins, higher levels of unbound drug may occur and can exert an exaggerated effect. Also, uremia may increase the unbound fraction of certain drugs and enhance their action, e.g., warfarin, phenytoin, phenylbutazone, salicylate, and diazepam.

Drug distribution is kinetically described by compartment models. If the drug is confined to the intravascular (central) space or is instantaneously distributed, it is described as a 'one-compartment model'. However, most drugs distribute to one or more peripheral compartments. When all compartments equilibrate, a steady-state drug level is reached, and the volume represented by this is termed the apparent volume of distribution. The mathematical representation of this is shown as:

$$V_d = \frac{fD}{C_p0}$$

where V_d = volume of distribution (l/kg); f = fraction of dose absorbed (intravenous administration = 1); D = dose administered (mg), and C_p0 = plasma concentration at zero time (mg/ml). The volume of distribution varies among healthy individuals and particularly among critically ill patients. Thus, a larger volume of distribution requires a larger dose to produce a comparable blood level.

Metabolism

The liver is the major organ of drug biotransformation, and most metabolites (active or inactive) are water soluble with a shorter half-life than the parent compound. Hepatic enzymes are primarily responsible for metabolism, and patients with impaired hepatic enzyme systems may exhibit a slower rate of metabolism. Certain drugs, such as cimetidine, may impair hepatic enzymes resulting in elevated serum drug levels. Conversely, some drugs and environmental factors induce hepatic enzymes (e.g., phenobarbital and cigarette smoking) and accelerate the rate of metabolism. Selected drugs affecting metabolic enzyme systems are listed in table III.

Excretion

Most drugs and/or their metabolites are eliminated from the body by glomerular filtration (unbound fraction) and tubular secretion (bound and unbound). If renal function is impaired, the elimination phase may be prolonged.

Table II. Selected drugs that are highly bound to plasma proteins

Drug	%	Drug	%
Warfarin	99	Diazepam	95
Thyroxine	99	Furosemide	91–98
Miconazole	98	Nifedipine	>90
Diphenhydramine	98	Amphotericin B	>90
Chlorpromazine	98	Verapamil	90
Spironolactone	98	Phenytoin	90
Digitoxin	90–97	Hydralazine	90
Prazosin	97	Quinidine	80–90
Tolbutamide	95–97	Valproate sodium	80–90
Chlordiazepoxide	95		

Table III. Selected drugs that affect metabolic enzyme systems

Inducers		Inhibitors
Alcohol	Griseofulvin	allopurinol
Antipyrine	Phenylbutazone	chloramphenicol
Barbiturates	Phenytoin	cimetidine
Carbamazepine	Rifampin	disulfiram
Diphenhydramine	Spironolactone	

Most drugs exhibit first-order kinetics, i.e., a constant *percentage* of drug is eliminated over time, irrespective of dose. A few drugs exhibit zero-order kinetics, i.e., a constant *amount* of drug is eliminated over time; thus the higher the dose, the longer the half-life. Doubling the dose of a first-order drug will approximately double the plasma level, while with a zero-order drug small changes in dose result in disproportionate changes in plasma levels. Drugs with first-order kinetics may become zero-order in overdose situations. Selected drugs with zero-order kinetics include salicylic acid, phenytoin, dicoumarol, heparin, and ethanol.

Urine pH also influences elimination for weak bases and weak acids. Amphetamine, a weak organic base, is more ionized (more water soluble) in an acid urine which facilitates elimination. Table IV lists selected drugs

Table IV. Selected drugs that are likely to be affected by changes in urinary and systemic pH

Weak acids	Weak bases
Aspirin	amphetamine
Phenobarbital	diazepam
Phenytoin	procainamide
Warfarin	quinidine

affected by changes in urinary and systemic pH. Total body clearance of a drug may be expressed as:

$$\text{total body clearance} = \frac{(0.693)\,(V_d)}{t_{1/2}},$$

where V_d = volume of distribution (l/kg); $t_{1/2}$ = half-life (min).

The fate of a drug in the body is complicated, and factors that distort normal kinetics are more likely to occur in critically ill patients. Changes in metabolic or urine pH, decreased plasma proteins, metabolic dysfunction, excretory dysfunction, and polypharmacy are all more prevalent. Thus, it is imperative to individualize drug dosage according to the desired response and the undesired effects.

Choosing an Appropriate Drug

Frequently it is necessary to initiate drug therapy while the disease etiology is still unknown. When a definitive diagnosis was made and the indicated drug is a unique pharmacologic entity, it is only necessary to tailor that therapy using sound pharmacokinetic principles. Adverse reactions, most of which are an extension of a known pharmacologic effect, can be anticipated and therapy adjusted.

When multiple drugs exist to treat a disease, there are certain questions that may aid in the decision-making process: (1) In renal dysfunction, which drug is least nephrotoxic? (2) Is the patient on a hepatic enzyme inducer or inhibitor? (3) In hypoalbuminemia, which drug is least protein bound? (4) Does congestive heart failure or liver dysfunction exist? A metabolized drug may need a decrease in dosage. (5) Are any of the drugs weak acids or bases and, therefore, more likely to be affected by shifts in metabolic and urinary pH? (6) If chronic therapy is anticipated, are any of the drug choices available in both parenteral and oral forms? (7) Do any of the drug choices have a lower therapeutic/toxic ratio? (8) Is one drug easier or more convenient for the nursing staff to administer?

When all these points are considered and the most optimal drug has been chosen, it is necessary to arrive at an appropriate dosage regimen.

Devising an Appropriate Dosage Regimen

After a drug is chosen, knowledge of its pertinent pharmacokinetic variables and the patient's condition will determine the proper dosing intervals.

Renal Failure

Patients with impaired renal function may require a dosage adjustment or a change in the dosing interval, and literature sources and nomograms are available for this purpose [5]. In general, the loading dose (if necessary) remains the same, and the maintenance dose is administered at longer intervals or reduced and administered at the usual intervals. When it is necessary to administer a nephrotoxic agent to a patient with compromised renal function, careful monitoring of renal function and possible reevaluation of existing treatment is self-evident.

Liver Failure

Impairment of the hepatic enzyme system's ability to metabolize drugs is unfortunately less quantifiable than is renal failure. Cimetidine-induced theophylline toxicity is well documented. However, no consistent changes in theophylline serum levels can be predicted. Therefore, clinical observations and laboratory monitoring for efficacy and toxicity in patients with impaired liver function are necessary in lieu of quantifiable pharmacokinetic changes.

Congestive Heart Failure

The patient with congestive heart failure has diminished hepatic blood flow and may metabolize drugs slower and require smaller doses to achieve therapeutic blood levels.

Hemodialysis

Characteristics that affect a drug's dialyzability are molecular weight, water solubility, and protein binding. The latter is most important, since it is inversely related to clearance. Therefore, drugs which are highly protein bound are nondialyzable. Drugs that are cleared by dialysis require dosage supplementation. Literature exists outlining drugs that are dialyzable.

Loading Dose

Without a loading dose, approximately five half-lives are required to achieve a steady-state plasma level. In the critical care setting, this is often unacceptable. The loading dose can be approximated by giving twice the amount you expect to administer during each half-life or may be calculated as follows:

$$LD = C_p0\ V_d,$$

where LD = loading dose (mg); C_p0 = desired plasma concentration (μg/ml); V_d = volume of distribution (liter/kg). An alternative method is to administer repetitive doses at peak effect intervals, until the desired response is achieved. For example, in severe hypertension, one may administer 0.2 mg of clonidine with repetitive doses of 0.1 mg every 1–2 h, until the desired or unacceptable undesired effects occur.

Dosing Regimen

An ideal dosing regimen provides satisfactory plasma levels and monitoring convenience. An antibiotic administered every 40 h may have sound pharmacokinetic basis, but is easily overlooked by the nursing staff. When precision dosing is mandatory, daily orders should be written rather than interval doses. Also, once-a-day drugs such as digoxin and warfarin should be administered in the afternoon to allow for the necessary laboratory work to be processed and appropriate dosage adjustment made. Regular dosing intervals are desirable to maintain constant serum levels. Three times a day and every 8th hour orders are, in most hospitals, quite different.

Intravenous Administration

Intravenous access is often most desirable because it provides complete bioavailability and a rapid onset of action. Also, discontinuing of therapy results in more rapid decline in serum levels. Intravenous administration may increase the number of complications, e.g., extravasation, excessive rate of administration, and unintended or unrecognized variation of the infusion rate. When a drug needs 'push' or 'bolus' administration, 3–5 min is recommended.

Intramuscular Administration

Absorption from this route may be erratic and incomplete. Any factor causing vasoconstriction will decrease muscle blood flow and retard the onset and peak of drug effect. Restoration of normal muscle perfusion may cause a surge in absorption with a pronounced effect. Chloramphenicol and chlordiazepoxide are ineffective when given by the intramuscular route. Also, some drugs are irritants and cause pain.

Nasogastric Administration

When available, elixirs and suspensions are ideal for administration through a nasogastric tube. However, when not available, other forms may be manipulated:

(1) Parenteral Administration. Most injectable products can be administered through a nasogastric tube, although acid-labile drugs may be degraded. Also, drugs subject to first-pass metabolism require dosage adjustments.

(2) Oral Capsules. Capsules may be emptied and mixed with a small amount of room temperature water. While solubilization is faster in hot water, heat-labile drugs will degrade prior to administration. Also, drug and water solutions should not be 'microwaved'.

(3) Oral Tablets. Tablets may be crushed to ease administration. Sustained release preparations should not be crushed because patients may receive a bolus of drug, far in excess of recommended, without the same duration of action. Sugar-coated tablets may be difficult to crush, but may dissolve if allowed to sit in water for a few minutes, and then the tablet formulation may be crushed and placed in water. Avoid mixing several drugs together in one solution. When all elixirs, crushed tablets, capsule contents, and parenteral products are combined, it is impossible to predict the net result of drug-drug incompatibilities and changes in pH and solubilities.

Monitoring Drug Therapy

To insure that therapy is adequate and to avoid toxicity, close monitoring is required. While the upper limit of a therapeutic level implies toxicity, it may not represent toxicity in an individual patient, and the urgency of the situation may require further increases in the dose, e.g., in severe arrhythmias.

Monitoring is done either through setting limits of clinical response or by direct laboratory measurement. For example, a dosage of propranolol may be titrated to heart rate, irrespective of serum levels. In the same way,

Table V. Selected drugs: pharmacokinetic data

Drug	Volume of distribution, l/kg	Half-life	Time to reach steady state[1]	Therapeutic plasma levels
Digoxin	5.1–7.4	36 h	7.5 days	0.9–2.0 μg/ml
Digitoxin	41	6 days	30 days	14–30 ng/ml
Quinidine	2.1–2.6	6–7 h	30–35 h	2–5 μg/ml
Procainamide	2	2.5–4.7 h	12–24 h	4–8 μg/ml
Propranolol	3–4.3	3.5–6 h	18–30 h	20–50 ng/ml
Disopyramide	0.6–1.3	4.4–8.2 h	22–41 h	3–6 μg/ml
Clonidine	not available	6–23 h	30–115 h	not available
Lidocaine	1.7	1.2–2.2 h	6–11 h	2–5 μg/ml
Phenytoin	0.5–0.8	dose dependent	5–15 days	10–20 μg/ml
Verapamil	6.5	3.7 h	18 h	not available
Nifedipine	not available	4–5 h	20–25 h	not available
Theophylline	0.3–0.7	3–10 h	15–48 h	10–20 μg/ml
Heparin	0.05–0.2	dose dependent	dose dependent	not available
Phenobarbital	0.5–0.6	2–5 days	10–25 days	15–45 μg/ml
Diazepam	0.7–2.6	20–50 h	100–250 h	100–200 μg/ml
Gentamicin	0.28	1.5–4 h	7.5–20 h	4–8 μg/ml
Tobramycin	0.28	1.5–4 h	7.5–20 h	4–8 μg/ml
Amikacin	0.19	1.5–3.2 h	7.5–16 h	< 30 μg/ml

[1] Without a loading dose (approximately five half-lives).

toxicity may be titrated to a target heart rate. Depending upon the availability and response of laboratory facilities, clinical end points may be the only available option.

Many drugs do not produce efficacy or toxicity early in the course of therapy, and serum levels compared to a desired therapeutic range may be helpful. Aminoglycoside antibiotics are an example where serum levels are invaluable in proper dosage calculations. Selected drugs and their pharmacokinetic data are presented in table V.

The question arises, if it is necessary to achieve therapeutic serum levels when a clinical response is seen. In most acute situations, such as infection, therapeutic serum levels are needed for quick and complete resolution of the disease. However, in chronic situations such as arrhythmia management, the lowest dosage necessary to clinically manage the disease state is the most desirable. This provides a wider range between therapeutic and toxic levels.

For example, a known interaction between aminoglycoside antibiotics and ticarcillin or carbenicillin occurs. When serum samples with both antibiotics are allowed to stand at room temperature, tobramycin is degraded and consequently results in lower serum levels than were actually present at the time the serum sample was drawn. This problem can be avoided by assaying the sample within the hour from the time it is drawn before this interaction can occur.

Some drugs are metabolized to potent compounds, and attention should be paid to active metabolites and their serum levels. One example is n-acetylprocainamide, an active metabolite of procainamide.

During the first couple of years after an acute myocardial infarction, patients are at high risk for sudden death or a subsequent fatal or nonfatal myocardial infarction. Besides risk factor modification, pharmacologic intervention may reduce the likelihood of a serious cardiac event.

The timing of serum levels and dosing intervals is essential for proper interpretation of drug levels. A random determination without regards to past doses is of little value and will probably be misleading.

Some drugs have a slow tissue distribution phase, e.g., digoxin, and blood levels should not be drawn until at least 6 h after the previous dose.

Drug level results often require a dosage adjustment. A thorough knowledge of the drug's pharmacokinetic properties is helpful to optimally increase or decrease a dosage regimen. If a dosage increase is needed, it may be advisable to administer a minimum loading dose to rapidly attain the desired steady state level. Without this additional dose, five half-lives are required to attain a new steady state.

Continuous observation of the drug effect is usually necessary to insure an adequate therapeutic response without undue toxicity. Monitoring clinical effectiveness and toxicity by patient inspection is always necessary, and monitoring of serum levels is a useful adjunct in selected circumstances.

Drug Therapy Failures

Although careful attention is given to drug choice and regimen, therapeutic failures occur. Early recognition that a prescribed regimen is ineffective or is producing unacceptable toxicity is important. In the event that a predicted clinical response does not occur, a checklist can be examined to determine the reason:

(1) Failure Due to Drug-Laboratory Test Interaction. Drugs may interfere directly with laboratory assays rendering the results inaccurate. For example, high concentrations of cephalothin or cefoxitin have caused false

results of creatinine levels performed by the Jaffe reaction. Serum samples should not be analyzed for creatinine if withdrawn within 2 h of drug administration.

(2) Failure Due to Inappropriate Timing of Serum Level. Correct timing of serum levels is essential for proper interpretation. Allow a drug to reach a steady state level before determinations are made, as interim levels may be difficult to interpret. Without a loading dose, three to five half-lives are necessary to approximate steady state conditions.

(3) Failure Due to Compliance. Because a drug was ordered does not necessarily mean that it was administered. Procuring delays, nursing time shortage, or the infusion of blood may interfere with administration. An inadequate clinical response or low serum levels need confirmation that ordered doses were administered. Also, a delay in stopping a discontinued drug may explain continued effect.

(4) Failure Due to Incomplete Drug Absorption. Verify the appropriateness of the route of administration. Intramuscular administration of phenytoin yields lower blood levels than either intravenous or oral administration.

(5) Failure Due to Inappropriate Drug Administration. Some dosage forms should not be manipulated, e.g., sustained release formulae. Do not crush Procan-SR® tablets for nasogastric tube administration, as a large initial dose with a shorter duration of action will result.

(6) Failure Due to Drug-Drug Interaction. Serum levels of digoxin may be elevated due to other concurrent therapy, e.g., quinidine and verapamil. Awareness of clinically significant drug interactions is important.

(7) Failure Due to Drug Inactivation. Drugs may be inactivated when mixed, if there are pH or chemical incompatibilities. Strongly acidic solutions degrade aminophylline preparations and should not be administered through the same infusion line.

(8) Failure Due to Change in Disease Status. A therapeutic failure may occur if a patient's renal function improves on an aminoglycoside antibiotic resulting in inadequate serum levels.

(9) Failure Due to Inappropriate Drug. Occasionally a therapeutic failure is due to a wrong choice of drug, e.g., with antibiotic therapy.

Discontinuing Drug Therapy

There are three reasons for discontinuing drug therapy: (1) ineffectiveness, (2) unacceptable toxicity, and (3) resolution of the problem. In regard to termination of therapy, the question arises: Should a drug be tapered or stopped immediately? An examination of pharmacokinetic parameters yields some guidelines.

Drugs with a long elimination half-life will remain in the circulation well after the drug is stopped. For example, the average half-life of lidocaine is 1–2 h. Therefore, if an infusion is abruptly stopped, 50% of the drug will remain in the circulation 2 h later. Therefore, the lidocaine infusion 'tapers' automatically without the immediate danger of 'rebound' arrhythmias.

Ideally, some drugs should be gradually withdrawn. Corticosteroids are best withdrawn gradually to avoid sequelae of adrenal suppression. With agents used to treat hypoperfusion, e.g., dopamine and nitroprusside, a gradual tapering of the infusion allows compensatory mechanisms to function and provides time for intervention, if untoward reactions occur.

Drugs used to treat unstable angina (nitrates, beta-adrenergic blockers, and calcium channel antagonists) are tapered when possible to avoid 'rebound' angina. Antibiotics are stopped abruptly with completion of a therapeutic course to avoid toxicity and unnecessary cost.

Suggested Reading

1 Evans, W.E.; Schentag, J.J.; Tusko, W.J.: Applied pharmacokinetics, principles of therapeutic drug monitoring. Appl. Ther. 99210 (Spokane, Washington 1984).

2 Avery, G.S.: Drug treatment (Adis Press, New York 1980).

3 Kostrup, E.K., et al.: Facts and comparisons (supplemental loose leaf references service; Mosby, St. Louis 1984).

4 Williams, R.L.; Mamelok, R.D.: Hepatic disease and drug pharmacokinetics. Clin. Pharmacokinet. *5:* 528–547 (1980).

5 Bennett, W., et al.: Drug therapy and renal failure: dosing guidelines for adults. Ann. intern. Med. *93:* 62–85, 286–325 (1980).

Thomas L. Whitsett, MD, Professor of Medicine, Clinical Pharmacology Program, V.A. Hospital, 921 NE 13th Street, Oklahoma City, OK 73104 (USA)

Prog. crit. Care Med., vol. 2, pp. 316–340 (Karger, Basel 1985)

Poisoning

Steven M. Barrett

Oklahoma Memorial Hospital, University of Oklahoma Health Sciences Center, Oklahoma City, Okla., USA

Introduction

The great multitude of ingestible, injectable, and inhalable substances guarantees a continuing therapeutic challenge to physicians and hospitals receiving poisoned patients. Over 1 million new chemical compounds were synthesized in the last decade alone [1]. Critically ill poisoned patients may require therapy for organ or system failure and therapy directed against the specific poisoning agent. In this chapter, the initial approach to the poisoned patient is reviewed, and certain toxic substances that may induce critical illness are discussed with emphasis on recent developments.

Diagnosis of Poisoning

The diagnosis of a toxic state may be elusive during the early treatment of the critically ill patient. Certainly the presence of poisoning should be suspected in the comatose or obtunded patient. The patient with an unexplained dysrhythmia or metabolic acidosis, the victim of multiple trauma, and the patient with psychiatric symptoms may also be suffering from the effects of toxic agents. Furthermore, the initial patient history is commonly inaccurate as to the presence of poisoning, the specific agent(s) involved (the majority of intentional overdoses involve multiple drugs), the amount of drug ingested, or the time of ingestion or exposure. For the above reasons, the toxicologic laboratory is quite useful in the diagnosis and management of a number of critical poisonings.

Table I. Odors associated with toxins [7]

Odor	Toxin
Acetone	chloroform, ethanol, isopropanol, lacquer (ketoacidosis)
Ammonia	(uremia)
Bitter almonds, silver polish	cyanide
Coal gas or stove gas	carbon monoxide (odorless but associated with coal or stove gas)
Disinfectants	creosote, phenol
Eggs (rotten)	disulfuram, hydrogen sulfide, mercaptans
Fruit-like	amyl nitrite, ethanol, isopropanol
Garlic	arsenic (breath and perspiration), dimethyl sulfoxide, malathion, parathion, phosphorus, selenium, tellurium, thallium
Peanuts	rodenticide (peanut flavoring agent) [8]
Pear-like	chloral hydrate, paraldehyde
Pungent, aromatic	ethchlorvynol
Shoe polish	nitrobenzene
Violets	urinary turpentine
Wintergreen	methyl salicylate

During the initial supportive management of the critically ill poisoned patient, certain signs and symptoms may identify the specific toxic agent before laboratory testing is completed. For example, fever may accompany salicylate, anticholinergic drug [9], or cocaine [2] toxicity. Bradycardia may indicate digitalis [93] or beta-blocker overdose and may accompany clonidine [3], verapamil, cyanide [164], and cholinergic drug toxicity [9]. Severe gastrointestinal symptoms may occur in poisoning with heavy metals, lithium, colchicine, theophylline, and certain mushrooms [9]. Pressure sores and bullae have been described in barbiturate, glutethimide, methaqualone [4], and carbon monoxide toxicity [5, 9]. Retinal hemorrhages suggest the possibility of subacute carbon monoxide poisoning (exposure for more than 12 h) [6]. Odors emanating from the patient may help identify the toxin (table I) Syndromes due to anticholinergic, cholinergic and opiate poisonings are well known. The appearance of symptoms after certain poisonings can be delayed for hours (table II).

While mydriasis is often nonspecific, miosis suggests toxicity from certain agents (table III). Noncardiogenic pulmonary edema may result from

Table II. Examples of poisonings that may present with delayed symptom onset

Delay in absorption from gastrointestinal tract (in overdose)	glutethimide, opiates, salicylate, tricyclic antidepressants [128]
Delay in metabolism to toxic compounds	ethylene glycol, methanol
Delayed organ failure	*Amanita phalloides,* hydrocarbon aspiration, organophosphate [187], toxic gas inhalation

Table III. Toxic agents that may cause miosis [9]

Barbiturates [10]	Clonidine [3]
Chloral hydrate	Opiates
Cholinergic agents	Phenothiazines

Table IV. Drugs and poisons that may cause noncardiogenic pulmonary edema

Barbiturates [11]	Insulin [18]
Colchicine [12]	Nitrofurantoin [19]
Ethchlorvynol [13]	Opiates [20, 21]
Glutethimide [14]	Paraldehyde [22]
Hydrocarbons [15, 16]	Paraquat [23, 24]
Hydrochlorothiazide [17]	Propoxyphene [25, 26]
	Salicylates [27–29]

poisonings by numerous substances which damage the alveolocapillary membrane directly by toxic effects or indirectly via central neurogenic or other mechanisms (table IV). The potential for pulmonary edema caused by these agents makes it mandatory to carefully monitor fluid administration. The collection of toxins that have caused metabolic acidosis with an increased anion gap requires a periodic update (table V).

A prolonged QRS interval may accompany tricyclic antidepressant, quinidine, or procainamide toxicity. Ingestible agents that may be radiopaque on abdominal X-rays include the following: heavy metals (e.g.

Table V. Toxins that may induce metabolic acidosis with increased anion gap [30]

Toxins that increase formation of lactic acid	Toxins that increase formation of other organic acids
Carbon monoxide (hypoxia)	Ethanol (lactic acidosis, ketoacidosis)
Colchicine [31]	Ethylene glycol
Cyanide [32, 33]	Formaldehyde [34]
Iron	Methanol
Isoniazid	Nalidixic acid
	Paraldehyde
	Salicylates
	Toluene [35–37]

arsenic, iron, lead); chloral hydrate, phenothiazine, and potassium chloride tablets [38].

Blood, urine, and gastric lavage effluent (emesis material should be sent to the laboratory separately) are routinely tested for presence of toxic substances. For many toxic agents, however, serum drug levels may not correlate with the severity of the patient's symptoms. For example, patients tolerant to alcohol or barbiturates may have high serum levels of these drugs without corresponding signs of toxicity. Serum levels of tricyclic antidepressants may not correlate with seriousness of symptoms [133]. Patients with chronic salicylate toxicity may be seriously poisoned with relatively low serum levels at the time of patient presentation [119].

Acute lithium ingestion may result in few symptoms despite high serum levels, probably because lithium diffuses slowly from the extracellular to the intracellular space [40, 41]. Chronic lithium toxicity can occur at therapeutic blood lithium levels, especially if the patient takes additional medications (e.g. thiazide diuretics, tetracyclines, and indomethacin) that impair lithium excretion [42, 43]. Severity of signs and symptoms from phencyclidine toxicity may not correlate with dose or serum levels [44, 45]. Quantitative serum drug levels are indicated, however, in acute poisoning with salicylate, acetaminophen, methanol, ethylene glycol, ethanol, iron, lead, digitalis, theophylline, and are frequently helpful in lithium and barbiturate poisoning. In addition, carboxyhemoglobin and methemoglobin levels, red cell or plasma cholinesterase activity (for organophosphate toxicity), and erythrocyte protoporphyrin levels (for lead poisoning) are useful blood tests.

Initial Therapy of Poisoning

Naloxone

Comatose patients should receive naloxone, dextrose, and other initial therapy as indicated. Naloxone can be administered by the intravenous, intramuscular, subcutaneous, or intraglossal routes, or down the endotracheal tube [46, 47]. Previous dosage regimens have caused frequent underdosage. If narcotic overdose is suspected, 2 mg of naloxone should be given intravenously to an adult [48]. In fact, for certain narcotic intoxicants (e.g. propoxyphene and pentazocine [49]), 2–4 or more times the above dose of naloxone may be required to reverse coma in an adult [48] and up to 0.1 mg/kg may be necessary in a child [50]. Naloxone is a surprisingly safe drug; up to 4 mg/kg has been administered intravenously to adult volunteers without inducing serious side effects [51]. A 2½-year-old child inadvertently received 20 mg of naloxone intravenously and experienced no ill effects [52]. Several sudden deaths possibly linked to naloxone occurred after naloxone reversal of anesthetic respiratory depression in postoperative patients. Such sudden reversal of anesthetic effect may precipitate a sympathetic storm with resulting dysrhythmias and pulmonary edema [48, 53]. Of course, naloxone may precipitate a withdrawal syndrome in the narcotic addict, but this is rarely medically serious.

Naloxone may reverse coma or respiratory depression from diazepam [54, 55], ethanol [56–58, 64] or clonidine [59, 60] overdose. Such salutary effects of naloxone, however, are controversial in diazepam-induced sedation [61, 62] and in ethanol [63] toxicity. Naloxone may antagonize central nervous system and circulatory depression due to nonopioid anesthetics [65, 156, 170]. Naloxone has clearly reversed hypotension in septic and other forms of shock in humans [66–69] and in hemorrhagic shock in animals [70–73]. In patients with decompensated chronic obstructive pulmonary disease (COPD), minute ventilation and oxygen saturation may increase after naloxone administration [74, 75]. In patients with a history of angina, naloxone may decrease the appearance time for ischemic myocardial pain [76].

Naloxone enhances functional neurologic recovery in animals with traumatized spinal cords [77] and has reversed neurologic deficits in patients with cerebral ischemia [78, 79] and in animals with surgically induced ischemic neurologic lesions [80]. The potential for prevention of cerebral infarction with naloxone therapy, however, is problematic and requires much more study [81]. Intravenous naloxone temporarily improved cognition in 7 patients with Alzheimer's dementia [82]. In a report of 2 patients, intravenous and oral naloxone reversed chronic idiopathic constipation, which had previously been responsive only to daily laxatives and additional suppositories and enemas [83]. The expanding list of naloxone effects indicates the physiologic and pathologic importance of endogenous opioids in the human body. Naloxone may also interact with receptors other than opioid receptors [65].

Gastric Evacuation

Gastric lavage and induction of emesis with syrup of ipecac are the two most common means of gastric emptying. The usual recommendation that ipecac be followed by 200 cc of water is controversial. Fluid boluses may hasten passage of gastric contents into the duodenum [84, 85] and do not enhance vomiting of soluble or particulate markers in animal studies [86]. Whereas ipecac emesis is the preferred method for stomach emptying in the awake child, gastric lavage is indicated in adults with serious overdoses [9]. Newer experimental emetics may be safer and more potent than ipecac [86]. Actually, induced emesis is not well-proven to beneficially affect patient morbidity and mortality [87].

Efficacy of gastric lavage may be enhanced by using warmed lavage fluid, which delays stomach emptying time [88]. Epigastric massage during lavage may facilitate return of toxic substances [89, 90]. Salicylates, barbiturates, glutethimide, meprobamate, carbamazepine [9], and iron [91] in overdose may form concretions in the stomach that may require removal by gastroscopy or gastrotomy to prevent persistent toxicity.

Although gastric evacuation is most useful within 4 h of drug ingestion [1], there is no specific time interval that makes poison recovery unlikely after large overdoses [92]. Gastric emptying may be useful 24 h or longer after overdose with certain drugs [1]. For example, intact Lomotil® tablets have been recovered from the stomach 27 h after overdose [52] and propoxyphene-aspirin tablets were spontaneously vomited 30 h after overdose [121]. Atropine administration prior to gastric evacuation procedures may prevent asystole or advanced block in patients suffering from digitalis toxicity with heart block or sinus bradycardia [93].

Activated Charcoal

Administration of activated charcoal should follow gastric emptying. The charcoal solution should be diluted, since aspiration of large chunks has caused respiratory compromise [94]. Activated charcoal adsorbs almost all ingested substances quite well; exceptions include alkali, boric acid, cyanide, DDT, ferrous sulfate, mineral acids [95], and alcohol [99]. Use of charcoal is not recommended in acetaminophen overdose, since charcoal will adsorb and inactivate the orally administered antidote, N-acetylcysteine. Nevertheless, this current contraindication may be short-lived, since intravenous administration of N-acetylcysteine may become the future route of choice [96, 97].

Multiple-dose charcoal therapy has recently been successfully used in numerous poisonings. Enterohepatic circulation of drug has been invoked as a rationale for multiple-dose charcoal treatment of toxicity from tricyclic antidepressants [98, 139], digitalis [92, 102, 103], Dapsone® [100, 101], methotrexate [115], and other substances. Removal of drugs that are continually secreted into the acid milieu of the stomach (phencyclidine [176], tricyclic antidepressants [139, 148] and others) may be hastened by multiple-dose charcoal therapy. Since there is no significant enterohepatic circulation or gastric secretion of phenobarbital [106], recent successful use of multiple-dose charcoal therapy for phenobarbital overdose [105] was followed by speculation about the existence of a phenomenon aptly termed 'gastrointestinal dialysis' [106, 107]. Many substances (including intravenously administered phenobarbital) may be 'dialyzable' across gastrointestinal mucosa from blood along a concentration gradient into intraluminal charcoal [106, 107].

This phenomenon may explain enhanced elimination of toxic amounts of drugs such as digitalis [103], phenylbutazone, carbamazepine [104], theophylline [106, 108], thallium [109], phenobarbital [106], and others after treatment with multiple doses of charcoal (e.g. 12- to 60-g boluses 2–6 times/day or more). For example, this therapy can decrease the elimination half-life of phenobarbital in overdose from 4 days to less than 2 days and may be as efficacious as forced alkaline diuresis (but less effective than hemoperfusion or hemodialysis) in barbiturate overdose [106]. Cathartics have less value than gastric evacuation and charcoal in the limitation of absorption of poisons from the gastrointestinal tract [110].

Forced Diuresis and Dialysis

Forced alkaline diuresis increases excretion of salicylate and phenobarbital. Forced acid diuresis enhances excretion of phencyclidine, amphetamines, and quinine [111]. Hemodialysis removes numerous drugs and poisons and is most effective for water-soluble compounds with low molecular weights, low protein binding, and small volumes of distribution (e.g., lithium) [111, 113]. Charcoal or resin hemoperfusion also removes certain substances and can increase clearance of lipid-soluble drugs [111, 114]. Actually, most supportive data for hemoperfusion are derived from uncontrolled observations, and the actual influence of hemoperfusion on morbidity and mortality after poisoning remains to be determined [112]. Furthermore, conservative management will suffice as therapy for the great majority of poisoned patients. Dialysis or hemoperfusion is indicated only in a small number of seriously toxic patients [114].

Specific Antidotes

Specific antibody Fab fragments can neutralize the toxic effects of digoxin and digitoxin [116]. Such immunopharmacologic therapy awaits an expanded clinical role in the management of the poisoned patient [116]. Antidotal therapy may be indicated for certain poisonings. For example, glucagon may circumvent beta-blockade in propranolol (and possibly other beta-blocker) overdoses, activate a 'non-beta' cardiac receptor, and enhance contractility even if isoproterenol is ineffective for inotropic support [117, 118]. Other well-known antidotes not discussed elsewhere in this chapter include atropine and pralidoxime (for organophosphate toxicity), methylene blue (for methemoglobinemia), ethanol (for methanol or ethylene glycol poisoning), and various chelators, such as deferoxamine for iron toxicity.

Specific Poisons

Salicylate

Acetylsalicylic acid is contained in many different prescription and over-the-counter medications and is responsible for a significant number of critical poisonings. Even so, the use of childproof safety caps since the early 1970s has helped to dramatically reduce the incidence of accidental pediatric poisoning [119]. According to reports from the National Clearinghouse for Poison Control Centers, 3.8% of all drug deaths in 1968 in the age group 5 years or older resulted from salicylate poisoning. In 1977, that percentage decreased to 2.2. The corresponding statistics for children under 5 years of age were 40.7% (1968) and 19.3% (1977).

In acute overdose, aspirin may slow gastric emptying. Especially if aspirin is taken with sedatives or narcotics, plasma salicylate levels may increase continually for as long as 24 h, and the appearance of toxic effects may thus be delayed [120, 121]. Serum concentrations of salicylate may not peak for 12 h or more after overdose with enteric-coated aspirin tablets [122]. Nevertheless, the salicylate nomogram [123] has been a useful predictor of toxicity after most acute (not chronic) aspirin poisonings. Chronic toxicity (ingestion over 12 h or more) is actually responsible for the majority of deaths and morbidity from aspirin poisoning in adults and children [119, 124, 188]. Children may die from chronic toxicity with serum salicylate levels as low as 15 mg/dl, although the level may certainly have been higher at another time [119].

The acutely poisoned patient classically presents with sweating, tachypnea, and vomiting. Unexplained hyperventilation or fever may be signs of aspirin toxicity. Agitation, convulsions, coma, noncardiogenic pulmonary edema, high anion gap metabolic acidosis, hypoprothrombinemia, subconjunctival hemorrhages and petechiae of the head and neck may occur [125]. These patients are commonly dehydrated, and therapy would include adequate fluid replacement. However, the presence of noncardiogenic pulmonary edema would mandate careful evaluation and management of the volume status.

The use of colloid for volume expansion has been advocated to reduce the risk of pulmonary edema in the salicylate-poisoned patient [126]. Nevertheless, volume overload is not a necessary predictive factor for the occurrence of noncardiogenic pulmonary edema [29]. Older patients who have multiple medical problems, a smoking history, and who have neurologic abnormalities, proteinuria, and a serum salicylate level higher than 40 mg/dl are at higher risk for aspirin-induced pulmonary edema. The pulmonary edema resolves in these patients as serum salicylate levels decline during therapy [29].

Forced alkaline diuresis or intravenous sodium bicarbonate therapy without forced diuresis [127] shortens the plasma half-life of salicylate. Systemic alkalinemia may also retard movement of salicylate from extracellular fluid into cells (including the CNS). Alkalinization of the urine (urine pH greater than 7.5) may be difficult to accomplish in some patients, especially children [119]. Administration of excessive sodium bicarbonate must be prevented by monitoring the blood pH. Hemodialysis is generally indicated in the severely poisoned patient (serum salicylate level greater than 100 mg/dl, CNS toxicity) who does not respond to bicarbonate therapy. Hemodialysis corrects acid-base, fluid, or electrolyte imbalance more rapidly than hemoperfusion [125]. Antacids, intravenous glucose, and vitamin K are administered as indicated.

Tricyclic Antidepressants

Therapeutic use of tricyclic antidepressants (TCAs) is truly a double-edged sword; these agents may be efficacious in patients with endogenous depression, but these same patients are at risk for suicide attempts from TCA overdose. The lethal dose in adults has varied; death has allegedly occurred after 500 mg [128] and survival after 10 g [129], and the half-life of TCAs in overdose may range from 25 to 81 h [135]. The incidence of serious complications increases when the plasma level of TCA exceeds 1,000 ng/ml, and that plasma level usually correlates with a QRS duration greater than 100 ms [130, 131]. However, in an occasional patient, the ECG may be normal despite a plasma level which exceeds 1,000 ng/ml [132–134], or cardiovascular toxicity may be present at lower levels [133].

Anticholinergic effects are almost always present in acute intoxications, unless these effects are masked by the influence of sedatives, seizures, anoxia, or myocardial depression [136]. Mydriasis is evident in half or more of these patients, and pupils may be poorly reactive or even nonreactive to light [39]. Transient hypertension occurs in about 25% of patients with TCA overdose and usually does not require treatment [137]. Systolic blood pressure less than 90 mm Hg is found in about 1/3 of patients [137]. Temperature elevation or hypothermia may be present [137]. Agitation, confusion, myoclonus, hallucinations, and seizures be prominent [137, 139]. Hyperreflexia occurs in about 50% of these patients, a positive extensor plantar response in about 30%, and clonus in 3% [137]. Nystagmus and dysarthria are uncommon findings, but about 20% of patients may be ataxic and 45% will be comatose [136, 137].

Cardiovascular toxicity is evident in the majority of serious TCA overdoses, and the most frequent sign of such toxicity is sinus tachycardia [131, 136, 139]. Other cardiovascular toxic effects include supraventricular tachycardias, premature ventricular complexes, ventricular tachycardia, ventricular fibrillation, prolonged QRS complex (40%), prolonged P-R and Q-T intervals, bradycardia, right or left bundle branch block, AV blocks, idioventricular rhythm, asystole, ST elevation, T-wave changes, elevated cardiac enzymes, and congestive heart failure [131, 133, 136, 137, 140–142]. Bradycardia is an ominous sign and is more common in massive overdoses [136].

Many patients with serious TCA overdose require tracheal intubation for protection of the airway and management of respiratory depression [136]. Hypotension often responds to careful administration of intravenous fluids [128, 133, 138, 145]. Otherwise, vasopressors are indicated [133].

Supraventricular and ventricular dysrhythmias, and bradycardia can often be abolished with alkalinization of the blood to a pH of 7.5 with sodium bicarbonate [136, 143, 145] or hyperventilation in the intubated patient [136, 144]. The success of alkalinization therapy is not well understood. An increase in plasma protein binding of TCA occurs in alkalemic blood, and this increase represents a significant decline in pharmacologically active TCAs [128]. Other hypotheses about the alkalinization effect require further experimental support [136].

Ventricular dysrhythmias may also respond to lidocaine [39, 136], phenytoin [139], or physostigmine [39], although convincing clinical supporting evidence is lacking for these drugs [39, 136]. Electrical countershock has usually been only temporarily successful [39, 139]. Quinidine, procainamide and disopyramide are contraindicated for treatment of ventricular dysrhythmias [136, 139]. Pacing may be necessary for bradycardia, heart blocks, and ventricular dysrhythmias refractory to drug therapy [136, 139]. Diazepam is more consistently effective than physostigmine (and phenytoin is relatively ineffective) for treatment of seizures induced by TCAs [136, 146]. Both gastric lavage and administration of activated charcoal every 6 h until the patient is stable may enhance elimination of TCAs, since these drugs are secreted back into the stomach and undergo enterohepatic circulation [139, 148]. Delayed and recurrent complications have been reported in patients after TCA overdose [39]. Plasma levels of TCA may remain elevated in these patients for days [135]. All reported patients with late death or recurrent or delayed dysrhythmias had initial cardiotoxicity, and none of these patients had been asymptomatic longer than about 12 h [39]. Therefore, monitoring for at least 24 h after the patient becomes symptom-free appears indicated [39].

Physostigmine has a nonspecific excitatory effect on the CNS apart from its ability to reverse coma from anticholinergic or TCA toxicity. Physostigmine has awakened patients from normal sleep [155, 156] and from coma or obtundation due to barbiturates, methyprylon, ethchlorvynol [136, 147], diazepam [149–151], phenothiazines [152, 153], cimetidine [154], and droperidol anesthesia [157]. Physostigmine can cause seizures and cholinergic crises in patients with TCA overdose [136, 158]. Furthermore, there is no convincing evidence that physostigmine decreases mortality, duration of hospitalization, or overall complication rate in TCA overdose [136].

Amoxapine is a tricyclic antidepressant with weak neuroleptic effects. Amoxapine is associated with a relative lack of cardiotoxic [159, 160] or anticholinergic [159] effects and has predominant CNS toxic effects after overdose [159, 161]. Acute renal failure [160] and coma [159, 161] may occur after amoxapine poisoning. Furthermore, over one-third of these patients experience seizures [161] and the mortality rate may prove to be higher after amoxapine overdose than after other cyclic antidepressant toxicity [161]. Tetracyclic antidepressants in overdose may be less cardiotoxic but as neurotoxic as the tricyclics [162], whereas the triazolopyridine antidepressants seem to be less toxic to all systems than the tricyclics [163]. However, the toxicologic experience with these newer drugs is still preliminary, and further reports are required to clarify early impressions.

Cyanide

Cyanide is one of the most rapidly acting of all poisons and is present in many materials in our environment. Cyanide compounds are used in fumigation of ships and warehouses, extraction of gold and silver metals from ores, electroplating and polishing of metals, case hardening of steel, and production of synthetic rubber. Cyanide is present in silver polishes, some fertilizers, rodenticides, and tobacco smoke [33, 164]. Gases from burning synthetic materials (e.g. polyurethane, nitrocellulose) and natural materials (e.g. wool, silk) may contain cyanide, and gas masks provide inadequate protection since hydrogen cyanide is absorbed through the skin [33, 165].

Prolonged use or excessive amounts of nitroprusside (especially if the dose chronically exceeds 8 [169] to 10 [33] μg/kg/min) may induce cyanide toxicity [166, 169]. Cyanide poisoning may occur in burn patients infected with pigmented forms of *Pseudomonas aeruginosa* [164]. Cyanogenic glycosides such as amygdalin are found in many plants and fruit seeds, including apple, apricot, peach, plum, pear, and cherry seeds, choke-cherries, cassava beans, and bitter almonds [33, 164, 167]. Laetrile is a synthesized form of amygdalin and has recently been responsible for numerous deaths from cyanide poisoning [33, 167, 168].

Cyanide induces cellular anoxia by binding with the cytochrome $a–a_3$ complex and thus inhibiting oxidative phosphorylation. Hydrogen cyanide gas can cause death within minutes after inhalation. Patients with oral cyanide ingestions are more likely to present to the hospital before irreversible toxicity has occurred [33]. The poisoned patient will generally progress rapidly through dizziness, tachycardia, palpitations, headache, dyspnea, combativeness, an occasional gasp or scream, stupor, seizures, and coma [164]. Sinus bradycardia, atrial fibrillation, premature ventricular complexes, pulmonary edema, and high anion gap metabolic (lactic) acidosis may occur [32, 164].

The early diagnosis of cyanide poisoning may be quite difficult. An odor of bitter almonds or silver polish on the patient's breath may identify cyanide toxicity. Unfortunately, 20–40% of people are unable to detect the cyanide odor [164]. Furthermore, the early symptoms of cyanide toxicity may erroneously suggest severe anxiety [171]. Occasionally, because of reduced oxygen utilization, venous blood in retinal vessels may retain the bright red color of arterial blood [173]. However, this physical finding may be present only in massive cyanide poisoning [32].

Some patients will survive potentially lethal doses of cyanide after nonspecific supportive therapy alone [32, 33, 172]. Supplemental oxygen therapy may have a specific salutary effect on the cellular toxicity of cyanide [32, 33]. Antidotal therapy with inhaled amyl nitrite and intravenous sodium nitrite will ideally produce a methemoglobinemia of near 40%. Methemoglobin competes with the cytochrome system for binding of the cyanide ion. Intravenous sodium thiosulfate provides sulfur groups, so that the enzyme rhodanese can convert cyanide into the less toxic thiocyanate which is excreted in the urine. Since thiosulfate and rhodanese are endogenous compounds, the body can detoxify itself from cyanide eventually (the rhodanese reaction is slow).

Convincing evidence for the clinical efficacy and safety of the nitrite-thiosulfate regimen does not exist [32, 33]. However, this regimen should definitely be tried if cyanide poisoning is suspected and if the patient is deteriorating despite supportive therapy [33]. Other antidotes may become clinically available in future years. Dicobalt EDTA (available in Europe) chelates cyanide to form a stable excretable compound (probably cobalticyanide) of low toxicity. However, the cobalt salts themselves are quite toxic and may cause vomiting and diarrhea, hypotension, and respiratory failure [33]. Like the nitrites, aminophenols induce methemoglobinemia. Aminophenols may act more rapidly and may decrease blood pressure to a lesser extent than sodium nitrite [33].

Possibly the most promising antidote is hydroxocobalamin (vitamin B_{12a}), which combines with cyanide to form cyanocobalamin (vitamin B_{12}). The two vitamin forms are relatively nontoxic [32, 33]. The combination therapy of hydroxocobalamin and thiosulfate may be especially efficacious in cyanide poisoning [32]. Hydroxocobalamin may be beneficial for prophylaxis against cyanide toxicity during prolonged or excessive nitroprusside treatment [33, 166]. Well-controlled studies are necessary to determine which antidotal regimen is safest and most effective [33].

Phencyclidine

Phencyclidine (PCP) is a modern-day drug of abuse whose great popularity somewhat defies understanding. PCP was used as a general anesthetic in humans in 1957, but a significant incidence of emergent delirium and dysphoria abolished interest in the role of PCP in anesthesia by 1965. In 1967, the drug was marketed as a veterinary anesthetic. Also in 1967, PCP surfaced as a drug of abuse in San Francisco, and later, in 1968, it appeared in the East Coast drug market. However, PCP vanished quickly from both illicit markets because of the unpredictable and frequently unpleasant nature of PCP 'trips'. Although PCP reappeared as an illicit drug in the early 1970s, it was frequently misrepresented as other more acceptable and more expensive substances, such as tetrahydrocannabinol, LSD, mescalin, psilocybin, cocaine, and amphetamine. During the 1970s, the popularity of PCP grew, and misrepresentations of the drug became less common [174, 175]. All manufacture and sale of PCP was declared illegal in 1978, and the drug as a veterinary anesthetic was voluntarily withdrawn from the market.

PCP may be purchased in tablets or capsules, as powder or a 'rock' crystalline form, as amorphous clumps, and occasionally as a liquid [174, 176]. PCP is usually snorted or smoked (as powder or liquid on marijuana, tobacco, parsley, mint, oregano, and other types of leaves) and can be administered orally or intravenously. The powder can be 'dusted' onto food, and the drug has been absorbed through conjunctival, rectal and vaginal mucosal surfaces [45, 175, 177]. Onset of drug effects occurs in 2–5 min after smoking PCP and in 30–60 min after oral ingestion [175].

PCP effects include involuntary isometric muscle activity of great intensity (with or without seizures) that may induce rhabdomyolysis (in about 2% of patients [44]) and myoglobinuric renal failure [45, 175, 180, 184]. PCP may also be directly toxic to muscle [181]. Restrained PCP-toxic patients may be more at risk for rhabdomyolysis, so that restraints should be used on these patients only if necessary [175, 180]. PCP also functions as a sensory blocking agent and interferes with the ability to integrate sensory input into appropriate behavior. The analgesic and dissociative properties of the drug may cause the patient to self-mutilate [175, 181] and to display surprising strength during violent behavior [44, 175, 181]. Furthermore, injured PCP-toxic patients may not complain of pain. PCP may induce sympathomimetic effects [174] and a hypertensive response. Although this response is usually mild and self-limiting, it may be severe (in about 4% of patients) and require antihypertensive medication [181].

PCP intoxication is associated with a challenging array of signs and symptoms. The most common signs, nystagmus (horizontal, vertical, or rotatory) and hypertension, are each found in only 57% of toxic patients. Behavioral effects are frequently the most dramatic manifestations of PCP toxicity. For example, disorientation and confusion, violent or bizarre behavior, agitation, hallucinations or delusions, catatonic states, coma, lethargy, and nudism may predominate. PCP intoxication may be misdiagnosed as mania, depression, or schizophrenia [179]. Cholinergic or anticholinergic signs, hypothermia or hyperthermia, tachypnea or respiratory arrest, tachycardia or cardiac arrest, generalized rigidity, seizures, or localized dystonias represent part of the strange spectrum of PCP toxic effects [181]. It is not surprising, therefore, that PCP intoxication in emergency patients is not recognized much of the time, even when experienced observers are involved in the initial patient evaluation. PCP qualifies as the 'great imposter' of toxicology [179].

Patients with acute brain syndrome, toxic psychosis, coma, or catatonia will generally require hospitalization, since most complications of PCP toxicity occur with these syndromes. Acute brain syndrome may persist for several weeks, psychosis for 1 month or more, coma and catatonia 6 days or more [44, 174]. Lethargic patients, and patients with violent or bizarre behavior, agitation, or euphoria (and who are oriented) often do not require hospital admission and can be discharged home from the Emergency Department after symptoms and signs of toxicity (excluding nystagmus) have abated [44]. Attempts to correlate signs and symptoms with the dose taken [176] may not be clinically useful, since PCP dosage is rarely known after the fact and patients may respond differently to similar doses of PCP [44, 175]. Likewise, PCP effects do not necessarily correlate with the serum or urine PCP levels [44, 45, 174, 179].

PCP is a weak base and is secreted into the stomach, in which the drug becomes ionized and thereby trapped [176]. PCP is then reabsorbed from the small intestine, and this enterogastric circulation may account for the prolonged or vacillating course of some patients [176]. As a result, continuous gastric suction [176] and multiple-dose charcoal therapy [182] may hasten the drug's elimination from patients with severe overdoses. Urine acidification may ionize and trap large amounts of PCP, and forced diuresis may further increase clearance of the drug [176]. However, about 90% of the PCP dose is metabolized by the liver, and only 10% of the active drug is excreted by the kidneys [45]. Therefore, only 10–13% of an ingested dose of PCP may be excreted during acid diuresis [183]. In addition, acid diuresis may exacerbate myoglobinuric renal damage and is contraindicated if rhabdomyolysis has occurred [184]. As a result, the issue of acid diuresis for management of PCP toxicity is quite problematic; many authorities [174, 176, 179, 183, 185], but not all [44, 45], advocate this therapy in serious overdoses. No controlled studies have yet been published that compare treatment with and without acid diuresis [175, 179].

Conflicting recommendations also exist for the use of chlorpromazine in PCP-induced psychosis. Phenothiazines may induce hypotension, lower the seizure threshold, and potentiate the anticholinergic effects of PCP and other drugs. Therefore, some authorities proscribe phenothiazines and recommend haloperidol for use in these psychotic patients [45, 174, 175]. However, chlorpromazine can be successfully employed in many PCP-toxic patients [179], especially if the blood pressure is elevated and the patient otherwise stable [44]. Other therapy for the PCP-toxic patient depends on the specific complications that develop. Nevertheless, most PCP toxicity is not severe, and 90% or more of these patients may do well with no treatment other than a quiet, supportive environment [183]. Most deaths after PCP intoxication actually result from trauma, drowning, suicide, and homicide. Sensory disturbances, ataxia, muscle rigidity, and judgement impairment may interfere with the patient's ability to swim, drive, climb at heights, flee from a fire, or sense imminent danger [186].

Conclusion

After new drugs or chemicals are introduced, knowledge about their human toxic effects develops directly from analysis of case report data. However, conclusions from initial case reports may be incomplete and misleading. Data from animal studies are quite helpful, but most reliable recommendations about therapy of poisoning and overdose must await a cumulation of experience with human toxicities. More large-scale controlled studies are needed to address the numerous controversies in toxicology.

The therapeutic role of naloxone and naloxone congeners in human disease will expand significantly in future years. Naloxone may prove to be an important adjunct to our treatment regimens for certain nonnarcotic drug toxicities, septic and other forms of shock, and neurologic disease and injury. The phenomenon of gastrointestinal dialysis can be exploited by multiple-dose charcoal therapy, so that toxicity from a growing list of substances may be reversed more expeditiously. The simplicity of multiple-dose charcoal therapy is attractive, and the number of poisoned patients that can be treated successfully with relatively uncomplicated and minimally invasive means will be increased even more. Nevertheless, the ultimate antidote for many seriously toxic substances may prove to be an antibody fragment.

References

1 Temple, A.; Mancini, R.: Management of poisoning; in Yaffe, Pediatric pharmacology, therapeutic principles in practice, pp. 391–406 (Grune & Stratton, New York 1980).

2 Gay, G.: Clinical management of acute and chronic cocaine poisoning. Ann. Emerg. Med. *11:* 562–572 (1982).

3 Anderson, R.; Hart, G.; Crumpler, C.; Lerman, M.: Clonidine overdose: report of six cases and review of the literature. Ann. Emerg. Med. *10:* 107–112 (1981).

4 Litovitz, T.: Methaqualone; in Haddad, Winchester, Clinical management of poisoning and drug overdose, pp. 466–469 (Saunders, Philadelphia 1983).

5 Nagy, R.; Greer, K.; Harman, L.: Cutaneous manifestations of acute carbon monoxide poisoning. Cutis *24:* 381–383 (1979).

6 Kelley, J.; Sophocleus, G.: Retinal hemorrhages in subacute carbon monoxide poisoning. J. Am. med. Ass. *239:* 1515–1517 (1978).

7 Goldfrank, L.; Weisman, R.; Flomenbaum, N.: Teaching the recognition of odors. Ann. Emerg. Med. *11:* 684–686 (1982).

8 Litovitz, T.: The 'sniffing bar' (Letter). Ann. Emerg. Med. *12:* 332–333 (1983).

9 Haddad, L.: A general approach to the emergency management of poisoning; in Haddad, Winchester, Clinical management of poisoning and drug overdose, pp. 4–18 (Saunders, Philadelphia 1983).

10 Winchester, J.: Barbiturates (including primidone); in Haddad, Winchester, Clinical management of poisoning and drug overdose, pp. 413–424 (Saunders, Philadelphia 1983).

11 Goodman, J.; Bischel, M.; Wagers, P.; Barbour, B.: Barbiturate intoxication: morbidity and mortality. West. J. Med. *124:* 179–186 (1976).

12 Hill, R.; Spragg, R.; Wedel, M.; Moser, K.: Adult respiratory distress syndrome associated with colchicine intoxication (Letter). Ann. intern. Med. *83:* 523–524 (1975).

13 Glauser, F.; Smith, W.; Caldwell, A.; Hoshiko, M.; Dolan, G.; Baer, H.; Olsher, N.: Ethchlorvynol (Placidyl)-induced pulmonary edema. Ann. intern. Med. *84:* 46–48 (1976).

14 Wright, N.; Roscoe, P.: Acute glutethimide poisoning: conservative management of thirty-one patients. J. Am. med. Ass. *214:* 1704–1706 (1970).

15 Eade, N.; Taussig, L.; Marks, M.: Hydrocarbon pneumonitis. Pediatrics *54:* 351–357 (1974).

16 Neeld, E.; Limacher, M.: Chemical pneumonitis after the intravenous injection of hydrocarbon. Radiology *129:* 36 (1978).

17 Steinberg, A.: Pulmonary edema following ingestion of hydrochlorothiazide. J. Am. med. Ass. *204:* 825–827 (1968).
18 Baruh, S.; Sherman, L.: Hypoglycemia, a cause of pulmonary edema: progressive fatal pulmonary edema complicating hypoglycemia induced by alcohol and insulin. J. natn. med. Ass. *67:* 200–204 (1975).
19 Murray, M.; Kronenberg, R.: Pulmonary reactions simulating cardiac pulmonary edema caused by nitrofurantoin. New Engl. J. Med. *273:* 1185–1187 (1965).
20 Frand, U.; Shim, C.; Williams, M.: Heroin-induced pulmonary edema. Ann. intern. Med. *77:* 29–35 (1972).
21 Sklar, J.; Timms, R.: Codeine-induced pulmonary edema. Chest *72:* 230–231 (1977).
22 Seyffart, G.: Paraldehyde; in Haddad, Winchester, Clinical management of poisoning and drug overdose, pp. 410–413 (Saunders, Philadelphia 1983).
23 Cooke, N.; Flenley, D.; Matthew, H.: Paraquat poisoning. Q. Jl Med. *42:* 683–692 (1973).
24 Raffin, T.; Robin, E.: Paraquat ingestion and pulmonary injury. West. J. Med. *128:* 26–34 (1978).
25 Bogartz, L.; Miller, W.: Pulmonary edema associated with propoxyphene intoxication. J. Am. med. Ass. *215:* 259–262 (1971).
26 Fisch, H.; Wands, J.; Yeung, J.; Davis, P.: Pulmonary edema and disseminated intravascular coagulation after intravenous abuse of *d*-propoxyphene (Darvon). Sth. med. J. *65:* 493–495 (1972).
27 Hrnicek, G.; Skelton, J.; Miller, W.: Pulmonary edema and salicylate intoxication. J. Am. med. Ass. *230:* 866–867 (1974).
28 Bowers, R.; Brigham, K.; Owen, P.: Salicylate pulmonary edema: the mechanism in sheep and review of the clinical literature. Am. Rev. resp. Dis. *115:* 261–268 (1977).
29 Heffner, J.; Sahn, S.: Salicylate-induced pulmonary edema: clinical features and prognosis. Ann. intern. Med. *95:* 405–409 (1981).
30 McAnally, J.: Acid-base disorders; in Haddad, Winchester, Clinical management of poisoning and drug overdose, pp. 108–124 (Saunders, Philadelphia 1983).
31 Stapczynski, J.; Rothstein, R.; Gaye, W.; Niemann, J.: Colchicine overdose: report of two cases and review of the literature. Ann. Emerg. Med. *10:* 364–369 (1981).
32 Graham, D.; Laman, D.; Theodore, J.; Robin, E.: Acute cyanide poisoning complicated by lactic acidosis and pulmonary edema. Archs intern. Med. *137:* 1051–1055 (1977).
33 Vogel, S.; Sultan, T.; Ten Eyck, R.: Cyanide poisoning. Clin. Toxicol. *18:* 367–383 (1981).
34 Eells, J.; McMartin, K.; Black, K.; Virayotha, V.; Tisdell, R.; Tephly, T.: Formaldehyde poisoning – rapid metabolism to formic acid. J. Am. med. Ass. *246:* 1237–1238 (1981).
35 Fischman, C.; Oster, J.: Toxic effects of toluene. A new cause of high anion gap metabolic acidosis. J. Am. med. Ass. *241:* 1713–1715 (1979).
36 Streicher, H.; Gabow, P.; Moss, A.; Kono, D.; Kaehny, W.: Syndromes of toluene sniffing in adults. Ann. intern. Med. *94:* 758–761 (1981).
37 Voigts, A.; Kaufman, C.: Acidosis and other metabolic abnormalities associated with paint sniffing. Sth. med. J. *76:* 443–447 (1983).

38 Done, A.: The toxic emergency – signs, symptoms, and sources. Emerg. Med. *14(i):* 42–77 (1982).
39 Callahan, M.: Tricyclic antidepressant overdose. J. Am. Coll. Emerg. Physns *8:* 413–425 (1979).
40 Mateer, J.; Clark, M.: Lithium toxicity with rarely reported ECG manifestations. Ann. Emerg. Med. *11:* 208–212 (1982).
41 Horowitz, L.; Fisher, G.: Acute lithium toxicity (Letter). New Engl. J. Med. *281:* 1369 (1969).
42 Speirs, J.; Hirsch, S.: Severe lithium toxicity with 'normal' serum concentrations. Br. med. J. *i:* 815–816 (1978).
43 Demers, R.; Rivenbark, J.: Lithium intoxication and its clinical management. Sth. med. J. *75:* 738–739 (1982).
44 McCarron, M.; Schulze, B.; Thompson, G.; Condor, M.; Goetz, W.: Acute phencyclidine intoxication: clinical patterns, complications, and treatment. Ann. Emerg. Med. *10:* 290–297 (1981).
45 Goldfrank, L.; Lewin, N.; Osborn, H.: Dusted PCP. Hosp. Physn *18:* 62–73 (1982).
46 Greenberg, M.; Roberts, J.; Baskin, S.: Endotracheal naloxone reversal of morphine-induced respiratory depression in rabbits. Ann. Emerg. Med. *9:* 289–293 (1980).
47 Tandberg, D.; Abercrombie, D.: Treatment of heroin overdose with endotracheal naloxone. Ann. Emerg. Med. *11:* 443–445 (1982).
48 Handal, K.; Schauben, J.; Salamone, F.: Naloxone. Ann. Emerg. Med. *12:* 438–445 (1983).
49 Stahl, S.; Kasser, I.: Pentazocine overdose. Ann. Emerg. Med. *12:* 28–31 (1983).
50 Moore, R.; Rumack, B.; Conner, C.; Peterson, R.: Naloxone, underdosage after narcotic poisoning. Am. J. Dis. Child. *134:* 156–158 (1980).
51 Cohen, M.; Cohen, R.; Pickar, D.; Weingartner, H.; Murphy, D.; Bunney, W.: Behavioral effects after high dose naloxone administration to normal volunteers (Letter). Lancet *ii:* 1110 (1981).
52 Rumack, B.; Temple, A.: Lomotil poisoning. Pediatrics *53:* 495–500 (1974).
53 Andree, R.: Sudden death following naloxone administration. Anaesth. Analg. *59:* 782–784 (1980).
54 Bell, E.: The use of naloxone in the treatment of diazepam poisoning. J. Pediat. *87:* 803–804 (1975).
55 Jordan, C.; Lehane, J.; Jones, J.: Respiratory depression following diazepam: reversal with high-dose naloxone. Anesthesiology *53:* 293–298 (1980).
56 Jefferys, D.; Flanagan, R.; Volans, G.: Reversal of ethanol-induced coma with naloxone (Letter). Lancet *i:* 308–309 (1980).
57 Barros, S.; Rodriguez, G.: Naloxone as an antagonist in alcohol intoxication (Letter). Anesthesiology *54:* 174 (1981).
58 Lyon, L.; Antony, J.: Reversal of alcoholic coma by naloxone. Ann. intern. Med. *96:* 464–465 (1982).
59 North, D.; Wieland, M.; Peterson, C.; Krenzelok, E.: Naloxone administration in clonidine overdosage (Letter). Ann. Emerg. Med. *10:* 397 (1981).
60 Kulig, K.; Duffy, J.; Rumack, B.; Mauro, R.; Gaylord, M.: Naloxone for treatment of clonidine overdose (Letter). J. Am. med. Ass. *247:* 1697 (1982).
61 Christensen, K.; Huttel, M.: Naloxone does not antagonize diazepam-induced sedation (Letter). Anesthesiology *51:* 187 (1979).

62 Bell, E.: Naloxone reversal of diazepam effect (Letter). Anesthesiology *53:* 264 (1980).
63 Mattila, M.; Nuotto, E.; Seppala, T.: Naloxone is not an effective antagonist of ethanol (Letter). Lancet *i:* 775–776 (1981).
64 Guerin, J.; Friedberg, G.: Naloxone and ethanol intoxication (Letter). Ann. intern. Med. *97:* 932 (1982).
65 Kraynack, B.; Gintautas, J.: Naloxone: analeptic action unrelated to opiate receptor antagonism? Anesthesiology *56:* 251–253 (1982).
66 Tiengo, M.: Naloxone in irreversible shock (Letter). Lancet *ii:* 690 (1980).
67 Peters, W.; Johnson, M.; Friedman, P.; Mitch, W.: Pressor effect of naloxone in septic shock. Lancet *i:* 529–532 (1981).
68 Swinburn, W.; Phelan, P.: Response to naloxone in septic shock (Letter). Lancet *i:* 167 (1982).
69 Higgins, T.; Sivak, E.; O'Neil, D.; Graves, J.; Foutch, D.: Reversal of hypotension by continuous naloxone infusion in a ventilator-dependent patient. Ann. intern. Med. *98:* 47–48 (1983).
70 Faden, A.; Holaday, J.: Opiate antagonists: a role in the treatment of hypovolemic shock. Science *205:* 317–318 (1979).
71 Vargish, T.; Reynolds, D.; Gurll, N.; Lechner, R.; Holaday, J.; Faden, A.: Naloxone reversal of hypovolemic shock in dogs. Circ. Shock *7:* 31–38 (1980).
72 Gurll, N.; Vargish, T.; Reynolds, D.; Lechner, R.: Opiate receptors and endorphins in the pathophysiology of hemorrhagic shock. Surgery *89:* 364–369 (1981).
73 Albert, S.; Shires, G.; Illner, H.; Shires, G.: Effects of naloxone in hemorrhagic shock. Surgery Gynec. Obstet. *155:* 326–332 (1982).
74 Santiago, T.; Remolina, C.; Scoles, V.; Edelman, N.: Endorphins and the control of breathing. Ability of naloxone to restore flow-resistive load compensation in chronic obstructive pulmonary disease. New Engl. J. Med. *304:* 1190–1195 (1981).
75 Ayres, J.; Rees, J.; Lee, T.; Cochrane, G.: Intravenous naloxone in acute respiratory failure. Br. med. J. *284:* 927–928 (1982).
76 Van Rijn, T.; Rabkin, S.: Effect of naloxone, a specific opioid antagonist, on exercise-induced angina pectoris. Circulation *64:* suppl. IV, p. 149 (1981).
77 Faden, A.; Jacobs, T.; Holaday, J.: Opiate antagonist improves neurologic recovery after spinal injury. Science *211:* 493–494 (1981).
78 Baskin, D.; Hosobuchi, Y.: Naloxone reversal of ischaemic neurological deficits in man. Lancet *ii:* 272–275 (1981).
79 Iselin, H.; Weiss, P.: Naloxone reversal of ischaemic neurological deficits (Letter). Lancet *ii:* 642–643 (1981).
80 Hosobuchi, Y.; Baskin, D.; Woo, S.: Reversal of induced ischemic neurologic deficit in gerbils by the opiate antagonist naloxone. Science *215:* 69–71 (1982).
81 Holaday, J.; D'Amato, R.: Naloxone in cerebral ischaemia (Letter). Lancet *i:* 1238 (1982).
82 Reisberg, B.; Ferris, S.; Anand, R.; Mir, P.; Geibel, V.; DeLeon, M.: Effects of naloxone in senile dementia: a double-blind trial (Letter). New Engl. J. Med. *308:* 721–722 (1983).
83 Kreek, M.; Schaefer, R.; Hahn, E.; Fishman, J.: Naloxone, a specific opioid antagonist reverses chronic idiopathic constipation. Lancet *i:* 261–262 (1983).

84 Henderson, M.; Picchioni, A.; Chin, L.: Evaluation of oral dilution as a first aid measure in poisoning. J. pharm. Sci. *55:* 1311–1313 (1966).
85 Chin, L.: Gastrointestinal dilution of poisons with water – an irrational and potentially harmful procedure. Am. J. Hosp. Pharm. *28:* 712–714 (1971).
86 Friday, K.; Powell, S.; Thompson, W.; Sunshine, I.; Groden, D.; Neumeyen, J.: Emetics in poisoned dogs: efficacy independent of ingested volume (Abstract). Crit. Care Med. *8:* 233 (1980).
87 Rumack, B.; Rosen, P.: Emesis: safe and effective? (Editorial). Ann. Emerg. Med. *10:* 551 (1981).
88 Ritschel, W.; Erni, W.: The influence of temperature of ingested fluid on stomach emptying time. Int. J. clin. Pharmacol. Biopharm. *15:* 172–175 (1977).
89 Bartecchi, C.: A modification of gastric lavage technique. J. Am. Coll. Emerg. Physns *3:* 304–305 (1974).
90 Bartecchi, C.: Removal of gastric drug masses (Letter). New Engl. J. Med. *296:* 282–283 (1977).
91 Lacouture, P.; Lovejoy, F.: Iron; in Haddad, Winchester, Clinical management of poisoning and drug overdose, pp. 644–648 (Saunders, Philadelphia 1983).
92 Goldfrank, L.; Flomenbaum, N.; Weisman, R.: General management of the poisoned and overdosed patient. I. Hosp. Physn *17:* 24–33 (1981).
93 Sharff, J.; Bayer, M.: Acute and chronic digitalis toxicity: presentation and treatment. Ann. Emerg. Med. *11:* 327–331 (1982).
94 Pollack, M.; Dunbar, B.; Holbrook, P.; Fields, A.: Aspiration of activated charcoal and gastric contents. Ann. Emerg. Med. *10:* 528–529 (1981).
95 Greensher, J.; Mofenson, H.; Picchioni, A.; Fallon, P.: Activated charcoal updated. J. Am. Coll. Emerg. Physns *8:* 261–263 (1979).
96 Prescott, L.; Illingworth, R.; Critchley, J.; Stewart, M.; Adam, R.; Proudfoot, A.: Intravenous N-acetylcysteine: the treatment of choice for paracetamol poisoning. Br. med. J. *ii:* 1097–1100 (1979).
97 Litovitz, T.: Acetaminophen overdose. Ear Nose Thrt. J. *62:* 28–39 (1983).
98 Crome, P.; Dawling, S.; Braithwaite, R.; Masters, J.; Walkey, R.: Effect of activated charcoal on absorption of nortriptyline. Lancet *ii:* 1203–1205 (1977).
99 Ipecac syrup and activated charcoal for treatment of poisoning in children; in Abramowicz, Med. Lett. Drugs Therap. *21:* 70–72 (1979).
100 Elonen, E.; Neuvonen, P.; Halmekoski, J.; Mattila, M.: Acute Dapsone intoxication: a case with prolonged symptoms. Clin. Toxicol. *14:* 79–85 (1979).
101 Reigart, J.; Trammel, H.; Lindsey, J.: Repetitive doses of activated charcoal in Dapsone poisoning in a child. Clin. Toxicol. *19:* 1061–1066 (1983).
102 Hansteen, V.; Jacobsen, D.; Knudsen, K.; Reikvam, A.; Skuterud, B.: Acute, massive poisoning with digitoxin: report of seven cases and discussion of treatment. Clin. Toxicol. *18:* 679–692 (1981).
103 Pond, S.; Jacobs, M.; Marks, J.; Garner, J.; Goldschlager, N.; Hansen, D.: Treatment of digitoxin overdose with oral activated charcoal (Letter). Lancet *ii:* 1177–1178 (1981).
104 Neuvonen, P.; Elonen, E.: Effect of activated charcoal on absorption and elimination of phenobarbitone, carbamazepine, and phenylbutazone in man. Eur. J. clin. Pharmacol. *17:* 51–57 (1980).
105 Goldberg, M.; Berlinger, W.: Treatment of phenobarbital overdose with activated charcoal. J. Am. med. Ass. *247:* 2400–2401 (1982).

106 Berg, M.; Berlinger, W.; Goldberg, M.; Spector, R.; Johnson, G.: Acceleration of the body clearance of phenobarbital by oral-activated charcoal. New Engl. J. Med. *307:* 642–644 (1982).
107 Levy, G.: Gastrointestinal clearance of drugs with activated charcoal (Editorial). New Engl. J. Med. *307:* 676–678 (1982).
108 Park, G.; Spector, R.; Roberts, R.; Goldberg, M.; Weisman, D.; Stillerman, A.; Flanigan, M.: Use of hemoperfusion for treatment of theophylline intoxication. Am. J. Med. *74:* 961–966 (1983).
109 Done, A.: The toxic emergency: thallotoxicosis – dated but deadly. Emerg. Med. *11(11):* 211–214 (1979).
110 Powell, S.; Van de Graaff, W.; Thompson, W.; Friday, K.; Sunshine, I.; Neumeyer, J.: Charcoals, emetics, and cathartics in care of poisoned patients (Abstract). Crit. Care Med. *8:* 233 (1980).
111 Winchester, J.: Active methods for detoxification: oral sorbents, forced diuresis, hemoperfusion, and hemodialysis; in Haddad, Winchester, Clinical management of poisoning and drug overdose, pp. 154–169 (Saunders, Philadelphia 1983).
112 Garella, S.; Lorch, J.: Hemoperfusion for acute intoxications: con. Clin. Toxicol. *17:* 515–527 (1980).
113 Winchester, J.; Gelfand, M.; Knepshield, J.; Schreiner, G.: Dialysis and hemoperfusion of poisons and drugs – update. Trans. Am. Soc. artif. internal Organs *23:* 762–842 (1977).
114 Gelfand, M.; Winchester, J.: Hemoperfusion in drug overdosage: a technique when conservative management is not sufficient. Clin. Toxicol. *17:* 583–602 (1980).
115 Gadgil, S.; Damle, S.; Advani, S.; Vaidya, A.: Effect of activated charcoal on the pharmacokinetics of high-dose methotrexate. Cancer Treat. Rep. *66:* 1169–1171 (1982).
116 Smith, T.; Butler, V.; Haber, E.; Fozzard, H.; Marcus, F.; Bremner, F.; Schulman, I.; Phillips, A.: Treatment of life-threatening digitalis intoxication with digoxin-specific Fab antibody fragments. New Engl. J. Med. *307:* 1357–1362 (1982).
117 Kosinski, E.; Malindzak, G.: Glucagon and isoproterenol in reversing propranolol toxicity. Archs intern. Med. *132:* 840–843 (1973).
118 Salzberg, M.; Gallagher, E.: Propranolol overdose. Ann. Emerg. Med. *9:* 26–27 (1980).
119 Done, A.: Aspirin overdosage: incidence, diagnosis, and management. II. Pediatrics *62:* suppl., pp. 890–897 (1978).
120 Ferguson, R.; Boutros, A.: Death following self-poisoning with aspirin. J. Am. med. Ass. *213:* 1186–1188 (1970).
121 Kaufman, F.; Dubansky, A.: Darvon poisoning with delayed salicylism: a case report. Pediatrics *49:* 610–611 (1972).
122 Todd, P.; Sills, J.; Harris, F.; Cowen, J.: Problems with overdoses of sustained-release aspirin (Letter). Lancet *i:* 777 (1981).
123 Done, A.: Salicylate intoxication: significance of measurements of salicylate in blood in cases of acute ingestion. Pediatrics *26:* 800–807 (1960).
124 Gaudreault, P.; Temple, A.; Lovejoy, F.: The relative severity of acute versus chronic salicylate poisoning in children: a clinical comparison. Pediatrics *70:* 566–569 (1982).

125 Proudfoot, A.: Salicylates and salicylamides; in Haddad, Winchester, Clinical management of poisoning and drug overdose, pp. 575–586 (Saunders, Philadelphia 1983).
126 Hormaechea, E.; Carlson, R.; Rogove, H.; Uphold, J.; Henning, R.; Weil, M.: Hypovolemia, pulmonary edema, and protein changes in severe salicylate poisoning. Am. J. Med. *66:* 1046–1050 (1979).
127 Prescott, L.; Balali-Mood, M.; Critchley, J.; Johnstone, A.; Proudfoot, A.: Diuresis or urinary alkalinisation for salicylate poisoning? Br. med. J. *285:* 1383–1386 (1982).
128 Manoguerra, A.; Weaver, L.: Poisoning with tricyclic antidepressant drugs. Clin. Toxicol. *10:* 149–158 (1977).
129 Burks, J.; Walker, J.; Rumack, B.; Ott, J.: Tricyclic antidepressant poisoning. J. Am. med. Ass. *230:* 1405–1407 (1974).
130 Biggs, J.; Spiker, D.; Petit, J.; Ziegler, V.: Tricyclic antidepressant overdose: incidence of symptoms. J. Am. med. Ass. *238:* 135–138 (1977).
131 Marshall, J.; Forker, A.: Cardiovascular effects of tricyclic antidepressant drugs: therapeutic usage, overdose, and management of complications. Am. Heart J. *103:* 401–414 (1982).
132 Marshall, J.: Tricyclic overdose (Letter). J. Am. med. Ass. *244:* 1900 (1980).
133 Nicotra, M.; Rivera, M.; Pool, J.; Noall, M.: Tricyclic antidepressant overdose: clinical and pharmacologic observations. Clin. Toxicol. *18:* 599–613 (1981).
134 Johnson, D.; Knepp, I.; Whelan, T.: Toxic tricyclic antidepressant levels and the ECG (Letter). J. Am. med. Ass. *250:* 1027 (1983).
135 Spiker, D.; Biggs, J.: Tricyclic antidepressants: prolonged plasma levels after overdose. J. Am. med. Ass. *236:* 1711–1712 (1976).
136 Jackson, J.; Bressler, R.: Prescribing tricyclic antidepressants. III. Management of overdose. Drug Ther. *12:* 175–189 (1982).
137 Noble, J.; Matthew, H.: Acute poisoning by tricyclic antidepressants: clinical features and management of 100 patients. Clin. Toxicol. *2:* 403–421 (1969).
138 Benowitz, N.; Rosenberg, J.; Becker, C.: Cardiopulmonary catastrophes in drug-overdosed patients. Med. Clins N. Am. *63:* 267–296 (1979).
139 Haddad, L.: Tricyclic antidepressants; in Haddad, Winchester, Clinical management of poisoning and drug overdose, pp. 359–371 (Saunders, Philadelphia 1983).
140 Brackenridge, R.; Peters, T.; Watson, J.: Myocardial damage in amitriptyline and nortriptyline poisoning. Scott. med. J. *13:* 208–210 (1968).
141 Rose, J.: Tricyclic antidepressant toxicity. Clin. Toxicol. *11:* 391–402 (1977).
142 Baldessarini, R.: Drugs and the treatment of psychiatric disorders; in Gilman, Goodman, Gilman, The pharmacological basis of therapeutics; 6th ed., pp. 391–447 (Macmillan, New York 1975).
143 Brown, T.: Tricyclic antidepressant overdosage: experimental studies on the management of circulatory complications. Clin. Toxicol. *9:* 255–272 (1976).
144 Kingston, M.: Hyperventilation in tricyclic antidepressant poisoning. Crit. Care Med. *7:* 550–551 (1979).
145 Hoffman, J.; McElroy, C.: Bicarbonate therapy for dysrhythmia and hypotension in tricyclic antidepressant overdose. West. J. Med. *134:* 60–64 (1981).
146 Starkey, I.; Lawson, A.: Poisoning with tricyclic and related antidepressants – a ten-year review. Q. Jl Med. *49:* 33–49 (1980).
147 Nattel, S.; Bayne, L.; Ruedy, J.: Physostigmine in coma due to drug overdose. Clin. Pharmacol. Ther. *25:* 96–102 (1979).

148 Gard, H.; Knapp, D.; Walle, T.; Gaffney, T.; Hanenson, I.: Qualitative and quantitative studies on the disposition of amitriptyline and other tricyclic antidepressant drugs in man as it relates to the management of the overdosed patient. Clin. Toxicol. *6:* 571–584 (1973).
149 Larson, G.; Hurlbert, B.; Wingard, D.: Physostigmine reversal of diazepam-induced depression. Anaesth. Analg. *56:* 348–351 (1977).
150 Avant, G.; Speeg, K.; Freemon, F.; Schenker, S.; Berman, M.: Physostigmine reversal of diazepam-induced hypnosis. Ann. intern. Med. *91:* 53–55 (1979).
151 Bidwai, A.; Stanley, T.; Rogers, C.; Riet, E.: Reversal of diazepam-induced postanesthetic somnolence with physostigmine. Anesthesiology *51:* 256–259 (1979).
152 Bernards, W.: Case history number 74: reversal of phenothiazine-induced coma with physostigmine. Anaesth. Analg. *52:* 938–941 (1973).
153 Wang, S.; Marlowe, C.: Treatment of phenothiazine overdosage with physostigmine. Pediatrics *59:* 301–303 (1977).
154 Mogelnicki, S.; Waller, J.; Finlayson, D.: Physostigmine reversal of cimetidine-induced mental confusion. J. Am. med. Ass. *241:* 826–827 (1979).
155 Spector, M.; Bourke, D.: Anesthesia, sleep paralysis, and physostigmine. Anesthesiology *46:* 296–297 (1977).
156 Roy, R.; Stullken, E.: EEG arousal by doxapram, naloxone, and physostigmine. Anesthesiology *51:* S47 (1979).
157 Bidwai, A.; Cornelius, L.; Stanley, T.: Reversal of Innovar-induced postanesthetic somnolence and disorientation with physostigmine. Anesthesiology *44:* 249–252 (1976).
158 Newton, R.: Physostigmine salicylate in the treatment of tricyclic antidepressant overdosage. J. Am. med. Ass. *231:* 941–943 (1975).
159 Kulig, K.; Rumack, B.; Sullivan, J.; Brandt, H.; Spyker, D.; Duffy, J.; Shipe, J.: Amoxapine overdose: coma and seizures without cardiotoxic effects. J. Am. med. Ass. *248:* 1092–1094 (1982).
160 Pumariega, A.; Muller, B.; Rivers-Bulkeley, N.: Acute renal failure secondary to amoxapine overdose. J. Am. med. Ass. *248:* 3141–3142 (1982).
161 Litovitz, T.; Troutman, W.: Amoxapine overdose: seizures and fatalities. J. Am. med. Ass. *250:* 1069–1071 (1983).
162 Done, A.: The toxic emergency: an update on antidepressants. Emerg. Med. *15(2):* 225–238 (1983).
163 Lesar, T.; Kingston, R.; Dahms, R.; Saxena, K.: Trazodone overdose. Emerg. Med. *12:* 221–223 (1983).
164 Arena, J.: Cyanide; in Haddad, Winchester, Clinical management of poisoning and drug overdose, pp. 744–747 (Saunders, Philadelphia 1983).
165 Symington, I.; Anderson, R.; Oliver, J.; Thomson, I.; Harland, W.; Kerr, J.: Cyanide exposure in fires. Lancet *ii:* 91–92 (1978).
166 Cottrell, J.; Casthely, P.; Brodie, J.; Patel, K.; Klein, A.; Turndorf, H.: Prevention of nitroprusside-induced cyanide toxicity with hydroxocobalamin. New Engl. J. Med. *298:* 809–811 (1978).
167 Dorr, R.; Paxinos, J.: The current status of Laetrile. Ann. intern. Med. *89:* 389–397 (1978).
168 Braico, K.; Humbert, J.; Terplan, K.; Lehotay, J.: Laetrile intoxication: report of a fatal case. New Engl. J. Med. *300:* 238–240 (1979).

169 Michenfelder, J.; Tinker, J.: Cyanide toxicity and thiosulfate protection during chronic administration of sodium nitroprusside in the dog. Anesthesiology *47:* 441–448 (1977).
170 Arndt, J.; Freye, E.: Opiate antagonist reverses the cardiovascular effects of inhalation anaesthesia (Letter). Nature, Lond. *277:* 399–400 (1979).
171 Editorial: Which antidote for cyanide? Lancet *ii:* 1167 (1977).
172 Edwards, A.; Thomas, I.: Cyanide poisoning (Letter). Lancet *i:* 92–93 (1978).
173 Buchanan, I.; Dhamee, M.; Griffiths, F.; Yeoman, W.: Abnormal fundal appearances in a case of poisoning by a cyanide capsule. Med. Sci. Law *16:* 29–32 (1976).
174 Sioris, L.; Skoutakis, V.: Phencyclidine (PCP) intoxication. Clin. Toxicol. Consult. *2:* 101–110 (1980).
175 Litovitz, T.: Phencyclidine (PCP); in Haddad, Winchester, Clinical management of poisoning and drug overdose, pp. 448–455 (Saunders, Philadelphia 1983).
176 Aronow, R.; Done, A.: Phencyclidine overdose: an emerging concept of management. J. Am. Coll. Emerg. Physns *7:* 56–59 (1978).
177 Brittain, J.: Some ABCs of PCP. Emerg. Med. *13(10):* 193–195 (1981).
178 Castellani, S.; Giannini, A.; Boeringa, J.; Adams, P.: Phencyclidine intoxication: assessment of possible antidotes. Clin. Toxicol. *19:* 313–319 (1982).
179 Aniline, O.; Allen, R.: Most PCP intoxication is missed. Contin. Educ. Fam. Physn *18:* 367–371 (1983).
180 Goode, D.; Meltzer, H.: The role of isometric muscle tension in the production of muscle toxicity by phencyclidine and restraint stress. Psychopharmacologia *42:* 105–108 (1975).
181 McCarron, M.; Schulze, B.; Thompson, G.; Condor, M.; Goetz, W.: Acute phencyclidine intoxication: incidence of clinical findings in 1,000 cases. Ann. Emerg. Med. *10:* 237–243 (1981).
182 Picchioni, A.; Consroe, P.: Activated charcoal – a phencyclidine antidote, or hog in dogs (Letter). New Engl. J. Med. *300:* 202 (1979).
183 Rumack, B.: Phencyclidine overdose: an overview (Editorial). Ann. Emerg. Med. *9:* 595 (1980).
184 Barton, C.; Sterling, M.; Vaziri, N.: Rhabdomyolysis and acute renal failure associated with phencyclidine intoxication. Archs intern. Med. *140:* 568–569 (1980).
185 Rappolt, R.; Gay, G.; Farris, R.: Emergency management of acute phencyclidine intoxication. J. Am. Coll. Emerg. Physns *8:* 68–76 (1979).
186 Burns, R.; Lerner, S.: Phencyclidine deaths. J. Am. Coll. Emerg. Physns *7:* 135–141 (1978).
187 Morgan, D.: Recognition and management of pesticide poisonings; 3rd ed., pp. 1–8 (US Environmental Protection Agency, Washington 1982).
188 Temple, A.: Acute and chronic effects of aspirin toxicity and their treatment. Archs intern. Med. *141:* 364–369 (1981).

Steven M. Barrett, MD, Oklahoma Memorial Hospital, University of Oklahoma Health Sciences Center, Oklahoma City, OK 73106 (USA)

Subject Index